Soft Tissue Rheumatic Pain:

Recognition, Management, Prevention

Soft Tissue Rheumatic Pain:

Recognition, Management, Prevention

ROBERT P. SHEON, M.D.

Clinical Associate Professor of Medicine
Medical College of Ohio at Toledo
Senior Rheumatologist, Toledo Clinic, Inc.
Director, Arthritis Progressive Care Unit
Flower Hospital, Sylvania, Ohio

ROLAND W. MOSKOWITZ, M.D.

Professor of Medicine
Chief, Division of Rheumatic Diseases
University Hospitals/Case Western Reserve University
Cleveland, Ohio

VICTOR M. GOLDBERG, M.D.

Associate Professor of Orthopaedics
Case Western Reserve University School of Medicine
Attending Orthopaedist
University Hospitals and Veterans' Administration Hospital
Cleveland, Ohio

Claire B. Kirsner
Medical Illustrator

Lea & Febiger   *1982*   Philadelphia

Lea & Febiger
600 Washington Square
Philadelphia, PA   19106
U.S.A.

Library of Congress Cataloging in Publication Data

Sheon, Robert P.
  Soft tissue rheumatic pain.

  Bibliography: p.
  Includes index.
  1. Rheumatism.   2. Pain.   I. Moskowitz, Roland W.
II. Goldberg, Victor M.   III. Title.   [DNLM:
1. Connective tissue diseases.   2. Rheumatism.
WE 544 S546s]
RC927.S49   1981   616.7'23   81-8167
ISBN 0-8121-0806-X   AACR2

PRINTED IN THE UNITED STATES OF AMERICA

Print No.   4   3   2   1

To

Irma,

Peta,

and Harriet

for their love and support

PREFACE

The need for a textbook of soft tissue rheumatism was perceived because responsibility for medical care for these disorders is diverse. These patients receive care from neurosurgeons, industrial physicians, orthopedists, rheumatologists, internists, generalists, osteopathic physicians, psychologists, physical therapists, or anesthesiologists. Many patients also seek relief from faith healers, charlatans, and others. The literature is similarly diffused; we have drawn our material from wide-ranging sources across the broad health field.

We spent the better part of a year deciding which disorders to include. Although many might argue over our selection, we have attempted to provide a meaningful working text of soft tissue rheumatic diseases; most have stood the test of time. Although objective determinants are often lacking, a constellation of characteristic signs and symptoms can be noted; more importantly, aggravating factors that can precipitate many of these conditions are known and described for each condition. The clinician can prevent recurrences if he is aware of these and gives this information to the patient.

These conditions often overlap or compound one another and the physician can feel overwhelmed by the myriad of complaints presented by these patients. Simple history-taking methods and physical examination maneuvers that reproduce the symptoms and aid in diagnosis are provided. Proper treatment that results in benefit to the patient further corroborates the diagnosis.

The continental approach with emphasis on enthesitis-enthesopathy (inflammation or disorders of the muscular or tendinous region of attachment to bone) has not yet added significantly to our understanding of these disorders; therefore, we have not categorized the disorders by that method. Rather, we approached the conditions by body regions because most patients with soft tissue pain disorders present with limited local complaints.

The textbook begins with a basic guide to diagnosis and management found in the Introduction. Often, diagnosis depends on the art rather than the science of practice. We have provided a technique for history and physical examination that can be used whenever soft tissue rheumatic pain is suspected. Because a favorable response to treatment may be important to corroborate a diagnosis, we have provided a detailed six-point management program in the Introduction. Further specific recommendations are then amplified for each condition in the chapters that follow.

The soft tissue pain disorders for each body region are then described in subsequent chapters. Approximately 150 entities are described. These disorders, beginning with the temporomandibular joint dysfunction syndrome and carotidynia and ending with the entrapment neuropathies of the foot, can be readily managed in an outpatient setting with an informed physician and a patient motivated to recover. We have provided a description of each disorder, possible etiologies, aggravating factors, and physical findings or maneuvers that aid in diagnosis, recommended laboratory and roentgenographic tests, and specific management recommendations. We further provide an expected outcome and additional suggestions if symptoms persist.

The problem of chronic persistent pain is presented in Chapter 13. Some of the current speculations on causation, including an update on the gate control theory, psychosocial factors, and a review of some of the pain management tools including oral drugs, transcutaneous nerve stimulators, biofeedback training, and acupuncture are described. (Spinal manipulation and the use of pain clinics are discussed in Chapter 7, "The Low Back and Pelvis.") The fibrositis syndrome was allotted a separate chapter.

Sites for local injection utilizing an anesthetic and a crystalline steroid suspension are described in each chapter where appropriate. In Chapter 14, the technique, indications, contraindications, and hazards associated with using these agents are discussed.

Physical therapy and exercise are perhaps the most important management factors, and are certainly more important than oral drug therapy. Chapter 15, "The Exercise Plan," discusses musculoskeletal flexibility, goals of therapeutic exercise, types of exercise, the pace of exercise, and adjuncts to the exercise plan.

Our purpose is to provide the reader with a textbook of disorders broadly considered as soft tissue rheumatic pain disorders; to provide useful descriptors and characteristic maneuvers that reproduce many of the syndromes; and to strongly emphasize those aggravating factors that often lead to recurrences. Treatment and prevention are available and often useful; they are rarely expensive, prolonged, or unsafe.

Toledo, Ohio   Robert P. Sheon
Cleveland, Ohio   Roland W. Moskowitz
Cleveland, Ohio   Victor M. Goldberg

ACKNOWLEDGMENTS

Perhaps the first description of soft tissue rheumatism should be ascribed to Hippocrates' description of the Scythians as "so loose-jointed that they were unable to draw a bowstring or hurl a javelin."*

Arthur Scherbel, M.D. of the Rheumatology Department, Cleveland Clinic, played a major role in igniting the interest of one of us (RPS) in these often ignored areas. Significant practical diagnostic and therapeutic modalities based on experience were gleaned from many colleagues over the years, including Drs. Allan Kirsner, Robert Finkel, Stephen Farber, Robert Gosling, Richard Baer, and numerous orthopedists, physical therapists, and patients.

Art and photography, under the direction of Claire B. Kirsner, Medical Illustrator, was ably assisted by the Medical Illustration Department at the Medical College of Ohio (Jerry Lubinski), the Department of Medical Illustration at Toledo Hospital, and by office assistants, Barbara Pearson and Beverly Jurek, who posed many evenings and weekends.

Secretarial, clerical, and library assistance was provided by Pat Jankowski, Sarah Sheon, Amy Sheon, Jody Glasser, Lucille Mundwiler, Linda Fankhauser, Susan Jacobs, Dorothy Ervin, Pat Gearig, Carol Coehrs, and Shannon Riley.

Bonnie Langevin, Administrative Assistant of the Division of Rheumatic Diseases at University Hospitals/Case Western Reserve University, provided invaluable assistance with communications and manuscript handling between co-authors in Cleveland and Toledo.

With appreciation for prompt, courteous, and professional assistance, we thank the staff of our publisher, Lea & Febiger. R. Kenneth Bussy, the Executive Editor, Janet B. Nuciforo, the Copy Editor, and

---

*Grahame R: Joint Hypermobility—clinical aspects. Proc Roy Soc Med 64:692–694, 1971.

Thomas J. Colaiezzi, the Production Manager, each provided patient and professional assistance to the authors throughout the past three years.

We wish to acknowledge and thank Flower Hospital and Toledo Hospital for use of facilities and for provision of library, photographic, and secretarial services.

Final preparation of the text, references, and legends was in the hands of Cathy Pompili and Irma Sheon, both of whom maintained amazing resilience throughout this period.

R.P.S.
R.W.M.
V.M.G.

CONTENTS

AN OVERVIEW OF DIAGNOSIS AND MANAGEMENT

This is a "What it is" and "How to treat it" book. The conditions discussed include localized disease problems that result from trauma, spasm, inflammation, degeneration, or congenital abnormalities. Included among the many entities discussed are tendinitis, bursitis, fasciitis, carpal tunnel and other nerve entrapment syndromes, disc and low back syndromes, other structural derangements of the musculoskeletal system, myofascial pain, and the fibrositis syndrome.

We have tried to detail each disorder or syndrome as the patients commonly present to the physician. Aggravating factors are stressed. Specific well-defined methods of management are given where available. In those entities where specific therapy is unavailable, empirical modes of treatment that appear to be effective and safe are described. In many cases treatment regimens may require extensive patient education and cooperation; therefore, we have tried to present an expected outcome. However, if further care is needed, guidelines are provided for additional diagnostic procedures and therapy. Most patients with these entities respond well to treatment if all the steps outlined are considered. A common mistake is to provide only one or two therapeutic modalities when a more comprehensive program is necessary. Furthermore, several causative mechanisms may coexist and must be discerned; therefore, the clinician must be thorough in his evaluation of the patient.

The pathogenesis of many of these disorders is poorly understood. The chapter on chronic pain (Chapt. 13) discusses a theoretic role for the central nervous system in any chronic pain state. The skeptical physician will find little objective data discussed in certain areas.

Prospective studies are hampered by the simultaneous occurrence of several disorders in one patient, with each contributing many variables to the problem.

Over 150 painful and disabling musculoskeletal disorders are described. No doubt, experienced physicians could add many more to those we have presented. For example:

*Back-pocket sciatica is caused by pressure on the sciatic nerve in the gluteal region [Gould]. We now record another related neuromuscular condition, ponderous-purse disease in shoulder-purseuses. Both disorders are highly sex-limited, back-pocket sciatica to men and ponderous-purse disease to women, although the latter can affect men of certain habit.

Ponderous-purse disease is manifest by pain, tenderness and spasm in upper shoulder and lateral neck muscles, especially trapezius, supraspinatus and rhomboideus, and is sometimes accompanied by radicular pains.

The pathogenic mechanism is neuromuscular. Constant contraction of the shoulder elevator and neck stabilizer muscles attempting to carry the load on the side of the shouldered purse results in pain, tenderness and focal spasms of those muscles. The muscle contractions can cause abnormal neck posture and provocation of cervical nerve radiculopathy. An informal assay of a series of feminine purse weights and contents revealed weights up to 5 kg. and internal milieus that can modestly and summarily, for the uninitiated, be pursimoniously likened to the contents of a goat's stomach. The profligate-credit-card factor and coins-for-coin-eating-machines factor are links with back-pocket sciatica, but the instruments, bottles, boxes, tubes, jars, packets, and spray cans of material necessary for natural beauty are unique to ponderous purses.

Prevention of ponderous-purse disease is so logical that to point it out may be considered purscilious. The physician's advice has almost no patient pursuance. An unfavored but sometimes patient-tried remedy is contralateral shifting of the shoulder purse, usually followed by contralateralling of the pain and needless pursponement of the cure. Switching to a hand-held purse is subjectively objectionable and objectively often complicated by purse partings, with resulting hot pursuits, purspirations and panic

*W.K. Engel, Editorial. Reprinted by permission of The New England Journal of Medicine, 299:557, 1978.

from loss of beauty aids (and credit cards). Another approach, reduction of the shoulder purse contents, is apparently more of a pain in the neck than the pain in the neck.

And so, like hookworms in unsanitary societies who won't wear shoes, ponderous-purse disease appears destined to remain endemic in ours.

One of our colleagues has labeled these disorders "wastebasket rheumatism"!* In our ignorance of the pathogenesis of many of the persistent musculoskeletal pain syndromes, classification has been difficult. "Nonarticular (soft tissue) rheumatism is a term embracing a large group of miscellaneous conditions with a common denominator of musculoskeletal pain and stiffness."[1]

Although systemic diseases can produce similar syndromes, we hope the physician will gain confidence in the early recognition and treatment of a *primary* soft tissue rheumatic pain disorder, thus preventing the establishment of a chronic pain-spasm-pain cycle.

The reader is encouraged to review the regional anatomy related to the syndromes described. Knowledge of anatomy and muscle function will aid the clinician in diagnosis and therapy of soft tissue rheumatism. The functional anatomy of the locomotor system is well described in Rene Cailliet's monograph, *Soft Tissue Pain and Disability*.[2] The reader is also encouraged to use an anatomy book or atlas as a companion to our text.

IMPACT OF MUSCULOSKELETAL PAIN ON SOCIETY

Musculoskeletal disorders, including soft tissue rheumatic pain disorders, are among the leading causes of time lost from work, and a major reason for disability payments in the United States. One third of these disabled persons are younger than 45 years of age. Chronic "medical absences from work" due to musculoskeletal disorders exceed medical absences due to circulatory, mental, and neoplastic disorders combined. Of the five leading diseases causing disability, four involve the musculoskeletal system.[3] The prevalence of musculoskeletal disorders has increased 24% in the past decade.[4] Of visits to practitioners of medicine, 15 to 25% are estimated to be due to complaints related to the musculoskeletal system.[5] The Mayo Clinic's Department of Physical Medicine reports that 30% of visits were the result of soft tissue musculoskeletal disorders.[6] Hopefully, early recognition of these disorders, recognition and avoidance of aggravating factors, and treatment will have a significant impact on the financial and emotional exhaustion that these patients experience.

---

*Courtesy of Allan B. Kirsner, M.D.

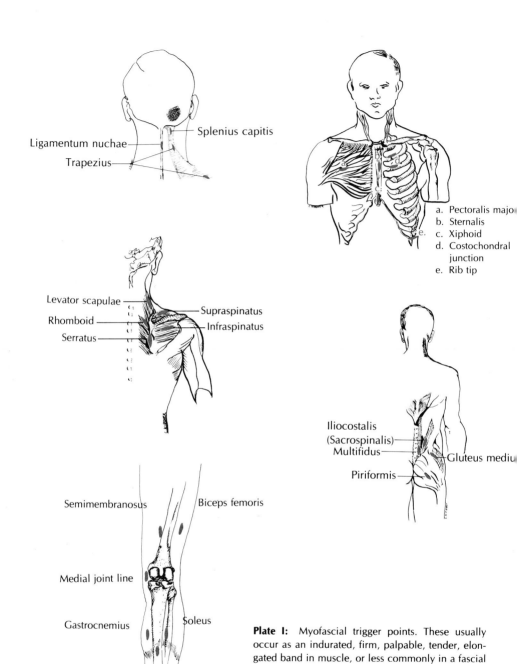

Splenius capitis
Ligamentum nuchae
Trapezius

a. Pectoralis major
b. Sternalis
c. Xiphoid
d. Costochondral junction
e. Rib tip

Levator scapulae
Rhomboid
Serratus
Supraspinatus
Infraspinatus

Iliocostalis (Sacrospinalis)
Multifidus
Piriformis
Gluteus medius

Semimembranosus
Biceps femoris

Medial joint line

Gastrocnemius
Soleus

Plate I: Myofascial trigger points. These usually occur as an indurated, firm, palpable, tender, elongated band in muscle, or less commonly in a fascial plane.

4

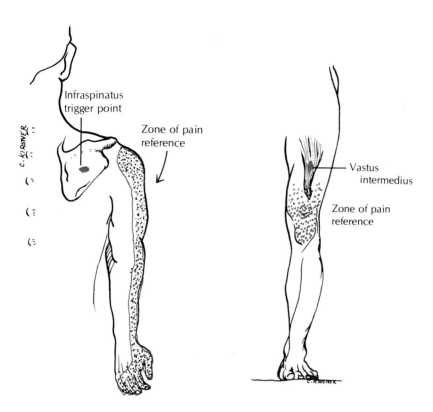

Infraspinatus trigger point

Zone of pain reference

Vastus intermedius

Zone of pain reference

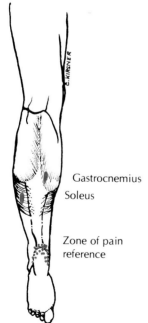

Gastrocnemius

Soleus

Zone of pain reference

Plate II: Zones of reference. Upon palpation of the trigger point, pain is produced in a target area or at some distance away. The zone of reference is characteristic for each trigger point.

RECOGNITION OF MYOFASCIAL SOFT TISSUE PAIN

Recognition and management of myofascial pain is an art as well as a science. The term "myofascial pain" implies regional musculoskeletal pain accompanying a *trigger zone*. The trigger zone, or *trigger point*, is a palpable, tender, indurated portion of muscle or fascia. Palpating the trigger zone causes pain in a target area or *zone of reference*, which may be within the same muscle bundle or at some distance.[7-9] (Plates I, II). The trigger zone may result from acute trauma or minor injury, repeated minor microtrauma of daily living, or chronic strain from sedentary living habits. Myofascial trigger points may also occur in systemic inflammatory disorders or infections. Visible swelling is rare. Travell[8] and Bonica[9] popularized trigger point identification and suggested that chronicity often resulted from a pain-spasm-pain cycle (see Chapt. 13).

Myofascial pain recognition requires that the clinician discern what pain the patient is experiencing throughout the day and night. The pain quality (aching, burning, numbness, throbbing) must be elicited; the physician should not prejudge the severity of the patient's pain.[10] Objective swelling must be distinguished from a *sensation* of swelling. Is "swelling" limited to a joint area, is it periarticular, or more diffuse? Is motion impaired, and if so, is the limited motion constant or intermittent?

What precipitating events preceded the pain? These may include injury from overstretching, a direct blow to the body, repetitive activity or prolonged inactivity from driving long distances or performing prolonged sedentary tasks. What therapeutic endeavors were tried by the patient and with what results?

The patient's general condition must be considered. Evaluation of the condition should proceed in an orderly, logical manner. Localized syndromes may reflect local limited areas of disease. Many local disorders result from "misuse injury."[11] Similar manifestations may result from a systemic disorder or may be drug-induced (e.g., drug lupus, serum sickness). If a systemic disease process is present, the physician must consider whether it is the cause of myofascial pain or coincidental. A comprehensive examination includes body development, posture, gait, movement, motivation, and emotional status in addition to the usual evaluation[12-13] (Fig. 1).

The physical examination of patients with nonarticular rheumatism includes special maneuvers unique to defining the syndromes described in this book. Each chapter describes the performance of these essential clinical tests; these tests often reproduce the symptoms.

The examining physician should observe the patient while sitting, when rising from a chair, or while bending and walking. In this manner, structural disorders can be recognized. Laying on of hands to palpate tender, indurated, trigger points of muscle, to determine joint passive range of movement, or to elicit joint hypermobility is particularly important. Careful joint palpation for synovial thickening or synovial effusion is essential to detect these subtle manifestations of various connective tissue diseases.

The diagnosis of myofascial origin of pain can be compared to the diagnosis of migraine headaches. The physician must first learn the specific features of such headaches. A careful history of the quality, location, and duration of the headache must be elicited. Associated characteristic symptoms include visual scotomata, nausea and vomiting, transient neurologic deficits, and personality features that occur with sufficient frequency to be recognized as a syndrome called

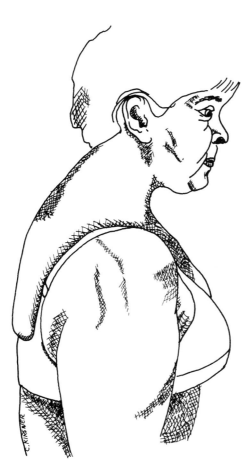

Fig. 1. The clinician observes the heavy breasts, improper brassiere with tight straps, heavy arms, forward sloping shoulder, and forward inclination of the neck. The patient is a good candidate for thoracic outlet syndrome, cervical fibrositis, or muscle contraction headaches.

"migraine." The possible aggravating features of bright light and mental stress are sought.[14] Treatment is specific, and is associated with a good response in most patients. *Relief from pain becomes a corroborative part of the syndrome recognition.* A majority of patients with nonarticular rheumatic disorders respond favorably to treatment, which often helps corroborate or establish the diagnosis.

Helpful Hints

1. Laying on of the examiner's hands often provides more useful information than do roentgenograms.
2. Osteoarthritis seen on roentgenograms is often unrelated to the pain syndrome.
3. Localized musculoskeletal pain disorders may be layered over another established disease process.
4. When morning stiffness does not *mainly* involve the hands and feet, rheumatoid arthritis is an unlikely diagnosis.
5. Pain so severe that the limbs cannot be touched (the touch-me-not syndrome), and with no discernible spasm, is usually of psychogenic origin.
6. Pain localized to a body quadrant seldom is due to a psychogenic cause.
7. Observing the patient while seated, while rising from a chair, while standing, and while bending forward can lead to recognition of basic *structural* alterations. "Misuse" of the musculoskeletal system may also be observed.
8. Drugs may be the least important part of treatment. Stretching exercises and avoiding aggravating factors often provide more sustained benefit than pills.

SIX POINTS FOR MANAGING MYOFASCIAL SOFT TISSUE PAIN

Six points of management can often be initiated during the patient's *first visit,* even before appropriate laboratory and radiographic findings are available.

1. Exclude systemic disease.
2. Recognize and eliminate aggravating factors.
3. Provide an explanation to the patient.
4. Provide instruction in self-help exercises.
5. Provide relief from pain.
6. Project an expected outcome.

Exclude Systemic Disease. Satisfy yourself and the patient that serious systemic disease is not present. Systemic inflammatory connective tissue disorders must be excluded as well as such entities as diabetes mellitus, thyroid dysfunction, occult neoplasm, and drug reactions. *Treatment need not wait for results from such tests* in many patients. If roentgenographs are likely to add little information to the findings, they may be deferred until results of the treatment program are evaluated a few weeks later. Expensive, time-consuming, and possibly hazardous procedures (e.g., angiography for a thoracic outlet syndrome) should only be considered if they are clinically justified. More often, such procedures can and should be reserved for patients who fail to benefit from the conservative therapy initiated on the first visit. We would certainly order appropriate screening tests, including complete blood counts, urinalysis, sedimentation rate, and appropriate serum chemistries. If radiographs have been done elsewhere recently, the results may be obtained by telephone.

Recognize and Eliminate Aggravating Factors. Events and activities preceding the pain state must be reviewed in an effort to

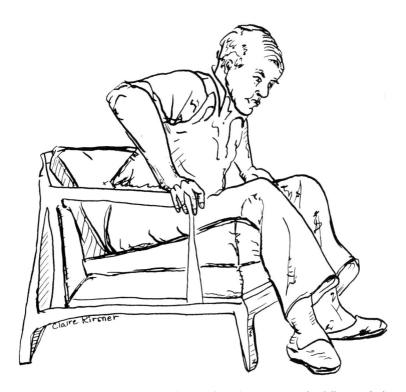

Fig. 2. Illustration of a patient arising from a chair demonstrating the following faults: (1) Hands and wrists used to push off from the side of the chair; this promotes quadriceps weakness and carpal tunnel syndrome. (2) The chair is too low; this impedes use of the quadriceps during the act of arising. (3) The neck is unsupported and the chair is overstuffed; this promotes muscular strain about the head and neck. (4) House slippers promote metatarsalgia.

recognize aggravating activities *that can cause recurrences*. Improper resting, sitting, or working positions are common precipitating factors (Fig. 2). Strain resulting from job performance, a new hobby, or repetitive tiring tasks should be recognized and altered. Strain resulting from structural disorders, such as flatfeet or heavy pendulous breasts, can also be altered with appropriate instructions. Chronic pain causes anxiety, depression, physical tension, and disturbed sleep. Let the patient know that emotional stress can be an aggravating factor, and may not only play a primary role in the pain syndrome, but may lower a patient's pain threshold and compound the pain-spasm-pain cycle. Similarly, secondary gain resulting in dependent interpersonal relationships can prolong treatment. Frank discussion usually leads to a satisfactory solution. Somatic delusions that accompany certain psychoses may confound the clinician. The need for psychiatric care in such patients soon becomes obvious.

Provide an Explanation to the Patient. The physican should provide the patient with a suspected cause for her symptoms. For example, if after the examination, a benign hypermobility syndrome (see Chapt. 5) is considered to be the cause of the patient's symptoms, this may be explained to the patient and she may be reassured immediately. Hypermobility syndrome is a more welcome diagnosis than systemic lupus erythematosus, or rheumatoid arthritis. When a myofascial pain syndrome such as gluteal fasciitis, or trochanteric bursitis, is superimposed upon another disorder, such as osteoarthritis of the hip, the patient's comprehension of the findings is vital to future care. The myofascial or bursitis pain may cause more suffering than the coexisting arthritis. Alternatively, nonarticular rheumatic pain may disrupt a physical therapy program that is essential for treatment of the accompanying arthritis. Treatment of the bursitis or fasciitis provides relief from pain, and furthermore allows the patient to follow conservative care necessary for the arthritis. If a myofascial pain syndrome has been found and trigger points identified, the patient can be informed that the pain is real, and that a pain-spasm-pain cycle may be prolonging the condition.

Provide Instruction in Self-Help Exercises. A prescription program of home physical therapy and exercises should be outlined on the first visit. Myofascial pain syndromes appear to respond best to a twice daily regimen performed first thing in the morning and last thing at night. Even if pain has subsided, twice daily stretching exercises should be continued until the involved region no longer tightens up during sleep. The ease or flexibility of morning stretching should be compared to the ease of stretching the preceding evening. The exercises should be continued until the morning and evening exercise regimens appear equally flexible (see "Therapeutic Exercises" in the Appendix).

Provide Relief from Pain. As mentioned, when pain is present, a vicious cycle may have occurred, promoting greater muscular spasm. The self-help therapy program can be more effective and results obtained more quickly when pain is relieved. If spasm is minimal, pain relief may be obtained by such time-honored therapy as heat or cold applications, and aspirin prior to performing the self-help exercises. Intense muscle spasm can usually be relieved by injecting the "trigger point" with a long-acting corticosteroid-local anesthetic mixture. Similarly, such an injection for treatment of a suspected bursitis, tendinitis, or carpal tunnel syndrome can provide prompt pain relief, and may help establish a nonarticular rheumatic disease diagnosis.[15] If pain chronicity suggests a vicious pain-spasm-pain cycle, using tricyclic antidepressant drugs, such as amitriptyline, may be helpful even in patients without apparent depression. Used at night, in a dose sufficient to cause a mild dry mouth, amitriptyline or other tricyclics may help interrupt the pain-spasm-pain cycle.[16-21]

Project an Expected Outcome. The physician should be familiar enough with soft tissue rheumatic pain disorders that the expected outcome and duration until benefits become evident can be projected. Relief from carpal tunnel syndrome, bursitis, or tendinitis may require only a few days, whereas symptoms due to hypermobility syndrome or disorders of other structural deficits may require several months before moderate or great improvement is seen. This should be told to the patient at the outset. The patient should also understand that the physician's diagnosis may depend upon the patient achieving symptomatic relief; this, in turn, often depends upon the patient performing the self-help program. The physician and the patient must work together.

Physicians concerned with cost effectiveness are recommending many of the treatment modalities described in this book.[22-24] We encourage the reader to try these measures, even though there is no proof of efficacy. Our 20 years of experience has established the safety of these measures in most disorders, and patient satisfaction that has resulted from the measures outlined here.

REFERENCES

1. Hench PK: Nonarticular rheumatism. *In* Rheumatic Diseases: Diagnosis and Management. Edited by WA Katz. Philadelphia, JB Lippincott, 1977.
2. Cailliet R.: Soft Tissue Pain and Disability. Philadelphia, FA Davis, 1977.
3. Reynolds MD: Prevalence of rheumatic diseases as causes of disability and complaints by ambulatory patients. Arthritis Rheum *21*:377–382, 1978.
4. Department of Health, Education and Welfare, Pub. No. (NIH) 78–318, 70–73 (Tables 1, 2) 1977.
5. Lipscomb PR: Foreword. *In* Musculoskeletal Disorders. Edited by RD D'Ambrosia. Philadelphia, JB Lippincott, 1977.
6. Stonnington HH: Tension myalgia. Mayo Clin Proc *52*:750, 1977.
7. Edeiken J, Wolferth CC: Persistent pain in the shoulder region following myocardial infarction. Am J Med Sci *191*:201–210, 1936.

8. Travell J, Rinzler SH: The myofascial genesis of pain. Postgrad Med *11*:425–434, 1952.
9. Bonica JJ: Management of myofascial pain syndromes in general practice. JAMA *164*:732–738, 1957.
10. D'Ambrosia RD (ed): Musculoskeletal Disorders. Philadelphia, JB Lippincott, 1977.
11. Fowler WM, Taylor RG: Differential diagnosis of muscle diseases. *In* Musculo-skeletal Disorders. Edited by RD D'Ambrosia. Philadelphia, JB Lippincott, 1977.
12. Kendall HO, Kendall FP, Boynton DA: Posture and Pain. Huntington, NY., Robert E. Krieger, 1970.
13. Sheon RP: Regional soft tissue pain syndromes. Postgrad Med 68:143–157, 1980.
14. Saper JR: Migraine I; classification and pathogenesis. JAMA *239*:2380–2383, 1978.
15. Kirsner AB, Sheon RP: Regional rheumatic syndromes (including bursitis, tenosynovitis, tendinitis and ganglia). Primer on the Rheumatic Disease, Eighth Ed. in press.
16. Raskin NH, Prusiner S: Carotidynia. Neurology 27:43–46, 1977.
17. Gomersall JD, Stuart A: Amitriptyline in migraine prophylaxis. J Neurol Neurosurg Psychiatry *36*:684–690, 1973.
18. Halpern LM: Analgesic drugs in the management of pain. Arch Surg *112*:861–869, 1977.
19. Duthie AM: The use of phenothiazines and tricyclic antidepressants in the treatment of intractable pain. S Afr Med J *51*:246–247, 1977.
20. Beaumont G: The use of psychotropic drugs in other painful conditions. J Int Med Res *4*:[Suppl (2)]56–57, 1976.
21. DeJong RH: Central pain mechanisms. JAMA *239*:2784, 1978.
22. Clark DD, Ricker JH, MacCollum MS: The efficacy of local steroid injection in the treatment of stenosing tenovaginitis. Plast Reconstr Surg *51*:179–180, 1973.
23. Phalen GS: Soft tissue affections of the hand and wrist. Hosp Med *7*:45–59, 1971.
24. Moskowitz RW: Clinical Rheumatology. Philadelphia, Lea & Febiger, 1975.

Chapter 1

THE HEAD AND NECK

Pain in the head or neck region may be due to many different structures and etiologies. Sometimes a combination of these occur and complicate the evaluation. Physical examination maneuvers and trigger point identification often provide diagnostically useful information. The disorders described in this chapter can be recognized and treated satisfactorily in the office without time-consuming or expensive investigation in most cases.

TEMPOROMANDIBULAR JOINT DYSFUNCTION SYNDROME

A common pain disorder, temporomandibular joint *dysfunction* syndrome may result from anxiety or stress associated with unconscious jaw closing movements.[1,2] Less often, similar distressing pain can result from *organic* diseases of the temporomandibular joint. Organic etiologies include subluxation and trauma, systemic inflammatory disease (e.g., rheumatoid arthritis, ankylosing spondylitis, or infection), and neoplasm.[3,4] As is often true of degenerative joint disease found elsewhere,[4-6] degenerative changes of the temporomandibular joint are poorly correlated with symptoms. Similarly, occlusal abnormalities correlate poorly with pain.[2]

Patients with temporomandibular joint dysfunction syndrome present with chronic pain in the jaw region with occasional pain radiating to the ear and neck. This syndrome is commonly seen in young to middle-aged females.[2,7] Temporomandibular joint noises, irregular mandibular movements, and limitation of jaw motion may accompany the pain. A sensation of pressure in the ear, or tinnitus sometimes delays recognition of the syndrome. Bruxism, grinding the teeth or clenching the jaw during sleep, is common. The pain is aggravated by chewing, by yawning, and sometimes by talking. Often the jaw deviates to one side during movement. Migraine headaches are ten times more frequent in this patient population.[2]

13

Physical examination of the patient with pain in the temporomandibular joint includes palpation of the medial pterygoid muscles located at the back of the mouth within the tonsillar pillars. A gloved finger is introduced into the mouth and gentle palpation causes mild to exquisite pain (Fig. 1–1). Before attempting the examination, the clinician should warn the patient not to bite.

Etiology. The temporomandibular joint dysfunction syndrome is often associated with malocclusion, which may be a cause for, or may result from, the chronic muscle tension compressing the joint.[4] The syndrome is common in edentulous elderly patients.[2] Costen's syndrome (temporomandibular joint pain, limited joint excursion, hearing

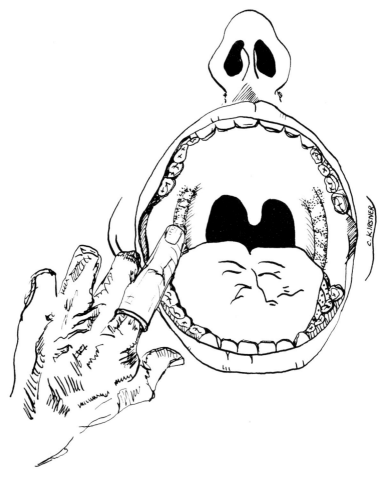

Fig. 1–1. Using a gloved finger, the examiner palpates the internal (medial) pterygoid muscle within the anterior pillar of the mouth. Each side is compared for pain reproduction. Tenderness is elicited on the symptomatic side.

deficits, and headaches)[8] has been reassessed in the light of myofascial pain mechanisms,[9] and this eponym has been abandoned. The temporomandibular joint dysfunction syndrome may result from the use of cervical traction, dental manipulation, trauma, or most often, from muscle fatigue due to jaw clenching.[4] Jaw clenching, in turn, is often due to anxiety and leads to a myofascial syndrome with a trigger point in the pterygoid musculature. However, psychologic investigation has yielded conflicting information.[10] Although these patients usually suffer from anxiety, the psychoneurosis apparently does not interfere with the response to treatment.

Radiographic changes, including erosions of the mandibular condyle or degenerative arthritis are difficult to relate to symptoms. Toller found no correlation of erosions to symptoms.[6] After 5 years of follow-up, 52% of patients with temporomandibular joint pain and *erosions* had relief from pain and radiographic *improvement*. This radiographic improvement of the erosion followed treatment that included a single corticosteroid injection of the temporomandibular joint. The relief from chronic joint compression may have allowed healing to occur.

The most severe degenerative joint changes were found in those patients who had the poorest results from therapy.[6] Persistent joint compression by the temporomandibular joint dysfunction syndrome may lead to degenerative arthritis.[4]

Laboratory and Radiographic Examination. Radiographic examination of the temporomandibular joint should be obtained if symptoms are persistent (rather than intermittent) or other features suggest tumor or infection. Erosions are not of prognostic significance.[6] The erythrocyte sedimentation rate is normal in the temporomandibular joint dysfunction syndrome. Leukocytosis, anemia, or an abnormal sedimentation rate suggests organic disorders.

Differential Diagnosis. Exclusion of organic disease as a cause for symptoms is essential. Inflammatory rheumatic diseases affecting the temporomandibular joint (such as rheumatoid arthritis or ankylosing spondylitis) rarely cause joint swelling.[5] Looking at the patient as a whole for evidence of other joint swelling is important to exclude systemic inflammatory disease and arthritis. Examination of the neck, teeth, tonsils, and cervical lymph nodes to exclude regional infection is necessary, but only a minority of patients have underlying organic disease.[11]

Management. Treatment obviously requires the exclusion of mechanical and inflammatory diseases. Patients with temporomandibular joint dysfunction syndrome may require dental evaluation for occlusive abnormalities and possible correction. Furthermore, a joint spacer (also called a bite plate or bite plate appliance) is helpful when used during sleep.[2,5,7,12] The acrylic bite plate appliance acts to gently stretch the pterygoid muscles and prevents jaw clenching during sleep (Fig. 1–2). Its use should be continued for at least several months. Some patients with accompanying neck pain can be helped by proper sleep instructions. The patient should sleep with a thin pillow that holds the neck in a neutral position. A neck contour pillow or a Jackson pillow (a soft tubular pillow) may assist the patient in attaining the proper sleep position.

Isometric jaw exercises are helpful. The patient, with her mouth open an inch, places her fist in front of the mandible (mentum) and tries to jut her jaw forward against the immovable fist; no motion actually occurs. She performs this exercise for 10 seconds and repeats it 6 times in succession. Then, in similar fashion, she places her fist to each side of and beneath the mandible while thrusting the jaw against the fist for 10 seconds, doing 6 repetitions in each position. Jaw

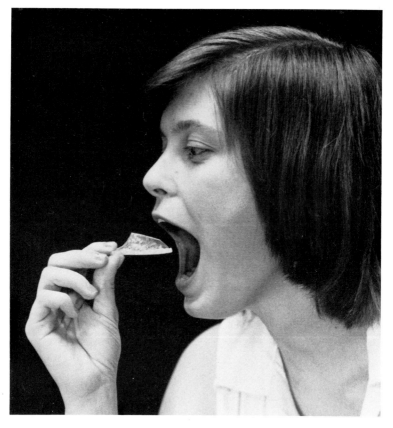

Fig. 1–2. One of several types of acrylic molded bite plate appliances used to prevent jaw clenching and to provide gentle stretching of the pterygoid muscle. (Courtesy Dr. Richard M. Klein.)

relaxation during the day may be provided by the acrylic bite plate appliance. Nocturnal sedation is helpful during the first few weeks.

Outcome and Additional Suggestions. The outcome is satisfactory in most patients with temporomandibular joint dysfunction syndrome.[2] The bite plate appliance should be worn for some time after symptoms are relieved.

If, in follow-up, the patient has not responded, a single injection of a corticosteroid-local anesthetic mixture into the temporomandibular joint (Fig. 1–3) may provide pain relief with subsequent relaxation of the pterygoid muscles and allow the rest of the treatment program to take hold. Biofeedback training has not proved useful in this disorder.[13] For the few patients who fail to benefit after these measures have been applied, reassessment of the patient, both from a mechanical and psychological standpoint, is indicated. The patient, obviously, will be concerned with coping with the chronic pain. Often, the addition of a tricyclic antidepressant is helpful (see Chapt. 13).

A special situation exists when temporomandibular joint pain occurs in a patient with previously established rheumatoid arthritis.

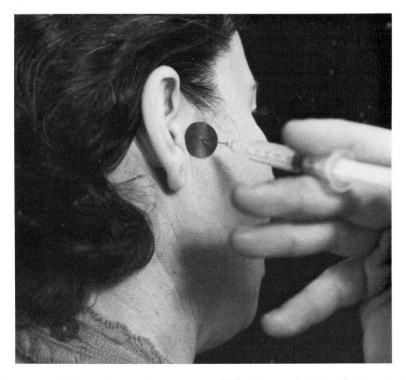

Fig. 1–3. With the mouth open, the temporomandibular joint may be injected using a No. 25 or No. 27 short needle with 1 ml of medication.

Rheumatoid synovitis of the temporomandibular joint produces constant muscle spasm, and the patient cannot fully open her jaw. The joint should be injected with a steroid-local anesthetic mixture on the first visit. Instead of an acrylic bite plate appliance, the patient should be instructed to obtain 3 or 4 corks, ranging in size up to 1½ inches in diameter. Several times a day the patient should insert the series of corks between the front teeth, beginning with the smallest cork. Each is held in place for 1 minute. Relief from pain and return to normal function is expected within 10 days.[5]

Management of
Temporomandibular Joint Dysfunction Syndrome

1. Exclude infections and inflammatory diseases.

2. Recognize aggravating factors (e.g., spasm, jaw muscle fatigue, dental malocclusion, anxiety, or stress).

3. Eliminate nocturnal jaw clenching with an acrylic bite plate appliance.

4. Provide dental care if indicated.

5. Provide jaw exercises.

6. Provide muscle relaxants, sedatives, and amitriptyline or similar tricyclic compounds at bedtime.

7. Perform local anesthetic-corticosteroid joint injections for persistent symptoms.

VASCULAR NECK AND FACE PAIN (CAROTIDYNIA)

Young and middle-aged men and women with this disorder, often with a past history or family history of migraine, present with persistent or intermittent aching pain over one temporomandibular joint, radiating forward along the mandible, up to the temple and into the ear.[14] The pain is described either as a dull ache or as an intermittent throbbing. Often, these patients have seen a dentist and otolaryngologist to no avail. Muscle contraction headache may coexist. Visual abnormalities do not occur. Jaw motion is normal. Physical examination reveals tenderness and sometimes palpable swelling of the external carotid artery.[15] Gentle pressure upon the external carotid artery often reproduces and intensifies the neck and facial pain (Fig. 1–4). Examination and comparison of the carotid vessels on each side of the neck may reveal unilateral swelling or tenderness of the

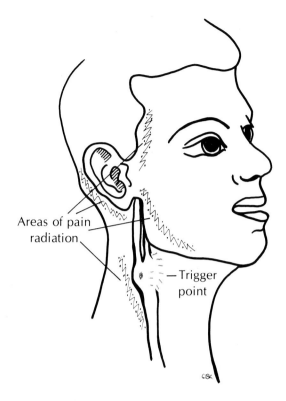

Areas of pain radiation

—Trigger point

Fig. 1–4. Palpation of the carotid artery just below the bifurcation accentuates pain referral forward along the mandible, up toward the temple, and occasionally into the ear.

involved vessel. Trigger points within the trapezius and posterior neck muscles commonly coexist. Tenderness and fullness within the temporal and masseter muscles may be found.[14–17]

Etiology. An elongated stylomastoid process probably is *not* a cause for this syndrome. Most current opinion suggests that carotidynia is a migraine equivalent.[15–17] Often, drugs useful in migraine prophylaxis appear effective in vascular neck and face pain.

Laboratory and Radiographic Examination. Laboratory and roentgenographic findings are not revealing. The normal Westergren sedimentation rate should exclude underlying sepsis or polymyalgia rheumatica or giant cell arteritis in the elderly. Radiographic evidence of cervical degenerative arthritis does not relate to this syndrome and should be considered a coincidental abnormality.

Differential Diagnosis. Differential diagnosis includes occult infection within the oropharyngeal structures, giant cell arteritis (only to be considered in the elderly), neoplasm, carotid body tumors, and the temporomandibular joint dysfunction syndrome.[18]

Treatment. Treatment begins with telling the patient to keep her hands off her neck. Once a patient realizes the pain is originating from the carotid artery, she has a tendency to stroke the area, thus exacerbating the condition. Often, we have found that these patients have coexisting myofascial trigger points in the trapezius and posterior neck muscles. In these cases, relaxing the trapezius muscle with a steroid-local anesthetic injection, performing exercises including

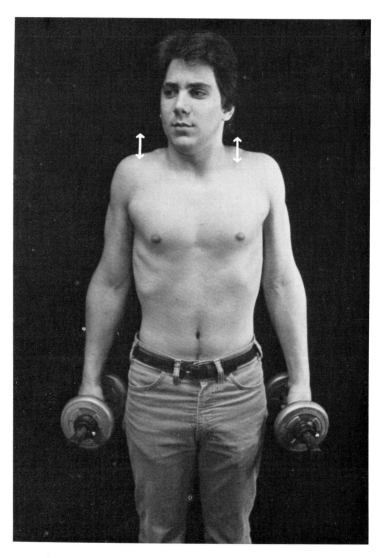

Fig. 1–5. Active-resistance shoulder shrugging: Using 5 to 10 pounds of weight placed upon each shoulder or held in each hand, the shoulders are shrugged and rotated upward and backward, and then slowly let down; the movement is repeated for 1 to 2 minutes.

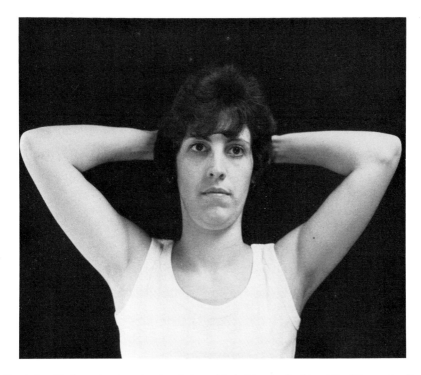

Fig. 1–6. Neck-erector strengthening: In isometric fashion, preferably while sitting or standing with back to wall, the head is pressed progressively into the hands, which act as a passive cushion.

shoulder shrugging and neck erector stengthening (Figs. 1–5, 1–6), and using a tricyclic antidepressant (amitriptyline) have been helpful.[15,16] Occasionally, ergot preparations or other drugs useful in the treatment of migraine are helpful.[15,17,19]

Outcome and Additional Suggestions. Most patients will be greatly improved following this treatment regimen. Therapy is continued for at least 3 months, and the exercises should be continued twice daily for several months. Patients should be instructed to avoid sleeping on their stomachs because neck hyperextension may intensify distress.

CERVICAL FIBROSITIS (THE CERVICAL SYNDROME)

Chronic pain in the muscles of the posterior neck worsens when sitting or upon arising in the morning. This pain improves with motion and may occur as an isolated complaint or as part of a more generalized fibrositis syndrome.[20] The aggravation of the pain *after rest* is a cardinal feature. Muscle contraction headaches often coexist. Numbness, tingling, weakness, and scotomata do not occur. Active neck motion may be restricted, but passive neck motion is normal. No neurologic abnormalities are noted. Trigger points within the trapezius and neck erector muscles are easily found by palpation. Sometimes a tight, tender ligamentum nuchae is noted during neck flexion[21] (Fig. 1–7). When the cervical syndrome occurs after trauma, several weeks often elapse before the onset of chronic diffuse neck pain.[22]

Laboratory and Radiographic Examination. Proper radiographic assessment must be obtained. Upright anteroposterior and lateral neck roentgenograms, in the neutral, flexion, and extension positions, and open-mouth odontoid views should be obtained to exclude cervical spine disease. Oblique views of the cervical spine are obtained for evaluation of the neuroforamina. Muscle spasm may lead to loss of the normal forward curve; skeletal injuries can be identified. Osteoporosis, neoplasm, and other diseases can also be ruled out. Degenerative changes, consistent with age, are often unrelated to symptoms.

Differential Diagnosis. Neck pain and stiffness that follow rest and improve during movement seldom result from more serious disease.

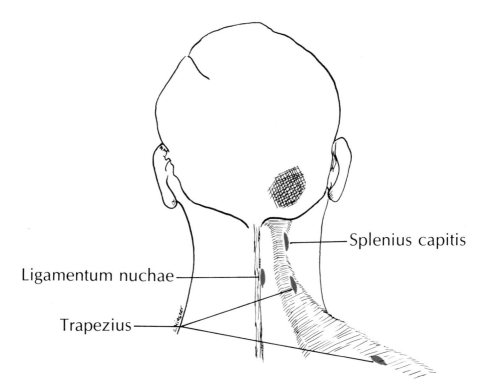

Fig. 1–7. Myofascial trigger points in the cervical region.

However, a careful history and physical examination, with exclusion of referred pain from the temporomandibular joint, diaphragm, and hiatus hernia, and with consideration for neurologic or cardiovascular disease, are necessary.[22] Psychogenic neck pain tends to occur episodically and does not improve with activity; pain is out of proportion to the physical findings, and palpation during the physical examination often reveals tenderness in excess of usual trigger point tenderness. Treatment of psychogenic pain requires the addition of helpful solutions to life problems. The floppy head syndrome, consisting of severe neck weakness and associated fatigue, strongly suggests hypothyroidism or polymyositis.[23]

Management. Treatment includes avoiding activities in which the head is held motionless for prolonged periods. Tasks requiring sitting or standing still should be interrupted every 30 minutes. Lying on a

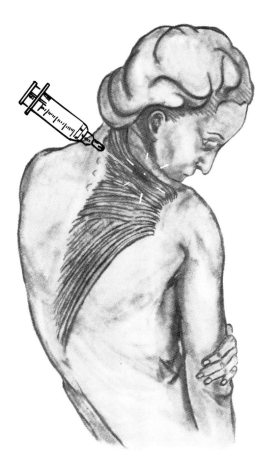

Fig. 1–8. Injection of trapezius trigger point with a 1-in. No. 23 needle.

sofa with the head propped up on the sofa arm induces neck strain, and should be avoided. Sleep position with the head preferably in a neutral position (with the patient lying on his back with legs elevated) is helpful[24] (see Fig. 7–7, p. 155). Injection of trigger points in the trapezius (Fig. 1–8) and neck erector (Fig. 1–9) muscles with a steroid-anesthetic combination may be performed on the first visit.[20]

Exercises to mobilize the trapezius and stretch the nuchal erectors are helpful to prevent recurrence.[25] Shoulder shrugging exercises are performed with 5- to 10-pound weights placed upon each shoulder or held by hand at each side. The shoulders are slowly raised upward and posteriorly, then let down slowly; this is repeated for 1 to 2 minutes (Fig. 1–5). Neck strengthening is helpful in our experience. This exercise is performed while the patient stands with his back to

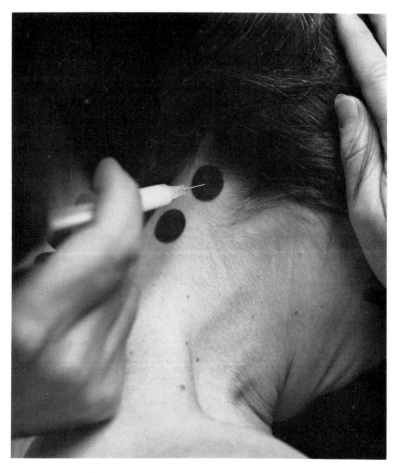

Fig. 1–9. Injection of cervical myofascial trigger points in the splenius capitus and upper cervical muscles using a No. 25 short needle and 1 to 2 ml of medication.

the wall, hands placed behind the head; the patient then distracts his head (head held vertically) posteriorly with as much force as tolerated, as if he were pushing his head through the hands and through the wall (Fig. 1–6). This is performed as an isometric exercise for 60 seconds at least twice daily.

Overhead cervical traction is frequently necessary (Fig. 1–10). Cervical traction should never be prescribed without first obtaining roentgenograms of the cervical spine. Note that 10 pounds of cervical traction produce no visible distraction of the vertebrae; 25 to 35 pounds of traction do distract the vertebrae, and furthermore, may free adhesions between dural sleeves.[22] Cervical traction should be performed at least twice daily (morning and evening) for 5 to 10 minutes.

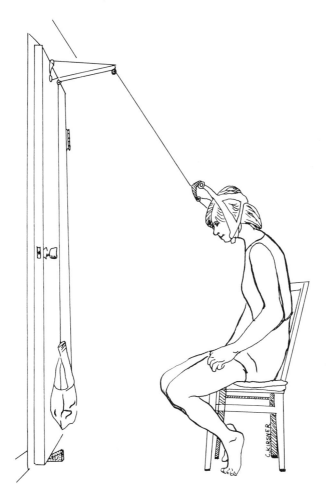

Fig. 1–10. Cervical traction is performed with the head flexed forward 15 to 25 degrees. Duration ranges from 5 to 15 minutes and traction is usually performed twice daily.

Beginning with 8 to 15 pounds, the weight is increased gradually until benefit results. Home traction of up to 20 pounds is usually well tolerated. Traction is then followed by neck strengthening exercises. **Outcome and Additional Suggestions.** After these therapeutic measures, relief from cervical fibrositis should begin within a week or two in the majority of patients. Whenever cervical traction is prescribed, the patient may have to continue the twice daily traction therapy for a prolonged period. Supervision by a physical therapist is desirable. A tricyclic antidepressant (amitriptyline), given at bedtime to relieve a pain-spasm-pain cycle, may be helpful. Biofeedback relaxation has also been advocated[13] (see Chapt. 13).

IMPINGEMENT OF THE FIFTH CERVICAL NERVE ROOT

Compression of the lower cervical nerve roots may result in shoulder region pain and disability. Dull aching about the shoulder, intermittent at first, later persistent, may be due to C-5 nerve root irritation resulting from such entities as disc degeneration, root sleeve injury, or trauma. Coughing, sneezing, or neck hyperextension may aggravate the pain. Neck and arm motion often are normal. Two helpful examinations are the Spurling maneuver and determination of vibratory sensation. The Spurling maneuver is an attempt to reproduce the pain by direct compression of the nerve.[26] The examiner places his hands on the seated patient's head, and rotates the head slightly to the painful side. In addition to turning the chin, the head is also slightly angled so that the patient's ear is tilted toward the painful shoulder. Pressure is then exerted downward on the patient's head with perhaps 20 pounds of force for 10 seconds (Fig. 1–11). Pain is reproduced or accentuated in the shoulder region if the Spurling test is positive. Vibration sense and pinprick sensation are usually diminished over the involved deltoid region. Atrophy is rare. Strength is usually preserved if the patient is seen soon after onset. Passive motion of the shoulder joint is normal. Swelling or the sensation of swelling does not occur.

Cervical spine roentgenograms must include oblique views to demonstrate the neuroforamina. Radiographic changes may not correlate with clinical features in some patients. Electrodiagnostic studies may not reveal abnormality, especially if performed within the first month of onset of symptoms.

Treatment begins with instructing the patient in proper sleep and sitting positions and avoidance of hyperextension of the neck.[27] A helpful sleep position is to have the patient lie flat on his back with thighs elevated on pillows, thus flattening the long spinal muscles. A rolled-up towel under the neck may be used.[24] Some patients prefer the use of a soft neck collar or neck pillow. Reducing cervical erector muscle spasm is imperative. Measures to do this include the applica-

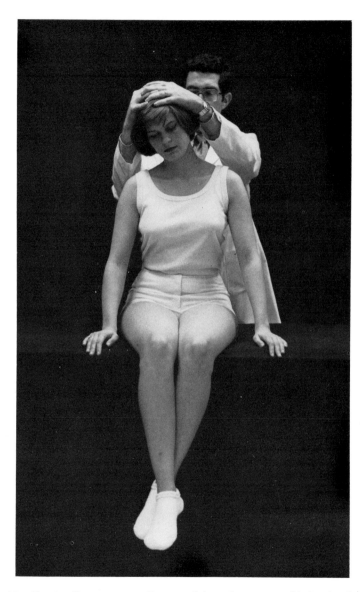

Fig. 1–11. The Spurling maneuver: Downward force for 10 seconds' duration is used to reproduce symptoms resulting from cervical nerve impingement.

tion of local moist heat, the injection of cervical muscle trigger points with a local anesthetic-corticosteroid mixture, and the use of neck-erector strengthening exercises. Cervical traction performed several times a day with a motorized intermittent traction machine or with a home traction kit is helpful.[22,28] Use of a mild muscle relaxant-analgesic preparation is beneficial only when used in conjunction with physical therapy measures. If cervical traction is necessary, the patient may need to use it daily for several months. Isometric neck exercises following each traction treatment can be helpful. Cervical collars are of value for protecting the neck from further injury especially while driving.

Most patients respond quickly and do not require electrodiagnostic (EMG) studies or consideration for a surgical procedure. As a rule, we treat patients initially with local heat and exercises, and if no benefit occurs in the first few weeks, we then add cervical traction. Never order cervical traction without performing a cervical spine radiographic examination to exclude malalignment or fractures. If traction fails, we then proceed to EMG and surgical consultation. In our experience, fewer than 1% of these patients require surgical intervention.

CERVICOTHORACIC INTERSPINOUS BURSITIS

Midline posterior cervical pain may result from formation of a bursa between the posterior spinous processes.[29,29a] The pain is dull, usually constant, and localized in the region between the posterior processes of C-7 and T-1. The patient usually has a dorsal kyphosis with a forward inclination of the neck in relation to the shoulders. The pain is worse with resting or sitting, but improves during movement. Often, the provoking cause is an activity requiring hyperextension of the neck and head, such as cleaning the upper shelves of a cupboard.

Physical examination reveals point tenderness directly at the midline of the lower cervical or upper thoracic spine. Rubbery swelling of the soft tissues may be palpated. Passive range of motion is normal. Roentgenographs to exclude osteoporosis and an erythrocyte sedimentation rate to exclude sepsis should be obtained.

Treatment includes injection of the interspinous space, approached from a lateral point of entry about ½ inch from the midline. A long-acting steroid-local anesthetic mixture is injected into each side of the bursa (Fig. 1–12). Proper sleep position, with the neck in a neutral position, is advised, and neck erector strengthening and shoulder shrugging exercises are provided. The patient is instructed to avoid hyperextension of the neck.

MUSCLE CONTRACTION HEADACHE

These patients describe a dull, aching, or occasionally throbbing pain in regions of the ocular orbit, forehead, temple, or scalp, pre-

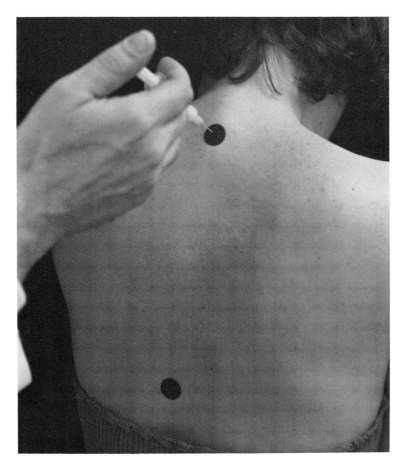

Fig. 1–12. Injection of intraspinous bursitis: A 1-in. No. 25 or No. 23 needle is used with a 45-degree angulated approach. Up to 2 ml volume is used.

ceded by a sensation of tightness in the neck erector muscles. Unlike migraine, these patients state that the headaches last for days or weeks. Often the headaches have been precipitated by working on a project while sitting for several hours at a time, going for a long drive, or falling asleep in a chair and allowing the head to fall forward. These patients often sleep on their stomachs, hyperextending their heads if a pillow is used.[24] Less often, nuchal muscles are strained during neck hyperextension from working overhead, such as painting a ceiling. Visual symptoms, if present, are described as a sensitivity to bright lights or foggy vision, but never scotomata.

Physical examination reveals a normal range of passive neck motion (when the examiner moves the patient's head laterally, forward, and backward, with the patient relaxed). Trigger points within the trapezius as well as the neck erector muscles are uniformly present. Other physical findings and tests for inflammation are normal.

Radiographic examination of the neck may reveal degenerative changes expected for age, but abnormalities are often unrelated. A Westergren sedimentation rate should be performed in elderly patients to exclude giant cell arteritis.[18]

Treatment includes instruction in proper sleep position, preferably with the patient lying on his back with a thin pillow or towel rolled up behind the neck.[24] Activities or tasks performed while sitting or standing should be paced, with no longer than 30 minutes at a time spent in sedentary activities. Exercises include neck erector strengthening[18] and shoulder shrugging (to loosen the trapezii) performed twice daily. (See "Cervical Fibrositis" in this chapter.) Women with pendulous breasts should use bras with wide elastic straps that prevent tugging on the trapezius (Figs. 1–13, 1–14). Injection of the cervical and trapezius trigger points with a steroid-local anesthetic mixture may be performed on the first visit.[20] Usually a relaxant or sedative is provided at bedtime for a few weeks.

The expected result is relief within a few days, but the exercises and preventive measures to avoid neck strain are continued for a prolonged period. Therapeutic failure is uncommon, but two additional

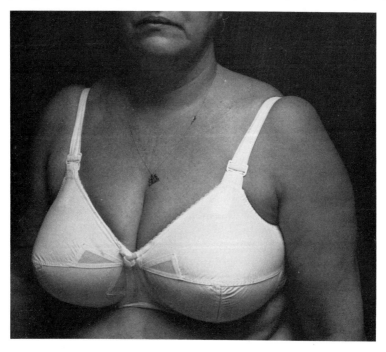

Fig. 1–13. Improper brassiere providing inadequate support and creating excessive traction on the shoulders.

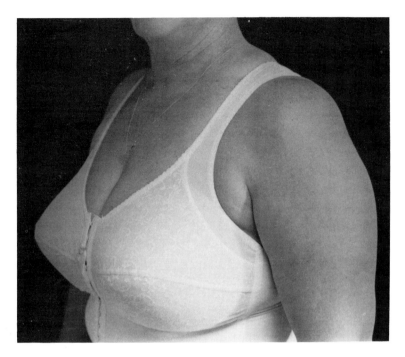

Fig. 1–14. Proper brassiere with wide elastic straps and good support.

helpful modalities are use of flexion cervical traction (Fig. 1–10) and amitriptyline.[19,30,31] Biofeedback relaxation may also be helpful[13] (see Chapt. 13).

OCCIPITAL NEURALGIA

Pain at the base of the skull posteriorly, with occasional bursts of pain and paresthesia traveling up the occiput, sometimes to the entire scalp, can be due to irritation of the sensory root of the second cervical nerve (the greater occipital nerve). Neck strain, from working with the head hyperextended, may have precipitated the pain. Occipital neuralgia may occur as a result of trauma, often in association with degenerative disease of the atlantoaxial joint.[32] Palpation at the base of the skull may reproduce or exacerbate the sensation.

Injection of cervical and trapezius trigger points with a steroid-local anesthetic mixture, instructions in sleep position (head and neck in line with trunk), and neck erector strengthening exercises should provide prompt relief. Proper radiographic assessment of the upper neck region should be obtained if symptoms persist. Lateral flexion and extension views and open-mouth odontoid views can identify underlying abnormalities, which may rarely require surgery.

REFERENCES

1. Schwartz L.: Disorders of the Temporomandibular Joint: Diagnosis, Management, Relation to Occlusion of Teeth. Philadelphia, WB Saunders, 1959.
2. Zarb, GA, Speck JE: The treatment of temporomandibular joint dysfunction: A retrospective study. J Prosthet Dent 38:420–432, 1977.
3. Sharav Y: The myofascial pain dysfunction syndrome—A common expression to various etiologies. Israel J Dent Med 26:11–15, 1977.
4. Guralnick W, Kaban LB, Merrill RG: Temporomandibular joint afflictions. N Engl J Med 299:123–129, 1978.
5. Mayne JG, Hatch GS: Arthritis of the temporomandibular joint. J Am Dent Assoc 79:125–130, 1969.
6. Toller PA: Use and misuse of intraarticular corticosteroids in treatment of temporomandibular joint pain. Proc R Soc Med 70:461–463, 1977.
7. Pinals RA: Traumatic arthritis and allied conditions. In Arthritis and Allied Conditions. 9th Ed. Edited by DJ McCarty. Philadelphia, Lea & Febiger, 1979.
8. Costen JB: A syndrome of ear and sinus symptoms dependent upon disturbed function of the temporomandibular joint. Ann Otol Rhinol Laryngol 43:1–15, 1934.
9. Freese AS: Costen's syndrome: A reinterpretation. AMA Arch Otol 70:33–38, 1959.
10. Small EW: An investigation into the psychogenic bases of the temporomandibular joint myofascial pain dysfunction syndrome. In Advances in Pain Research and Therapy. Vol. 1. Edited by JJ Bonica, D Albe-Fessard. New York, Raven Press, 1976.
11. Marbach JJ: Arthritis of the temporomandibular joints. Am Fam Physician 20:131–139, 1979.
12. Greene, CS, Laskin DM: Splint therapy for the myofascial pain dysfunction syndrome: A comparative study. J Am Dent Assoc 84:624–628, 1972.
13. Peck CL, Kraft GH: Electromyographic biofeedback for pain related to muscle tension. Arch Surg 112:889–895, 1977.
14. Lovshin LL: Vascular neck pain—a common syndrome seldom recognized. Cleve Clin Q 27:5–13, 1960.
15. Lovshin LL: Carotidynia. Headache 17:192–195, 1977.
16. Fay T: Atypical facial neuralgia, a syndrome of vascular pain. Ann Otol 41:1030–1062, 1932.
17. Raskin NH, Prusiner S: Carotidynia. Neurology 27:43–46, 1977.
18. Goodman BW Sr: Temporal arteritis. Am J Med 67:839–852, 1979.
19. Couch JR, Seigler DK, Hassanein R: Amitriptyline in the prophylaxis of migraine. Neurology 26:121–127, 1976.
20. Moskowitz RW: Clinical Rheumatology. Philadelphia, Lea & Febiger, 1975.
21. Cyriax J: Textbook of Orthopaedic Medicine. I. Diagnosis of Soft Tissue Lesions. 7th Ed. London, Bailliere Tindall, 1978.
22. Jackson R: The Cervical Syndrome. Springfield, IL, Charles C Thomas, 1978.
23. Katz AL, Pate D: Floppy head syndrome. Arthritis Rheum 23:131–132, 1980.
24. Kraus H: Clinical Treatment of Back and Neck Pain. New York, McGraw-Hill, 1970.
25. Brown BR: Diagnosis and therapy of common myofascial syndromes. JAMA 239:646–648, 1978.
26. Spurling RG, Scoville WB: Lateral rupture of the cervical intervertebral discs. Surg Gynecol Obstet 78:350–358, 1944.
27. British Association of Physical Medicine: Pain in the neck and arm: A multicentre trial of the effects of physiotherapy. Br Med J 1:253–258, 1966.
28. Honet JC, Puri K: Cervical radiculitis: Treatment and results in 82 patients. Arch Phys Med Rehabil 57:12–16, 1976.
29. Anderson JE: Grant's Atlas of Anatomy. 7th Ed. Baltimore, Williams & Wilkins, 1978.
29a. Bywaters EGL: Tendinitis and bursitis. Clin Rheum Dis 5:883–927, 1979.
30. Gomersall JD, Stuart A: Amitriptyline in migraine prophylaxis. J Neurol Neurosurg Psychiatry 36:684–690, 1973.
31. Saper JR: Migraine. II: Treatment. JAMA 239:2480–2484, 1978.
32. Turek SL: Orthopaedics: Principles and Their Application. 3rd Ed. Philadelphia, JB Lippincott, 1977.

Chapter *2*

THE THORACIC OUTLET REGION

When the classic triad of numbness, weakness, and a sensation of swelling occurs in one or both upper limbs, a diagnosis of a neurovascular entrapment disorder is strongly suggested. More often, symptoms are vague and physical findings are lacking. Physical examination maneuvers often clarify the disorders that arise in the thoracic outlet. Sometimes a therapeutic trial of the treatment measures described in this chapter assists in diagnosis by providing symptomatic relief.

THE THORACIC OUTLET AND RELATED SYNDROMES

Intermittent obstruction of the neurovascular bundle of the upper extremity results in both neurologic and vascular symptoms. Paresthesia, pain, and often a *sensation* of swelling of the arm and hand on one or both sides occur. Occasional complaints include weakness of the hands, chest wall pain,[1] and less often, discomfort of the entire shoulder girdle. Intermittent pain and paresthesia occur in nearly all patients, and usually follow the ulnar nerve distribution, or involve the entire hand and lower arm.[2,3] Vascular disturbances, which accompany neurologic symptoms, include a sensation of coldness, congestion of the entire hand (rings feel tight in the morning), and distension of the veins of the hand. The symptoms represent compression of the neurovascular bundle as it traverses the cervico-axillary canal, comprising three potential spaces. These are the triangular space between the scalene muscles, the costoclavicular space, and the pectoralis minor space under the pectoralis minor muscle[4,5] (Fig. 2–1). In the past, multiple terms were used for this syndrome. Terminology was based upon a presumed site of obstruction, and included the costoclavicular syndrome,[6] the hyperabduction or Wright's syn-

33

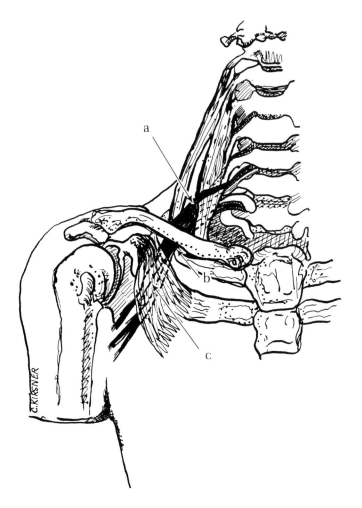

Fig. 2–1. The thoracic outlet: The neurovascular bundle passes through 3 potential spaces, which are (a) the triangular space between the scalene muscles, (b) the costoclavicular space, and (c) a space beneath the pectoralis minor muscle.

drome,[7,8] the scalenus anticus syndrome, and the cervical rib syndrome. In recent years, observations made at the time of operation demonstrated *multiple sites* of obstruction in individual patients.[3,7] Therefore, the more general term, thoracic outlet syndrome, is preferred.

Etiology. Anatomic anomalies include cervical ribs with or without radiolucent cervical bands, first rib anomalies, elongation of a cervical transverse process, hypertrophy of the omohyoid or the scalenus anticus muscles, and poststenotic aneurysms of the subclavian artery.[7] Roos described surgical findings in 232 patients who required surgical decompression.[9] Of these, 27 cases were associated with cervical ribs or clavicle anomalies; other anatomic anomalies found included cervical bands (22 cases), and hyperplastic first ribs (3 cases). Roos found no anatomic anomalies in the remaining 81% of his cases.

Cervical ribs are common, and may, or may not, contribute to thoracic outlet syndrome. Often, the cause is a functional change in the thoracic outlet due to aging (sagging muscles from sedentary activities) with no significant anatomic fault.[3,4,8]

A carpal tunnel syndrome may coexist.[3,10] Retrograde neurologic symptoms from a carpal tunnel syndrome are common and may be confusing diagnostically. Patients may complain of hand congestion, arm weakness, shoulder pain, and nocturnal paresthesia relieved only by elevating and hyperabducting the arm—all due to a carpal tunnel syndrome.[10] Positive tests for median nerve compression at the wrist, or relief following a corticosteroid injection into the carpal tunnel, will help resolve the cause of symptoms in most patients. Thus, the carpal tunnel syndrome can accompany a thoracic outlet syndrome, or can cause similar symptomatology.

The Examination. A careful history and physical examination are essential. Of 149 patients reviewed by Dale and Lewis,[3] all had reported painful upper extremities; 58% suffered intermittent paresthesia, 23% reported motor incoordination, and only 16% had edema of the upper extremities.

Occupational and other aggravating causes should be elicited. Painters, welders, mailmen, and auto mechanics who frequently work with their arms overhead may acquire the syndrome during hyperabduction. Poor sleep position, with the arms hyperabducted, leads to neurovascular compression. Sedentary activities that allow the shoulders to drop down and forward may provoke symptoms.

The important factor in the physical examination is to *look at the patient*. Is there a postural problem? In the female with heavy pendulous breasts, tight brassiere, and deep strap marks, drooping shoulders will be evident (Fig. 1, p. 7). Is the patient's thorax unusually narrow at the apex? Does the patient have poor muscle tone with drooping clavicles? Palpation and auscultation of the costoclavicular space for the presence of a cervical rib, tumor, aneurysm, or malformation of the body structures are quick, simple, and necessary procedures.[3] Therefore, laying on of hands is essential in the art of dealing with nonarticular rheumatism.

Physical maneuvers, to determine the presence of compression of the neurovascular bundle, include the Adson test, the costoclavicular maneuver,[11] and the hyperabduction maneuver.

The modified *Adson test* is performed with the patient seated, arms at her side; the pulse is palpated at the wrist, and auscultated for a bruit in the supraclavicular space.[12] During the Adson maneuver, the patient performs a Valsalva maneuver with the neck fully extended, arm elevated and the chin turned toward the side being examined, or away from the involved side[7,8] (Fig. 2–2). The purpose of this test is to tense the scalenus anticus muscle. A positive test results in diminished pulsation of the radial artery and a bruit over the axillary vessels; the patient becomes aware of increased paresthesia.

The *costoclavicular maneuver* is performed by having the patient's shoulder rotated backward and downward, with neurovascular features similar to Adson's test becoming evident (Fig. 2–3). The *hyperabduction maneuver* reproduces symptoms when the patient

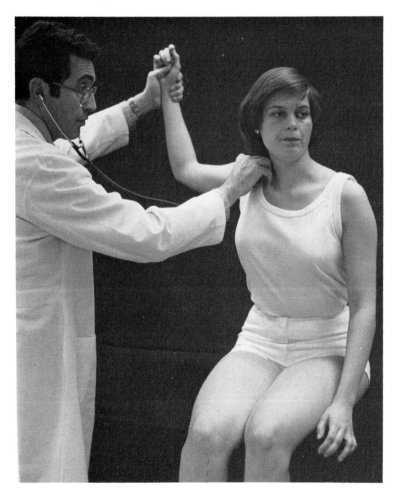

Fig. 2–2. The modified Adson maneuver for neurovascular compression by scalenus anticus muscle. A positive test includes reproduction of symptoms, diminution of the pulse at the wrist, and the development of a bruit over the axillary vessels.

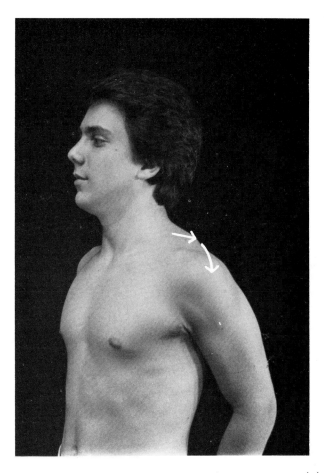

Fig. 2–3. The costoclavicular maneuver (arrows) reproduces symptoms and decreases the pulse amplitude at the costoclavicular space. Backpacking is a common cause for the costoclavicular syndrome.

laterally circumducts the arms and clasps the hands over the head (Fig. 2–4). This results in compression of the neurovascular bundle beneath the insertion of the tendon of the pectoralis minor muscle at the coracoid process.[7]

The *Spurling maneuver,* discussed in Chapter 1, helps to exclude the presence of a cervical nerve root impingement as a cause of symptoms[13] (Fig. 1–11). Of normal asymptomatic persons, 38% have a positive Adson's test, 68% have a positive costoclavicular maneuver, and 54% have a positive hyperabduction maneuver.[10] The reproduction of the patient's symptoms with these tests is valuable in making the diagnosis.

Taking a complete history, observing for neurovascular compres-

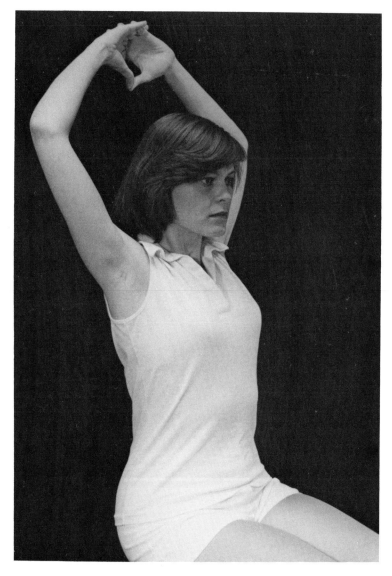

Fig. 2–4. The hyperabduction maneuver reproduces symptoms when compression occurs beneath the insertion of the pectoralis minor tendon at its insertion upon the coracoid process.

sion, reproducing symptoms with one or another of the test maneuvers, and determining any occupational or positional aggravating causes for thoracic outlet compression certainly helps the clinician.[3] A good response to therapy is excellent support for the diagnosis.

Laboratory and Radiographic Examination. Roentgenographs of the chest and cervical spine are necessary to exclude the presence of tumors, cervical ribs, or other skeletal anomalies. An erythrocyte sedimentation rate should be performed to exclude inflammatory and neoplastic conditions. Special tests, including nerve conduction or invasive vascular studies, can be withheld as long as vascular features are not objectively present at the time of the first visit. Stress electrocardiograms may be necessary to exclude other causes if chest pain is a prominent feature.[3] If the patient does not respond to initial therapy, nerve conduction velocities can sometimes provide prognostic information. In normal persons, the ulnar nerve conduction velocity ranges from 68 to 75 m/sec; however, patients with thoracic outlet syndrome usually have delayed conduction levels. Urschel reported that patients whose ulnar nerve conduction velocity was less than 60 m/sec generally required surgical intervention.[2] Electromyogram (EMG) findings were diagnostically supportive in only 40% of patients tested; the chief value of EMG determination may be the recognition of a carpal tunnel syndrome.[3] Vascular studies, including

---

Diagnostic Workup for
Thoracic Outlet Syndrome

History
1. Intermittent pain, paresthesia, and swelling of part or all of an upper extremity.
2. Aggravating factors, such as hyperabducting arms, at work or during sleep.
3. Absence of specific features of carpal tunnel syndrome, cervical disc disease, or other systemic disease.

Physical Examination
1. Check for masses in supraclavicular fossa.
2. Perform special maneuvers (e.g., Adson's, hyperabduction, costoclavicular maneuvers).
3. Absence of objective swelling or atrophy in most patients.

Routine Tests
1. Cervical spine and chest roentgenograms.
2. Tests for inflammation.
3. Electrocardiogram if chest pain coexists.

A Beneficial Response to Treatment May Be the Best Test

Special Tests (rarely needed)
1. Ulnar nerve conduction.
2. Vascular studies, including venography, venous flow rates, or angiography.

arteriography and venography, are indicated when physical findings suggest a vascular disorder, such as an aneurysm or venous thrombosis,[10] but otherwise help little in making the diagnosis. When symptoms suggest the presence of a carpal tunnel syndrome, nerve conduction tests of the ulnar and median nerves can be helpful. Cervical myelography may have to be considered in order to exclude cervical disc disease. We must emphasize that all tests may be normal and careful assessment of each patient is essential.

Differential Diagnosis. Conditions outside of the thoracic outlet rarely cause intermittent neurologic and vascular symptoms in the upper extremity. One should consider the possibility of tumors of the superior pulmonary sulcus (Pancoast's syndrome; see "Pancoast's Syndrome" in this chapter), impingement of a cervical nerve, cervical cord tumor, brachial plexus paralysis, carpal tunnel syndrome with retrograde symptomatology, peripheral neuropathies, syringomyelia, progressive muscle atrophy, reflex sympathetic dystrophy, and thrombosis or inflammation of the vascular tree.[2,14]

Complaints of a purely vascular obstruction, with objective swelling of the upper limb or Raynaud's phenomenon, are rare. Inflammatory diseases, such as giant cell arteritis, Takayasu's arteritis, and thrombosis of the subclavian vein (also called effort thrombosis or Paget-Schroetter's syndrome) must be considered.[2,4]

Management. On the first visit, if the examination is suggestive of a thoracic outlet syndrome, the patient may be told that the diagnosis is probably a benign neurovascular compression syndrome. Aggravating factors can be remedied. For example, women with heavy pendulous breasts should obtain brassieres that support properly. Sleep position should be reviewed with each patient. Patients should avoid sleeping with their arms hyperabducted or elevated. Some patients can be trained to avoid hyperabduction by tying their wrists with a stocking. This, in turn, is safety-pinned to the bed sheet to allow some arm motion, but will restrict hyperabduction of the arms during sleep. (If the patient maintains her sanity, this can work. Most patients break the hyperabduction habit quickly.) During sedentary activities, patients should learn to roll their shoulders up and backward to prevent drooping of the clavicle. Hyperabduction required by employment may necessitate consultation with an occupational therapist.

Trigger points are frequently present along the trapezius ridge, and if palpable, can be relieved with injection of a nonaqueous steroid-anesthetic mixture (see Fig. 1–8). Of paramount importance are exercises to strengthen and correct postural deficits.[3,15] The following exercises should be prescribed: shoulder elevation with resistance, isometric neck strengthening, and if symptoms of chest-wall pain are evident, chest-wall stretching. These exercises correct the forward inclination of the neck and stretch the pectoral musculature.

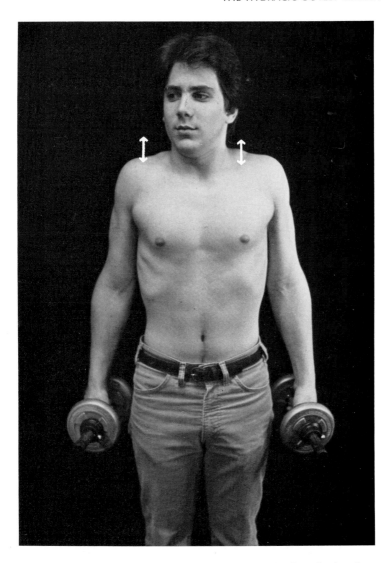

Fig. 2–5. The shoulder shrugging exercise: Using 5 to 10 pounds of weight placed upon each shoulder or held in each hand, the shoulders are shrugged and rotated upward and backward, and then slowly let down; the movement is repeated for 1 to 2 minutes.

The exercises for shoulder elevation can be performed with a 5- to 10-pound weight in each hand or across each shoulder; the patient may be seated or standing. The shoulders are rotated backward, and shrugged slowly up and down while the arms hang at the sides (Fig. 2–5). This exercise is repeated slowly for a few minutes twice daily. An isometric neck-strengthening exercise that seems helpful is performed with the patient backed up to a wall. The patient's heels are 6 to 8 inches out from the wall, the torso lies back against the wall, and the hands are placed loosely behind the vertex of the head. The elbows may be pointed at a 45 degree forward angle from the wall, and the chin is kept neutral (face held perfectly vertical, parallel to the wall). The patient presses her head backward with increased vigor, and feels a stretching and contracting of the neck musculature (Fig. 2–6). This position is held for 10 to 30 seconds, with 3 to 10 repetitions, and is performed twice daily. Chest-wall stretching is accomplished by having the patient stand facing a corner of a room. The patient stands approximately 2 feet out from the corner and places her hands on each wall with the fingers pointed toward the corner.

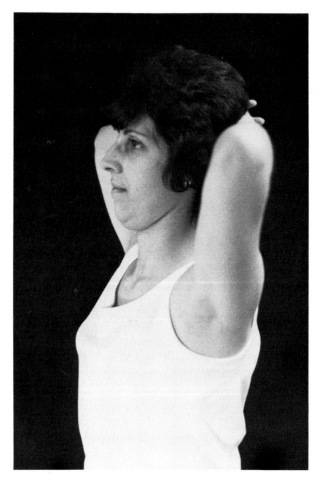

Fig. 2–6. Isometric neck exercise with the chin kept neutral. The hands should *not* press the head forward, but should only meet the backward thrust of the head and hold it from further motion.

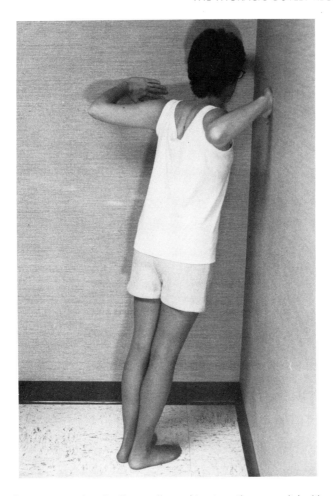

Fig. 2–7. The corner "push up": Chest wall stretching is easily accomplished by standing 2 feet out from a corner, with each hand approximately 18 to 24 inches away from the corner, hands pointed toward the corner and held at shoulder height. With the chin held neutral, the chest wall is gently forced in toward the corner, until a stretching sensation is perceived in the pectoral muscle region.

The shoulder, arm, elbow, and hand are held at shoulder height. She then thrusts her chest slowly into the corner with her head held in the neutral position (the chin neither raised nor lowered).[16] The patient should experience a feeling of stretching in the pectoral muscles (Fig. 2–7). This position is held for 10 to 30 seconds and repeated 3 to 10 times at least twice daily. If sleep is disturbed, a relaxant or sedative may be prescribed at bedtime for the first week or two.[3]

Outcome and Additional Suggestions. Physical therapy and exercise, instructions in proper sitting, and proper work and sleep positions, should provide relief in 50 to 80% of patients[3,7,9,10] usually within 6 weeks.[3] Morning stiffness, hand congestion, paresthesia are the first symptoms to improve. Fewer than 5% of our patients require surgical treatment.

Before surgical exploration, check out the following:
1. Has carpal tunnel syndrome or cervical disc lesion been excluded?
2. Has chest roentgenogram for tumor been reviewed recently?
3. Were aggravating factors eliminated (sleep position, sitting positions, improper work habits)?
4. Did the patient comply with the exercise program?

Vascular studies and nerve conduction tests may be normal, yet surgical intervention is still undertaken because of persistent symptoms. At operation, compression has been found as low as the second rib,[9] and the current surgical procedure of choice is resection of the first rib to provide more space for the neurovascular bundle. Unfortunately, we have seen surgical failures. The symptoms have returned when the patient resumed work requiring hyperabduction. A change in jobs should have preceded operation. We have found that if cases are properly selected, first rib resection through the transaxillary approach gives good results in 85% of operated patients.[17] Others reported somewhat less surgical success.[18]

REFLEX SYMPATHETIC DYSTROPHY (RSD)

The essential features of reflex sympathetic dystrophy (RSD), which may occur in either the upper or lower extremity, include *throbbing, burning pain,* diffuse uncomfortable aching, sensitivity to touch or cold, altered color or temperature of the involved extremity, localized edema, and erythema. Three stages in the course of RSD may occur. In the earliest stage, the presentation consists of hyperesthesia, hyperalgesia, localized edema, erythema, and altered skin temperature. In the second stage, 3 to 6 months from the time of onset, progression of the soft tissue edema, thickening of the skin and articular soft tissues, muscle wasting, and brawny skin develop. In the third and most severe stage, the shoulder-hand syndrome manifestations of limitation of movement, contractures of the digits, waxy trophic skin changes, and brittle, ridged nails appear.[19-23]

Terminology has included causalgia, minor causalgia, shoulder-hand syndrome, shoulder-hand syndrome variant, Sudeck's atrophy, and acute atrophy of bone. Often the syndrome follows injury, surgical intervention, or vascular accidents, such as heart attack or stroke. Pak, in a study of 140 patients, reported that 40% of cases of RSD occurred following soft tissue injury, 25% followed fractures, 20% occurred postoperatively, 12% followed myocardial infarction, and 3% followed cerebral vascular accidents.[24] Of patients with RSD, 37% had significant emotional disturbances at the time of onset.[24] Myofascial trigger points are common in the area of trauma or about the shoulder girdle and trapezius.[25,26] Although only one extremity may appear involved, careful inspection may reveal symmetric synovitis.[22,27] The elbow is usually spared.

Etiology. The probability that central nervous system (CNS) disturbance plays a role in RSD causation is supported by the finding that unilateral sympathetic nerve blocks result in improvement in bilateral skin potential variations (pain thresholds).[25] This improvement lasts 48 hours, long after the pharmacologic effect of the anesthetic has worn off. Furthermore, myofascial trigger points also disappear (even in the limb contralateral to the sympathetic nerve block). A feedback loop with involvement of skin, afferent input into the CNS, then feeding back via a sympathetic output to the skin is proposed as the method for CNS involvement.[25] Changes in the "gate controls" of Melzack and Wall are probable[20,21,28,29] (see Chapt. 13). A self-perpetuating "short circuiting" between pain fibers and sympathetic nerves is then established.

Laboratory and Radiographic Examination. In the early stage, reflex sympathetic dystrophy may reveal no abnormal findings on laboratory testing. After 6 weeks' duration, scintigraphy, using technetium 99m pertechnetate (99m TcO$_4$), may reveal increased uptake in the peripheral joints of the involved extremity.[30,31] Sedimentation rate and other tests of inflammation may increase in the later stages. In the third stage, roentgenographs of the involved extremities may reveal patchy osteoporosis, presumably due to increased blood flow to the involved extremity.[30] A valuable test is the use of regional sympathetic nerve blocks, for both therapy and diagnosis. Abrupt relief from pain and dysesthesia, although transient, is suggestive of a diagnosis of reflex dystrophy. Tests to rule out insidious onset of a connective tissue disease should include rheumatoid and antinuclear factor determinations. A chest roentgenogram for an occult neoplasm at the apex of the lung, on the involved side, should be performed. EMG with nerve conduction velocity may be helpful if thoracic outlet syndrome or carpal tunnel syndrome is a consideration.

Differential Diagnosis. In the earliest stages, reflex sympathetic dystrophy is a difficult diagnosis. However, the quality of *throbbing, burning* pain, *paresthesia*, and *altered skin temperature* is suggestive. Cervical nerve root impingement, Pancoast's syndrome, vasculitis, rheumatoid arthritis, peripheral neuropathy, migratory osteolysis, venous thrombosis, arteriovenous fistulae, progressive systemic sclerosis, and angioedema might be confused with early features of various presentations of RSD.

Management. Four modes of therapy are available, depending on the stage of the dystrophy at the time of the first visit. These are (1) myofascial trigger point injection and physical therapy, (2) sympathetic nerve blocks, (3) oral corticosteroids, and (4) sympathectomy.[32] In the first stage, trigger-point injections with a corticosteroid-local anesthetic mixture, followed by physical therapy, including heat and exercise, may abort progression of the dystrophy. Use of sedation or antidepressive medication may be helpful. Consideration for any possible missed diagnosis (e.g., a missed fracture) is important.

In second stage dystrophy, with beginning induration of the skin of the hand, resting hand and wrist splints may be helpful. At this point, stellate ganglion blocks performed at intervals of 1 to 4 days and repeated 6 to 12 times have been useful. If an immediate response (improved temperature, lessened pain) does not occur following the first or second nerve block, this treatment is abandoned.[21,27] An alternative therapy is using oral corticosteroids in divided doses, ranging from 30 mg per day[23] to 80 mg per day.[27] The dose of corticosteroids is tapered quickly as the patient responds; continued low-dose corticosteroid treatment may be necessary for a prolonged period in severe cases. In all patients, at all stages of the disease, physical therapy should be performed twice daily at home, and use of resting splints should be maintained. Sympathectomy is indicated if progression is apparent, and a positive response to sympathetic nerve blocks occurs. Patients with advanced dystrophic hands should have consultations with physical and occupational therapists. Patients, on occasion, have both reflex sympathetic dystrophy and thoracic outlet syndrome, and may require surgical treatment for both conditions (resection of the first rib and cervical sympathectomy).[3]

Outcome and Additional Suggestions. Our experience with treatment of reflex dystrophy prior to contracture has been excellent with either stellate ganglion blocks or corticosteroid therapy. As mentioned, if seen early after onset, trigger-point injections may break the cycle. We have seen patients have an exacerbation several months after treatment, either upon exposure to cold or following emotional trauma. Small doses of amytal (30 to 60 mg qid) for several weeks, or use of tricyclic antidepressants (amitriptyline) for a recurrence has been helpful in our experience. In late-stage dystrophy, with a practically immobilized hand, aggressive physical therapy is essential, and sympathectomy must be considered. We have seen late-stage dystrophy significantly improve without resorting to sympathectomy. Oral corticosteroids have not proven as helpful in late-stage dystrophy.

PANCOAST'S SYNDROME

Tumors within the superior pulmonary sulcus that compress the lower roots of the brachial plexus, the intercostal nerves, the stellate

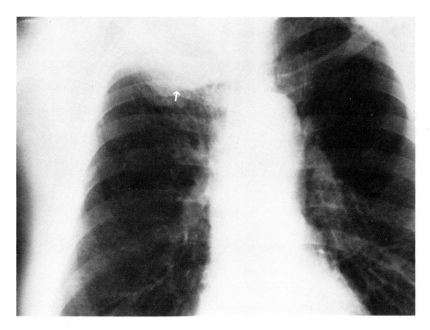

Fig. 2–8. A lung tumor (arrow) associated with Pancoast's syndrome. Although such lesions may be clinically silent until late, chest roentgenograms with apical lordotic views should be performed if symptoms are at all suggestive.

ganglion, and the sympathetic nerve chain comprise Pancoast's syndrome. Features include constant pain, at first in the shoulder region, and later along the ulnar distribution to the arm and hand. Still later, Horner's syndrome and anhidrosis of the ipsilateral face and upper extremity occur, and atrophy of the intrinsic muscles of the hand may be noted.[33]

Careful study of the superior pulmonary sulcus with standard and apical lordotic roentgenographs is essential (Fig. 2–8). Treatment obviously depends upon finding the nature of the mass, since the vast majority are malignant.

We must again emphasize that discomfort of the thoracic outlet syndrome is intermittent, whereas Pancoast's syndrome of pain, burning, and numbness is constant. The constancy of symptoms (present day and night) must stimulate the physician to order appropriate roentgenographs and study them carefully. In one report, 34% of patients treated surgically for superior sulcus tumors survived 5 years, and 29% survived 10 years.[34]

REFERENCES

1. Urschel HC, Razzuk MA, Hyland JW, et al: Thoracic outlet syndrome masquerading as coronary artery disease (pseudoangina). Ann Thorac Surg 16:239–248, 1973.

2. Urschel HC, Razzuk MA: Management of the thoracic-outlet syndrome. N Engl J Med 286:1140–1143, 1972.
3. Dale WA, Lewis MR: Management of thoracic outlet syndrome. Ann Surg 181:575–585, 1975.
4. Bertelsen S: Neurovascular compression syndromes of the neck and shoulder. Acta Chir Scand 135:137–148, 1969.
5. Keshishian JM, Smyth NPD: Thoracic outlet syndrome: Diagnosis and management. Ann Thorac Surg 9:391–400, 1970.
6. Winsor T, Brow R: Costoclavicular syndrome; Its diagnosis and treatment. JAMA 196:109–111, 1966.
7. Tyson RR, Kaplan GF: Modern concepts of diagnosis and treatment of the thoracic outlet syndrome. Orthop Clin North Am 6:507–519, 1975.
8. Steinbrocker O: The painful shoulder. *In* Arthritis and Allied Conditions. 8th Ed. Edited by JE Hollander and DJ McCarty Jr. Philadelphia, Lea & Febiger, 1972.
9. Roos DB: Experience with first rib resection for thoracic outlet syndrome. Ann Surg 173:429–442, 1971.
10. Conn J: Thoracic outlet syndromes. Surg Clin North Am 54:155–164, 1974.
11. Roos DB, Owens JC: Thoracic outlet syndrome. Arch Surg 93:71–74, 1966.
12. Jackson R: The Cervical Syndrome. Springfield, IL, Charles C Thomas, 1978.
13. Spurling RG, Scoville WB: Lateral rupture of the cervical intervertebral discs. Surg Gynecol Obstet 78:350–358, 1944.
14. Duthie RB, Ferguson AB: Mercer's Orthopedic Surgery. 7th Ed. Baltimore, Williams & Wilkins, 1973.
15. Peet RM, Henriksen JD, Anderson TB, Martin GM: Thoracic outlet syndrome: Evaluation of a therapeutic exercise program. Proc Staff Meet Mayo Clin 31:281–287, 1956.
16. Swezey RL: Arthritis: Rational Therapy and Rehabilitation. Philadelphia, WB Saunders, 1978.
17. Goldberg VM: The results of first rib resection in thoracic outlet syndrome. Orthopedics 4:1025–1029, 1981.
18. Fairbairn JF, Clagett OT: Peripheral Vascular Diseases. 4th Ed. Philadelphia, WB Saunders, 1972.
19. Homans J: Minor causalgia: A hyperesthetic neurovascular syndrome. N Engl J Med 222:870–874, 1940.
20. deJong RH, Cullen SC: Theoretical aspects of pain: Bizarre pain phenomena during low spinal anesthesia. Anesthesiology 24:628–635, 1963.
21. Bonica JJ: Causalgia and other reflex sympathetic dystrophies. Postgrad Med 53:143–148, 1973.
22. Steinbrocker O, Argyros TG: The shoulder-hand syndrome: Present status as a diagnostic and therapeutic entity. Med Clin North Am 42:1533–1553, 1958.
23. Mowat AG: Treatment of the shoulder-hand syndrome with corticosteroids. Ann Rheum Dis 33:120–123, 1974.
24. Pak TJ, Martin GM, Magness JL, Kavanaugh GJ: Reflex sympathetic dystrophy. Minn Med 53:507–512, 1970.
25. Procacci, P, Francin F, Zoppi M, et al: Role of sympathetic system in reflex dystrophies. *In* Advances in Pain Research and Therapy. Vol. 1. Edited by JJ Bonica, D Albe-Fessard. New York, Raven Press, 1976.
26. Edeiken J, Wolferth CC: Persistent pain in the shoulder region following myocardial infarction. Am J Med Sci 191:201–210, 1936.
27. Kozin F, McCarty DJ, Sims J, Genant HK: The reflex dystrophy syndrome. I. Clinical and histological studies: Evidence for bilaterality, response to corticosteroids and articular involvement. Am J Med 60:321–331, 1976.
28. Bonica JJ: Neurophysiologic and pathologic aspects of acute and chronic pain. Arch Surg 112:750–761, 1977.
29. Melzach R, Wall PD: Pain mechanisms: A new theory. Science 150:971–979, 1965.
30. Kozin F, Genant HK, Bekerman C, McCarty DJ: The reflex sympathetic dystrophy syndrome. II. Roentgenographic and scintigraphic evidence of bilaterality and of periarticular accentuation. Am J Med 60:332–338, 1976.

31. Carlson DH, Simon H, Wegner W: Bone scanning and diagnosis of reflex sympathetic dystrophy secondary to herniated lumbar disks. Neurology 27:791–793, 1977.
32. Moskowitz RW: Clinical Rheumatology. Philadelphia, Lea & Febiger, 1975.
33. Hepper NGG, Herskovic T, Witten DM, Mulder DW, Woolner LB: Thoracic inlet tumors. Ann Intern Med 64:979–988, 1966.
34. Paulson DL: Carcinomas in the superior pulmonary sulcus. J. Thorac Cardiovasc Surg 70:1095–1104, 1975.

Chapter 3

THE SHOULDER GIRDLE REGION

When presented with a shoulder problem, the physician must take a careful history to determine whether the complaint is an *intrinsic* shoulder problem (e.g., osteoarthritis, bursitis), an *extrinsic* shoulder problem reflecting pain from other structures (e.g., reflex dystrophy, referred pain arising from cholecystitis), or part of systemic disease.[1-3] A *pain pattern* may delineate the nature of the specific shoulder problem.[1] Furthermore, the clinician should seek aggravating factors that might cause recurrences.

The History. Pain quality, location, duration, and frequency are important. For example, axillary pain of a constant undulating quality should raise suspicion of a mediastinal lesion. Pain over the deltoid region is frequently referred from the subacromial bursa, but can also arise from a myofascial trigger point in the infraspinatus muscle; and pain in the triceps area may be referred from the serratus posterior superior muscle.[4]

Intermittent pain and disability suggest tendon injury or myofascial disturbances. Pain that is present both day and night suggests capsular involvement, true shoulder synovitis, or tumor. Pain that is intermittent, throbbing, or burning suggests reflex sympathetic dystrophy (shoulder-hand syndrome). Abrupt onset of pain accompanied by limitation of movement suggests tissue disruption, such as a capsular tear or a shoulder joint dislocation.

What about the rest of the body? Are there complaints in other parts of the same extremity, or is there a history of systemic inflammatory rheumatic disease? For example, a patient with carpal tunnel syndrome occasionally has retrograde nerve involvement to the shoulder,[5] and cervical radiculopathy pain is often noted at the shoulder. Knowledge of the patient's past history may suggest intra-abdominal or intrathoracic problems with referral of pain to the shoulder or scapular regions. Diaphragmatic irritation from intrathoracic or intraabdominal structures has specific patterns of pain referral. For example, irritation of the anterior portion of the diaphragm may refer pain to the clavicle or to the front of the shoulder, pain from the posterior diaphragm may refer to the supraspinatus region of the shoulder, pain from the dome of the diaphragm may refer to the acromioclavicular joint area, and irritation of the central portion of the diaphragm may refer pain into both shoulder regions.[6]

Therefore, systemic rheumatic diseases, metabolic disorders (e.g., hyperparathyroidism, hypothyroidism, hyperthyroidism, diabetes), neurologic disturbances, and cardiovascular diseases involve the shoulder.[7-9] Fortunately, fewer than 5 to 10% of shoulder afflictions are due to true arthritis.[3,10]

Aggravating factors can range from activities on the job, sports, hobbies, or sleep position. Most important are activities in which the arm is held in close to the body for prolonged periods (e.g., typing or needlepoint). Next in importance are work habits with repetitive motions, particularly while the arm is raised over the head. A middle-aged person taking up tennis, carpentry, or starting a new calisthenic program may become symptomatic. Sleeping with the arms held overhead may be a factor in developing shoulder pain.

The Shoulder Examination. Examining a patient with a shoulder problem is an art. The examiner must know the accepted normal ranges of shoulder motion, something about the dynamics of shoulder function, and something about innervation of the shoulder structure. Shoulder function depends on a scapulohumeral rhythm, an unhampered gliding motion, integrity of the musculotendinous cuff, normality of the bursae, integrity of the long head of the biceps, and mobility of the joint capsule.[3] The sternoclavicular joint is the pivot on which the shoulder girdle moves on the trunk.[11]

It is important that the clinician examines the whole patient. We have already demonstrated the importance of postural disturbances, and have stressed that shoulder problems arising from involvement of distant structures (e.g., the neck, the carpal tunnel, or systemic inflammatory disease) may be apparent on gross inspection. Note the *symmetry* of acromioclavicular joints of the scapulae and muscle bulk, and observe scapular movement during active shoulder and neck motion.

When the patient performs a movement, the movement is called *active movement*; when the examiner moves the patient's arm, it is called *passive movement*; and when the patient attempts active movement against the examiner's resistance, the movement is called *active resistive motion*.

First, the patient performs an active motion, shoulder abduction, which should be observed from the rear. The patient swings his arm away from his side, out and up. *Abduction* occurs from zero degrees (arm handing dependently at the side) outward and upward to 90 degrees; *elevation* proceeds from 90 to 180 degrees. Next, the shoulder, used as a hinge, is observed from the side view as *forward* and *backward extension*. Motion is next observed with the shoulder used as a rotary or ball-and-socket joint. With his arm at his side, the patient bends his elbow to 90 degrees and rotates his elbow internally (hand

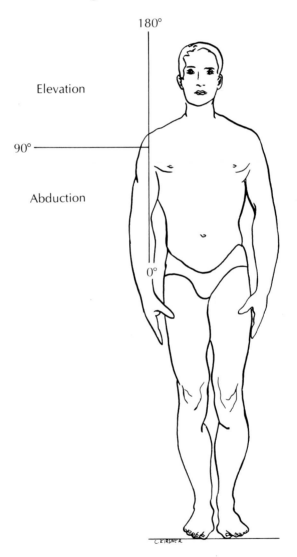

Fig. 3–1. Active shoulder motion during *abduction* from 0 to 90 degrees. Further raising of the arm, *elevation*, proceeds from 90 to 180 degrees.

to chest), or externally (hand away from chest). This rotation may also be observed with the arm abducted to 90 degrees; this time external rotation brings the hand up, and internal rotation brings the hand down. Thus, *internal* and *external rotation* refer to the direction of movement of the humerus (Figs. 3–1, 3–2, 3–3).

Active shoulder motion may be limited either from pain or from intrinsic shoulder disturbances. With the patient as relaxed as possible, *passive* shoulder motion is attempted by the examiner to determine the presence of intrinsic shoulder disease. The examination should be performed slowly in each direction to prevent muscle guarding. The examination for passive range of movement includes abduction-elevation and internal-external rotation, while keeping scapular movement to a minimum. The examiner should keep a hand upon the suprascapular ridge, to identify scapular movement and to demonstrate true glenohumeral motion, while performing passive arm motion.

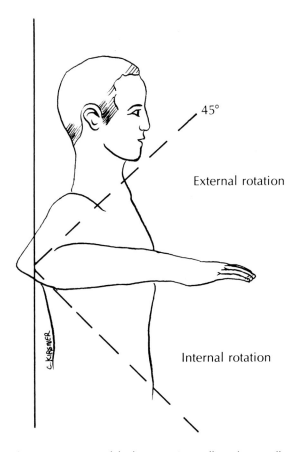

Fig. 3–2. Rotation of the humerus, internally and externally.

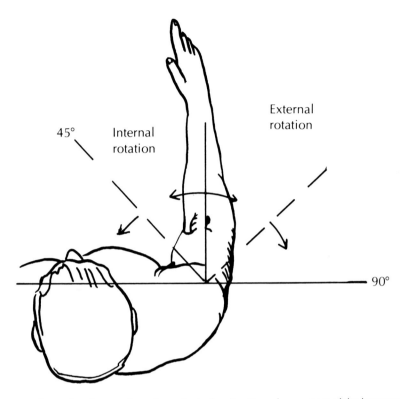

Fig. 3–3. Internal and external rotation refer to the direction of movement of the humerus.

Bursitis and tendinitis may interfere with active movement, but usually allow passive movement. Adhesive capsulitis restricts both active and passive shoulder motion. Furthermore, loss of motion in only one direction suggests a single tendon injury or bursitis, whereas loss of passive motion in two or more planes suggests capsule or true shoulder joint disease. Generally, myofascial disorders or nerve root impingement interfere little, if at all, with passive shoulder motion.

The examiner palpates for synovitis, bicipital tenosynovitis, acromioclavicular joint swelling, sternoclavicular joint swelling, and shoulder joint crepitus. The examiner palpates posteriorly for myofascial trigger points in the serratus, rhomboid, trapezius, teres minor, and supraspinatus muscles, and along the medial border of the scapula while the scapula is drawn laterally (by having the patient adduct the arm across the chest to rotate the scapula laterally) (Fig. 3–4). Firm pressure over these structures in obscure shoulder pain problems may establish the presence of a myofascial trigger point, which will then reproduce the pain in the "target zone." A common example is an

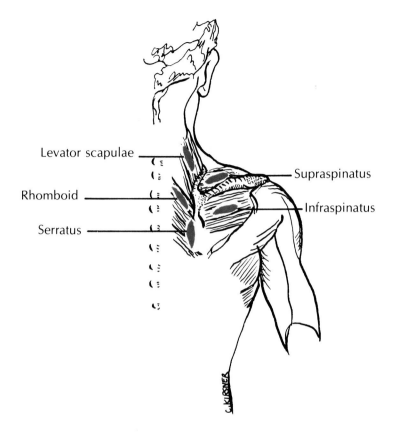

Levator scapulae

Rhomboid

Serratus

Supraspinatus

Infraspinatus

Fig. 3–4. While the scapula is drawn laterally by having the patient bring his arm across the chest, palpation in the region of the supraspinatus, infraspinatus, serratus, rhomboideus, and levator scapulae muscles may establish the presence of myofascial trigger points with reproduction of pain in the "target zone."

infraspinatus trigger point with a target zone over the deltoid area of the shoulder (Fig. 3–5).

We have already mentioned performing the Spurling maneuver in patients with suspected cervical nerve root impingement (see Chapt. 1). Patients with bicipital tenosynovitis may have palpable swelling of the biceps tendon sheath; tenderness and swelling are detected by rolling a finger across the biceps tendon and comparing this with the uninvolved biceps tendon of the opposite shoulder (Fig. 3–6). Active resistant motion is performed by having the patient abduct and elevate the arm from 80 to 100 degrees against the examiner's resistance.[1,12] The examiner searches particularly for a tear of the shoulder capsule. Shoulder pain in a patient with a normal shoulder

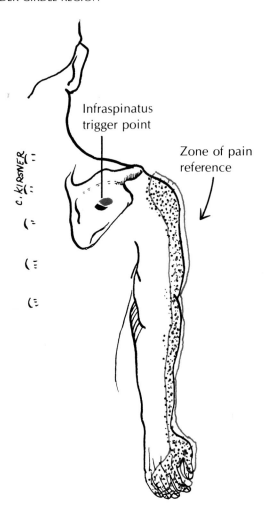

Infraspinatus
trigger point

Zone of pain
reference

C. KIRSNER

Fig. 3–5. Infraspinatus trigger point with target zone radiating from the deltoid region down as far as the hand.

examination should raise the suspicion of referred shoulder pain. The physician should develop a patterned habit of shoulder examination, and should no longer simply label a shoulder problem "arthritis."

MUSCULOTENDINOUS ROTATOR CUFF DISORDERS

Shoulder injury and morbidity are second only to back injury in industrial-related injuries.[13] The conditions included as "rotator cuff" disorders are often overlapping, and are initially the result of tendon injury and degeneration. The musculotendinous rotator cuff portion of the shoulder capsule is the conjoint tendon of the supraspinatus,

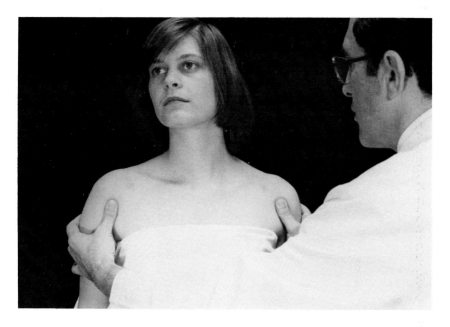

Fig. 3–6. Detection of bicipital tendinitis by rolling across the long head of the biceps and comparing one side to the other.

infraspinatus, and teres minor muscles, which insert onto the greater tuberosity, and the subscapularis, which inserts onto the lesser tuberosity.[1] Injury generally occurs in patients over the age of 40, following stressful activities of the shoulder, or in young patients after a severe injury.

Types of Rotator Cuff Disorders. The most common rotator cuff disorders are supraspinatus tendinitis, the impingement syndrome, calcific tendinitis, subacromial and subcoracoid bursitis, and rotator cuff tears. Rotator cuff tendinitis is seldom isolated to a single musculotendinous structure, and unless promptly recognized and treated, the tendinitis can progress to a frozen shoulder. The *impingement syndrome* refers to supraspinatus tendinitis or bicipital tendinitis, which results from these tendons being pinched between the head of the humerus and the acromion[14] (Fig. 3–7).

Tendinitis and the Impingement Syndrome. The supraspinatus muscle and tendon are the most common sites of shoulder disease.[7] The patient complains of painful motion of the shoulder in an arc from 60 to 75 degrees of abduction. Forward motion is generally unimpaired. Night pain is usually troublesome. This pain is distributed generally throughout the shoulder region, and may vary from day to day or become constant. The impingement syndrome usually results

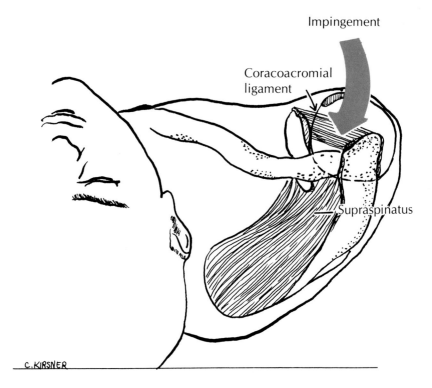

Fig. 3–7. The impingement syndrome: Pinching the supraspinatus or bicipital tendons between the head of the humerus and the acromion.

from injury to the supraspinatus and upper-end of the biceps tendons, during repetitive elevation and forward motion of the arm, in work or sports. The supraspinatus and biceps tendons become impinged by the head of the humerus pressing against the acromion process or the coracoacromial ligament[14,15] (Fig. 3–7). Occasionally, the neurovascular bundle can also be impinged at this site,[16] in an area of relatively decreased blood supply. At this point, ischemic degenerative disruption of the rotator cuff can occur.[17]

Calcific tendinitis usually involves the supraspinatus or biceps muscles and tends to occur in younger individuals, and in particular, white collar workers.[11,18] Calcific tendinitis can mimic gout with acute attacks not only in the shoulder, but in other periarticular sites.[8,19] Calcific tendinitis tends to have an acute onset that reaches maximum severity within several days, and then has a rapid spontaneous improvement as the calcium ruptures into the subacromial bursa. Calcium deposits, as seen on roentgenogram, frequently correlate poorly with shoulder symptoms. Only 35% of patients with radiographic evidence of soft tissue shoulder calcification develop symptoms (Fig. 3–8). However, if the deposits are greater than 1.5 cm in diameter, most patients develop shoulder symptoms.[8,20] Conversely, calcific deposits are not generally seen in patients who have tears of the musculotendinous cuff, and are not usually symptomatic in the elderly.[21] Nevertheless, calcific tendinitis can occur as a specific syndrome.

Bicipital tendinitis may occur as an isolated condition. The patient notices discomfort in the anterior upper area of the bicipital tendon.

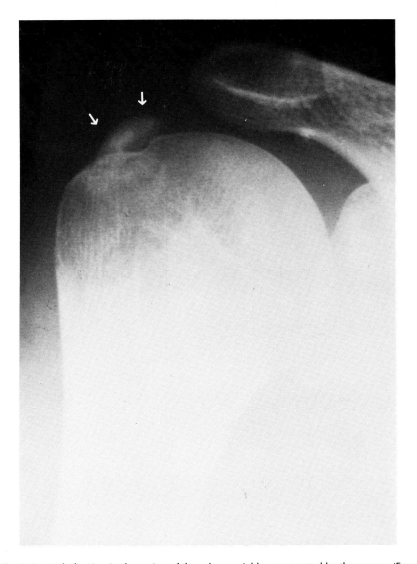

Fig. 3–8. Calcification in the region of the subacromial bursa as noted by the arrows. (From the ARA Clinical Slide Collection, 1972. Used by permission of the Arthritis Foundation.)

This area is frequently injured during forced resistance to the flexed elbow while the forearm is supinated (palm turned upward).[6] Repetitive movement, as in tightening jar lids, is a common cause. Bicipital tendinitis may be a part of the *impingement syndrome*, and the patient may complain of pain in the anterior shoulder and over the coracoacromial ligament.

Physical examination of patients with supraspinatus tendinitis may reveal tenderness over the greater tuberosity while the arm is hanging downward (Dawbarn's sign). Pain elicited while the examiner pulls downward on the patient's arm may also suggest supraspinatus tendinitis. Scapulohumeral rhythm (see "Scapular Region Disorders" on p. 74) during active shoulder movement may be altered as the patient splints the glenohumeral joint and uses the scapula to provide shoulder motion. This results in a shrugging-type motion of the shoulder.[1] Bicipital tendinitis is usually accompanied by swelling of the biceps tendon sheath; the enlargement is palpable as the examiner rolls his fingers across both the involved and uninvolved biceps tendons at the same time, and compares the two sides (Fig. 3–6). Tenderness is usually exquisite over the involved biceps tendon. The test for Yergason's sign for bicipital tendinitis is performed by flexing the elbow and having the patient forcefully supinate (turn the palmar aspect upward) the forearm against resistance (Fig. 3–9). In the presence of bicipital tendinitis, the patient feels pain in the area of the

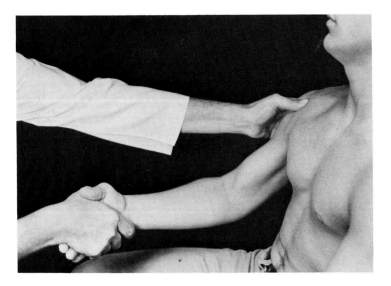

Fig. 3–9. Yergason's sign for bicipital tendinitis: Patient forcefully turns the palmar aspect of the hand upward (supination) while the elbow is held in a flexed position. Supination is performed against the examiner's resistance. Pain is produced if bicipital tendinitis is present.

bicipital groove. Most important, in tendinitis of the long head of the biceps or the musculotendinous cuff, *passive range of movement is normal*.

Rupture of the biceps tendon, following a fall on the shoulder, results in visible swelling of the biceps muscle belly rolled up in the distal one third of the arm, and weakness of elbow flexion is apparent.[11]

To test for the impingement syndrome, the examiner attempts to force the humerus against the anterior acromion while elevating the arm to reproduce impingement pain. Pain relief with injection of a local anesthetic agent beneath the acromion is a helpful diagnostic sign.[14]

Bursitis. The onset of subacromial bursitis may be acute or chronic. The attack often follows injury to the musculotendinous cuff, particularly the supraspinatus tendon. The pain is often exquisite, may be present day and night, and is aggravated by active abduction of the arm. *The pain frequently is referred to the insertion of the deltoid muscle at the junction of the upper third and middle third of the arm,*[6] *and may be the prominent site of the patient's complaint.*

Subacromial and subcoracoid bursitis are frequently secondary to adjacent tendon injury.[1] Bursitis may occur following tendinitis of the musculotendinous cuff, biceps tendon, or impingement of the bursa. A tear of the musculotendinous cuff may involve the floor of the subacromial bursa with a buildup of pressure by the fluid.[1] The subcoracoid bursa, which is between the coracoid process and the joint capsule, may be irritated by pressure from the coracoid against the head of the humerus during excessive arm use. Pain is noted over the coracoid process and medial shoulder.[6] The presenting symptom of bursitis is seldom swelling, unless a systemic disease has caused true joint synovitis with spread to the communicating bursae. Physical examination of patients with acute bursitis requires absolute patient relaxation before *passive* range of movement can be determined to be normal. If muscle splinting prevents passive range of movement in a patient with bursitis, the loss of range of movement occurs in only one plane, *abduction*.

Rotator Cuff Tear. In the younger individual, rupture or tear of the musculotendinous cuff causes acute pain following trauma; it is less noticeable and easily missed in the elderly.[11] A history of falling on the shoulder joint or on the outstretched arm should raise suspicion of a tear of the musculotendinous cuff. Physical examination to elicit a shoulder cuff tear is important in evaluating any patient with shoulder pain. In a cuff tear, the patient may be able to actively abduct the arm to slightly less than 90 degrees. When the patient attempts further abduction and elevation against the examiner's resistance, the arm gives way and drops (the Moseley test), yet the shoulder is capable of normal passive motion.[1,11] This discrepancy should quickly raise concern for a musculotendinous tear.

In summary, examination of the shoulder joint requires the following rules: (1) think of the whole patient, (2) consider aggravating factors, such as poor posture or injurious work habits, activities, hobbies, or sports, (3) examine the entire arc of shoulder motion actively, passively, and against resistance, (4) inspect scapulohumeral "rhythm" during active motion of the shoulder. "Laying on of hands" is essential.

Etiology. The etiology of soft tissue shoulder disturbances is obscure, but probably is biochemical and traumatic in origin.[21] Some degeneration of the musculotendinous cuff occurs in all of us after the fifth decade.[11] The "critical zone" of the musculotendinous cuff at its insertion on the humerus is vulnerable to injury. Ischemia of the cuff in this region may play a role in rupture. Incomplete tears of the musculotendinous cuff have been noted in 30% of cadavers.[6] The supraspinatus tendon is under constant friction against the acromion during motion, and degeneration of this tendon is a constant feature of shoulder cuff disorders.[6]

Impingement of the biceps and supraspinatus tendons between the anterior edge of the acromion and the coracoacromial ligament results in injury. Three stages are recognized: edema and hemorrhage, fibrosis and tendinitis, and bone spurs with tendon rupture.[14] The biceps tendon is often noted to be eroded at operation; it can completely disappear or remain fixed and scarred in the bicipital groove in patients over the age of 50.[11]

Dislocation of the biceps brachii may occur when the joint capsule is stretched, allowing the tendon to slip over the lesser tuberosity, resulting in bicipital tendinitis.[6] The biceps tendon is covered by a transverse humeral ligament that crosses the bicipital groove, and the tendon is enveloped by a synovial extension from the true joint capsule. A supratubercular ridge of Meyer or a shallow bicipital groove (both of which are congenital) may be found in patients with chronic bicipital tendinitis. Tenosynovitis of the biceps may occur in systemic disease, particularly rheumatoid arthritis. Any shoulder joint inflammation may communicate with the bicipital tendon sheath, and cause tenosynovitis, as may infection of the true shoulder joint.[11]

Patients with a shallow glenoid are subject to subluxation or dislocation following trauma. In contact sports, acute subacromial bursitis may result from hemorrhage into the bursa from adjacent tendon tears; rupture of the musculotendinous cuff must be considered.[14] Impingement syndrome frequently occurs in sports enthusiasts over 40 years of age; biceps tenosynovitis may be the presenting problem. Bicipital tendon subluxation can also occur in the older athlete when the musculotendinous cuff is torn.

In calcific tendinitis, histopathologic studies reveal calcific deposits, infiltration with chronic inflammatory cells, and giant cells in dystrophic fibrillation of tendons. This suggests that calcification is secondary to dystrophic changes within the tendon.[13] Tendon rupture is rarely seen in surgical examination of patients with calcific tendinitis. Calcium deposits with a toothpaste consistency commonly occur about the tendocapsular structures and tendon insertions.[22] Specific identification of the calcific deposits, as hydroxyapatite, may be difficult due to their small crystal size, but shiny, globular coin-like bodies, which appear to represent crystals in clumps, provide a clue to their presence.[8,23,24] Electron microscopic and electron probe analysis techniques can corroborate crystal identification as apatite.[22-24] If the calcium deposit is deep in the tendon body, no symptoms result; pain occurs when the deposit irritates the bursa, and is relieved when the deposit ruptures into the bursa.[6] A metabolic disorder resulting in calcium hydroxyapatite deposition may be primary to the etiology of calcific tendinitis. Radiographic examination for deposits in other periarticular structures is helpful.

In summary, the etiology of musculotendinous rotator cuff disorders is mechanical and biochemical. Impingement of bony structures upon tendons may occur, and degenerative change is a constant finding. Biochemical processes, particularly those involving hydroxyapatite deposition, may be involved. Consideration of aggravating repetitious microtrauma should be in the clinician's mind. When the aggravating factors are alleviated, most patients enjoy longstanding improvement. The history of job, sports activities, hobbies, and sleep position must be considered to recognize and prevent future repetition of the musculotendinous injury.

Laboratory and Radiographic Examination. Erythrocyte sedimentation rate, roentgenograms of the chest, and routine, rotational, trans-scapular, or axillary roentgenographic views of the shoulder should be obtained. These may be deferred if the problem appears straightforward and the patient agrees to obtain roentgenograms on the first follow-up visit if relief has not occurred. Radiographic examination of the chest, with lateral view and with particular reference to the mediastinum, should be obtained in every patient with axillary pain.

Roentgenograms of the shoulder may reveal the presence of calcification with a "skull cap" appearance in the soft tissues about the lateral shoulder tip (Fig. 3–8). This is suggestive of calcium that has ruptured into the subacromial bursa,[21,25] and which, as a rule, will be absorbed spontaneously. However, if the calcium deposit is greater than 1.5 cm in diameter, irrigation of the bursa should be considered. This will be discussed under "Management," in this chapter.

The roentgenogram may reveal osteoporosis or patchy cysts of the head of the humerus in the presence of supraspinatus tendinitis. The outer border of the clavicle may have disappeared in patients with malignancy. Degenerative arthritis of the glenohumeral joint or the acromioclavicular joint may be seen. These findings must be correlated with the clinical features.

An arthrogram of the shoulder is indicated when physical findings suggest a shoulder cuff tear, or when further information is required. This may be deferred until a follow-up visit after conservative therapy has been attempted. However, if the Moseley test is positive, an arthrogram should be obtained immediately. Repair of a torn muscular cuff is difficult if the tear is not recognized promptly. In other musculotendinous cuff disorders, an arthrogram may be of some diagnostic help, but it is invasive and may not change the treatment program.

Differential Diagnosis. The differential diagnosis of shoulder pain includes referred pain from diaphragmatic irritation, neurovascular compression, systemic inflammatory diseases, and tumor. Patients with diffuse shoulder pain, without objective tenderness or limitation of movement, may have diaphragmatic irritation with referred pain. In such patients the pain may be reproduced by gentle but firm pressure over the epigastrium. When this is found, roentgenography of the upper gastrointestinal tract for hiatus hernia, reflux esophagitis, gastric ulcer, or peptic ulcer should be considered. A careful neurologic examination for cervical disc disease or studies to exclude hypothyroidism may be rewarding.

Management. Management begins with the recognition of one or more of the musculotendinous rotator cuff disturbances, and exclusion of systemic or referred pain conditions. The clinician should explain the problem to the patient, in order to have the patient and the physician together try to recognize and avoid aggravating factors. In the case of sport-induced injury, correction of improper shoulder use can often alleviate future recurrences.[14] Work habits, particularly overhead arm use,[25] may require evaluation by an occupational therapist.

Pain relief in tendon problems about the shoulder may be obtained in dramatic fashion if a corticosteroid-anesthetic mixture is injected into the correct tendon site (Figs. 3–10, 3–11). A local anesthetic alone may be administered to test whether pain is relieved before adding the corticosteroid. Relief from the injection provides diagnostic value in bicipital tendinitis, supraspinatus tendinitis, subacromial and subcoracoid bursitis, and the impingement syndrome.[1,6,14,21] After the injection, the patient should be discouraged from participating in stressful shoulder activities for 2 to 3 weeks, although the pain has been relieved.

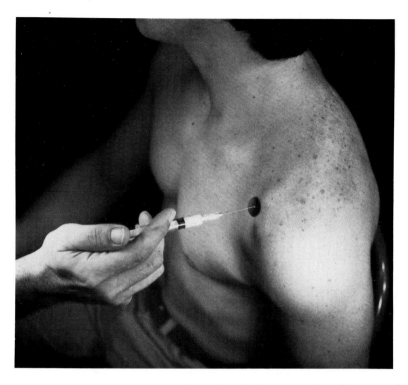

Fig. 3–10. Having located the site of tendinitis beneath the acromioclavicular joint, a short No. 23 needle is threaded into the supraspinatus tendon and a corticosteroid-anesthetic mixture administered.

Every patient with a musculotendinous cuff problem should have a home exercise program directed toward the involved site. In the case of bursitis and supraspinatus tendon inflammation, pendulum exercises should be initiated as soon as acute symptoms are relieved, followed by gentle stretching of the shoulder capsule (Figs. 3–12, 3–13). Bicipital tendinitis in particular requires a gentle stretching out of the biceps tendon to release adhesions between the tendon and its sheath. This can be performed with a wand exercise (Fig. 3–14). In general, it is wise to perform the exercises twice daily, and continue them for several weeks after the pain has been relieved.

When calcific tendinitis is present and the deposit is greater than 1.5 cm in diameter, aspiration and irrigation (with a large No. 16 to No. 18 bore needle) may be helpful if initial corticosteroid injection does not provide relief. Following corticosteroid injection, pain may be aggravated for the first 24 hours. Ice can be applied, particularly during the night following injection. Relief generally occurs within a few days.

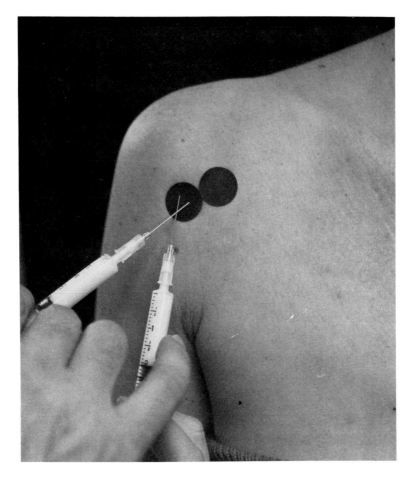

Fig. 3–11. In performing injection for biceps tendinitis, the needle should be directed parallel to the tendon after puncturing the skin.

Rarely is more than one injection necessary. If a tendon requires two or more injections, orthopedic consultation should be considered.[1,26] On occasion, use of ultrasound to disperse the steroid crystals is helpful, and is performed immediately following injection of a steroid anesthetic mixture.

When calcific tendinitis occurs in a young adult, calcium apatite deposition disease should be suspected. The use of colchicine (0.6 mg, 2 to 4 times daily)[19] or nonsteroidal anti-inflammatory drugs may be prescribed for long-term use.

Outcome and Additional Suggestions. Richardson reported that prognosis of musculotendinous rotator cuff disorders correlated with passive range of movement. A good result was seen in nearly all

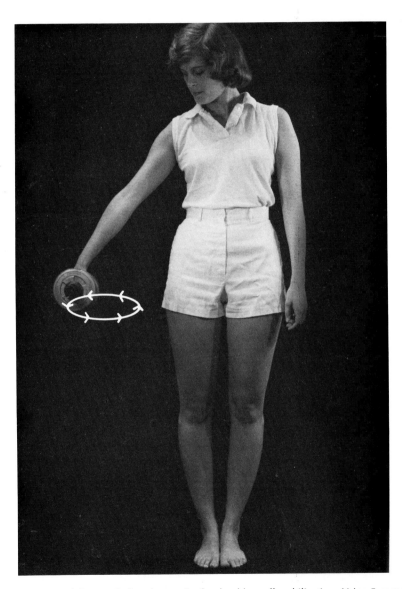

Fig. 3–12. Pendulum or Codman's exercise for shoulder cuff mobilization: Using 5 or more pounds, the patient rotates the arm in a 12-in. diameter circle while leaning slightly to the side. This is performed for a minute in each direction.

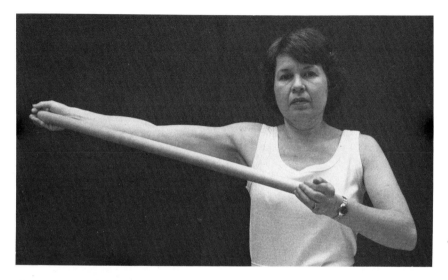

Fig. 3–13. Wand exercise in which the good arm gently forces the arm on the bad side out and away, thus stretching the shoulder capsule. After a minute or so, the good arm draws the bad arm back toward the midline.

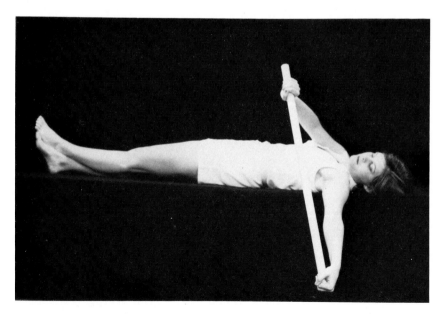

Fig. 3–14. Wand exercise: Performed off the side of the bed to stretch the long head of the biceps. The arm of the good side gently forces the shoulder into posterior extension, thus stretching the biceps tendon.

patients following injection and exercise, if there was a good passive range of motion of the shoulder at the start of treatment.[27] Of patients with these disorders, 90% will obtain satisfactory recovery within 3 to 6 weeks.[1,14,21] Only 10% of patients with musculotendinous disorders require surgical consideration.[21] Patients who do not respond to conservative therapy, or young or middle-aged patients with a definite injury history and features of a rotator cuff tear, should have orthopedic consultation.[11,14]

Prolonged immobilization for a tear of the musculotendinous cuff may promote adhesive capsulitis (frozen shoulder). Early use of assisted passive range of movement exercise is the best preventive program. A trial of assisted passive exercises followed by active exercises should be undertaken.

FROZEN SHOULDER (ADHESIVE CAPSULITIS)

The term "frozen shoulder" aptly describes a common disturbance of the shoulder with a *limitation of shoulder motion*. Described as periarthritis, adhesive capsulitis, frozen shoulder, adhesive bursitis, check rein disorder,[1] and DuPlay's disease,[21] this disorder may involve one or both shoulders. This disorder often occurs in women with cardiovascular disease,[11] but is frequently seen in men as well. It is rare in persons under the age of 40.

Onset usually begins on one side and is insidious. The usual presenting complaint is pain at night in a shoulder that has lost range of motion.[28] The earliest motion lost may be that which is necessary when reaching backward to fasten a brassiere or slip into a coat. Later, shoulder elevation is lost. The ache is described in the anterolateral aspect of the shoulder, the anterolateral arm, and the flexor portion of the forearm; occasionally the pain radiates to the chest wall. Throbbing discomfort or neuritic symptoms seldom occur. The condition may follow any underlying shoulder disorder. Untreated, a frozen shoulder develops in three stages: "freezing," "frozen," and "thawing."[1] However, it is uncommon for an untreated frozen shoulder to dissipate completely and return to normal function.[29,30] More commonly, pain improves, but motion remains limited. The pain may fluctuate from day to day, depending upon physical activity.

Physical examination usually reveals abnormalities. *Active* and *passive* motion are both restricted. At first, only elevation and internal rotation are lost; later, all ranges of movement are lost, with the exception of forward extension. As the examiner puts the patient through passive movement, limitation of movement is noted even in the most relaxed patient. Tenderness is elicited regularly upon palpation of the tendons that form the musculotendinous rotator cuff.[11] Upon palpation, the humeral head may be felt higher in the shoulder joint, approximating the acromion, when compared to the uninvolved side. Patients with long-standing limitation of motion may have atrophy of the entire shoulder girdle musculature. Dystrophic changes in the remainder of the upper extremity are rare.

Etiology. Frozen shoulder has been considered the result of an extension of inflammation of adjacent tendon structures,[11] or of work in which the arm is kept abducted and motionless, as in typing.

Insulin-dependent diabetes has been linked to frozen shoulder. In one study of patients with frozen shoulder, 5 to 10% had diabetes.[9] No increased frequency of diabetic neuropathy was noted, and a third of the patients were insulin-dependent. Of patients with adhesive capsulitis and diabetes, 6% also had Dupuytren's contracture of the hand.[9] A relation to ischemic heart disease was also noted. [9,31,32]

Neviaser described the pathology of the shoulder capsule as thickened and contracted, with a chronic inflammatory infiltration.[33] The capsule appeared to suffer from a "glueing down," particularly in the region of the long head of the biceps.

Immunologic abnormalities have recently been noted in patients with frozen shoulder. The HLA B27 determinant was present in 21 of 28 patients with frozen shoulder.[34] Also noted was a decreased immunoglobulin A level, and a decreased lymphocyte transformation.[35] Bulgen speculates that in the genetically susceptible host, an autoimmune inflammatory reaction follows supraspinatus tendon degeneration and leads to the frozen shoulder.[35] Drugs implicated in some patients include phenobarbital, iodine, and isoniazid.[36]

Laboratory and Radiographic Examination. In the early stages of an adhesive capsulitis, the erythrocyte sedimentation rate may be elevated. Tests for diabetes should be performed. An arthrogram will seldom be necessary. Differential diagnosis from capsular tear is not difficult, and the presence of any remote underlying tear is unimportant clinically. However, Reeves has demonstrated the radiographic features of decreased volume with arthrography.[37]

Differential Diagnosis. If the result of the erythrocyte sedimentation rate is greater than 70 mm/hr by the Westergren test, one must consider polymyalgia rheumatica and giant cell arthritis. Rheumatoid arthritis can produce a frozen shoulder. Careful evaluation during follow-up visits is necessary. A general examination of the patient with a frozen shoulder should be undertaken to observe for subtle features of systemic rheumatic disease.

Management. The patient can be informed that pain-free motion should occur but may take many months to achieve. Normal routine activity can be maintained during this time. However, until complete recovery occurs, active arm use should be limited so as not to precipitate severe pain. The exercise program for frozen shoulder must be progressive. Beginning with pendulum exercises, the patient should progress to wand manipulation,[3,38] and finally to overhead-pulley exercises.[11] Wall-ladder exercises can be used from the beginning if the patient has at least 60 degrees of abduction (Fig. 3–15). The duration of therapy depends on the patient pursuing an exercise program *despite pain*. Pain is the patient's worse enemy in trying † recover from frozen shoulder. As the patient attempts to perform ᷆ exercise program, the muscles comprising the musculotendinous cuff of the involved shoulder must be kept relaxed while stretching. This

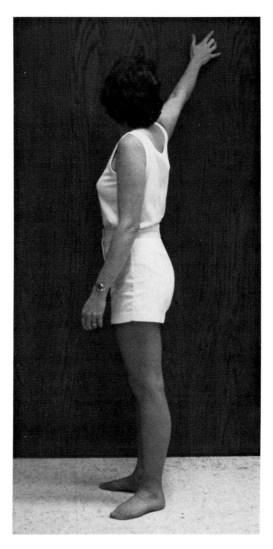

Fig. 3–15. Wall-ladder exercise for shoulder mobilization. The patient stands approximately 3 feet from a wall at a 90-degree angle. The fingers reaching for the wall "walk" in an upward and slightly posterior direction. Once the highest point possible has been reached, the hand is slowly lowered.

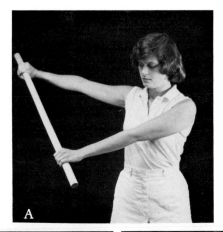

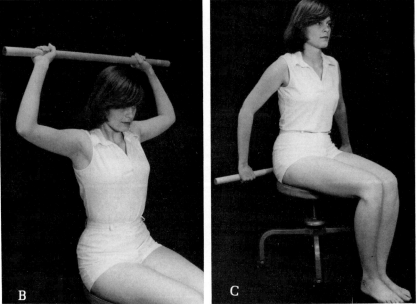

Fig. 3–16. Wand exercises to mobilize the frozen shoulder. The good arm is used to, *A*, force the arm on the involved side straight away, *B*, up and over head, and *C*, back and upward. Each position is performed as a single continuous movement or with short repetitions for 1 minute before going on to the next movement.

is accomplished by performing wand exercises (Fig. 3–16). The patient should be encouraged to gently, but persistently, stretch *beyond pain* to her tolerance. The wand is grasped with hands wide apart across the front of the body. The good arm is used to push the bad arm out and straight away slowly (Fig. 3–16A). After several repetitions, the wand is raised up and overhead (Fig. 3–16B). Lastly, the wand is placed behind and across the low back and raised backward slowly (Fig. 3–16C).

Most authors currently recommend corticosteroid injections of the shoulder cuff, as well as intra-articular administration. A nonaqueous crystalline steroid suspension and local anesthetic mixture, injected into multiple locations about the shoulder capsule and into the joint, may be the best method of relieving pain. Equal aliquots of the mixture are injected into each site: the supraspinatus tendon insertion area, the subacromial bursa anterolaterally, the bicipital tendon sheath, the joint capsule posteriorly in the region of the teres minor muscle, and the glenohumeral joint[3] (Fig. 3–17). The injection may be repeated if night pain recurs and if the first injection did provide some relief.[39]

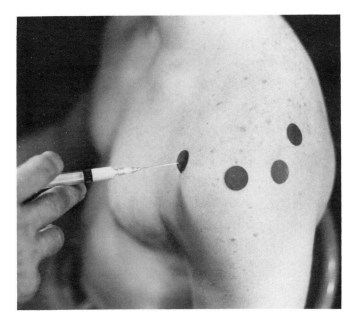

Fig. 3–17. The four points for injection of the frozen shoulder: Utilizing a suspension of a corticosteroid and local anesthetic, equal aliquots are injected into the supraspinatus tendon region, the subacromial bursa, the bicipital tendon sheath, and the joint capsule posteriorly in the region of the teres minor muscle. The latter site may be utilized also to inject the shoulder articulation.

Outcome and Additional Suggestions. Of patients who benefit, 60 to 95% return to normal, or at least near normal range of motion.[30,36,38] In our experience, the multiple shoulder injections, followed by immediate use of the wand exercises and wall-ladder exercises, provide relief from night pain in at least 90% of patients within 2 weeks. Once the patient has achieved 90 degrees of passive abduction (with the examiner assisting abduction), the shoulder motion nearly always returns to normal with home exercises alone. Some residual loss of motion can be seen in the elderly, but this may be "normal" for age.[29,30] The few who fail to respond can be referred to a physical therapist for stretching *manipulation*, and must continue to perform home exercises while under the therapist's care. In our experience, fewer than 1% of frozen shoulders need be manipulated under *anesthesia*. Of interest, insulin-dependent diabetic patients have the most intractable frozen shoulders, but the clinician cannot predict outcome just on this basis. If patients have failed to show progress following these maneuvers, infiltration brisement under anesthesia (injecting an anesthetic and steroid suspension under pressure into the shoulder capsule), followed by manipulation under anesthesia, has been recommended.[21] Manipulation under anesthesia must be considered a last resort in the case of a frozen shoulder.[11]

SCAPULAR REGION DISORDERS

Normal scapular motion is an integral part of upper extremity movement. The "setting phase" of the scapula occurs during arm abduction or forward flexion. Then scapulothoracic motion contributes significantly to shoulder motion.[11] The rhomboids, serratus anterior, levator scapulae, and pectoralis minor are important stabilizers of scapular movement, and may be the source of pain in and about the scapula. Three painful disorders of the scapula are described: snapping scapula, scapulocostal syndrome, and winging of the scapula.

Snapping Scapula

Audible and palpable sounds with discomfort may be due to alterations in the scapulothoracic articulations. Causes include anterior angulation of the superior scapular angle, rib deformities, the tubercle of Luschka (an enlarged bony nodule on the anterior aspect of the superior scapular angle), and scapular osteochondromatosis or tumors.[11] Scapular bursitis is an uncertain entity.[40] Oblique roentgenographic views of the scapula are necessary. The most common disturbance is an osteophyte on the superior medial border of the scapula.[41] The snapping scapula, which necessitates surgery, has been rare in our experience.

Scapulocostal Syndrome

The patient has insidious onset of pain in the superior and posterior aspects of the shoulder girdle radiating to the neck, upper triceps, deltoid insertion, and around the chest wall. Numbness and tingling of the hand occasionally accompany the scapulocostal syndrome.[11] Physical examination reveals diminished scapular motion on the involved side. Palpation reveals a trigger point located on the chest wall, medial and *beneath* the scapula. In order to locate the trigger

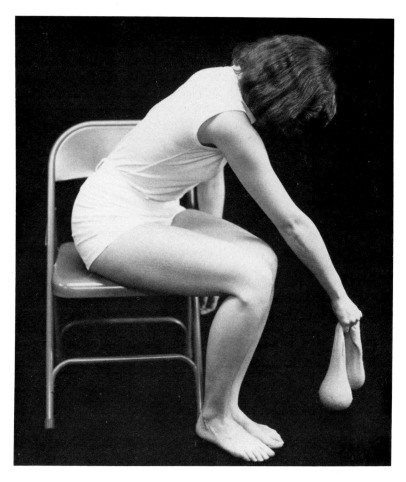

Fig. 3–18. Scapular stretching. Grasping a 2- to 5-pound weight, the patient slowly thrusts the arm forward; then leaning forward while keeping the trunk straight, she brings the arm on the involved side across the chest. The weight is allowed to approach the floor (but should not rest on the floor), in front and to the side of the foot, stretching the parascapular muscles. A pulling feeling in the area of pain will be noted. The position is held for 10 to 20 seconds and repeated 3 to 6 times twice daily.

point, the patient must draw the scapula laterally by reaching across her chest, placing her hand on the uninvolved shoulder, and rotating the involved shoulder forward. The trigger point is obviously tender, and palpation of the trigger point reproduces pain. Relief following infiltration of the lesion with an anesthetic and steroid injection confirms the diagnosis. The cause may include friction between the scapula and the thoracic cage, myofascial strain from poor posture, disuse, trauma, or tumors about the scapula. Treatment includes posture exercises, scapular stretching (Fig. 3–18), and one or two sequential injections of a crystalline steroid-local anesthetic mixture.[11]

Other Myofascial Scapular Region Pain

Travell reports the serratus posterior superior muscle medial to the superior pole of the scapula as the most frequent source of parascapular pain.[4] However, it seldom acts alone as the source of myofascial pain. The infraspinatus trigger point may cause local and referred pain to the outer and anterior upper arm. The supraspinatus and trapezius muscles commonly have trigger points located approximately ½-inch from each other in the center of the belly of the muscles. The trigger point is palpable as an indurated, elongated muscle band that rolls under the examiner's finger and is quite tender. Treatment includes injecting the trigger point with a crystalline nonaqueous steroid anesthetic mixture (Fig. 3–19), stretching and postural correction exercises, and avoiding strain. Reaching from the front seat of a car across to the back seat, and then pulling a briefcase forward, is a common strain. Traveling salesmen are often seen with a myofascial scapular pain syndrome.

OTHER SHOULDER REGION DISORDERS

Winging of the Scapula

The patient with paresis or paralysis of the serratus anterior muscle may present with painless limitation of shoulder elevation, particularly the last 30 degrees of overhead-arm extension. There may be parascapular discomfort. As the physician observes the patient going through active shoulder motion, the scapula may be seen to draw away from the thoracic cage. While the patient presses his outstretched arms against a wall, the physician observes the involved scapula project from the thorax. This condition is the result of neurogenic paralysis of the serratus anterior muscle. Paralysis may result from injury to the long thoracic nerve or brachial plexus from a direct blow to the suprascapular region, and has been described in army recruits carrying heavy packs with resultant nerve injury. Tetanus antitoxin, typhoid, measles, or influenza vaccination may result in brachial plexitis and lead to winging of the scapula.[6] Electromyography can

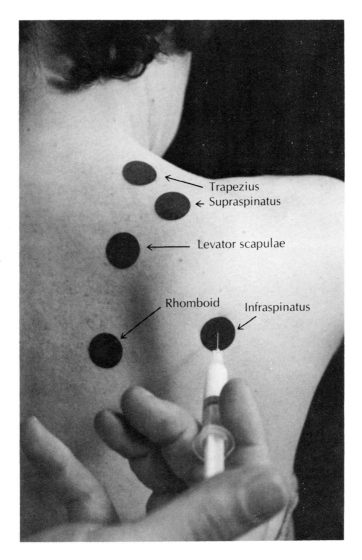

Fig. 3–19. The scapular myofascial trigger points are injected with a nonaqueous steroid-anesthetic mixture.

demonstrate nerve injury as the cause, and may be useful in following the progress of the condition, which often requires a year or two for recovery. Treatment is expectant with exercises to preserve normal glenohumeral joint motion. Transcutaneous nerve stimulation may help alleviate discomfort.

Acromioclavicular Joint Pain

Pain in the region of the acromioclavicular joint may result from trauma with subluxation or separation of the acromioclavicular joint, from a tear or strain of the coracoclavicular ligament,[15] or from tendinitis of the musculotendinous cuff of the shoulder. Osteoarthritis of the acromioclavicular joint may cause joint swelling and tenderness following excessive shoulder action. Synovitis of the acromioclavicular joint should alert the physician to the presence of a systemic inflammatory process, such as rheumatoid arthritis, spondyloarthritis, or giant cell arteritis.[42] Degenerative joint disease with bony enlargement is seldom the only cause of pain in the region of the acromioclavicular joint. A more likely cause is nearby tendinitis or bursitis. Careful palpation is essential. Frequently, acromioclavicular pain can be relieved by injecting a local anesthetic-corticosteroid mixture beneath the joint in the vicinity of the supraspinatus tendon (Fig. 3–10).

Soft Tissue Enlargement of the Shoulder

This unusual complaint is mentioned for completeness. Soft tissue thickening about the point of the shoulder may occur in amyloidosis (shoulder pad sign) or acromegaly, and from massive synovitis in patients with rheumatoid arthritis. Also, lipomas may occur about the shoulder. Amyloid infiltration has a rubbery feel upon examination. No fluctuance is noted. The enlargement is diffuse and does not follow any tendon-sheath pattern. The physician encountering such a disturbance should check the erythrocyte sedimentation rate, complete blood count, and serum protein electrophoresis. Features of acromegaly will be obvious, if it is kept in mind.

Abduction Contracture of the Shoulder

The inability to return the raised arm back down to the side of the body may result from repeated injections of any medication in large volume into the deltoid muscle. A band of dense scar tissue forms in the intermediate part of the deltoid and leads to contracture; permanent arm abduction follows. Surgical excision of the band may be required for relief.[43]

REFERENCES

1. Bland JH, Merrit JA, Boushey DR: The painful shoulder. Semin Arthritis Rheum 7:21–46, 1977.

2. Boyle AC: Joints and their diseases. Br Med J 3:283–285, 1969.
3. Kozin F: Painful shoulder and the reflex sympathetic dystrophy syndrome. In Arthritis and Allied Conditions. 9th Ed. Edited by DJ McCarty. Philadelphia, Lea & Febiger, 1979.
4. Travell J, Rinzler, S, Herman M: Pain and disability of the shoulder and arm. JAMA 120:417–422, 1942.
5. Kummel BM, Zazanis GA: Shoulder pain as the presenting complaint in carpal tunnel syndrome. Clin Orthop 92:227–230, 1973.
6. Duthie RB, Ferguson AB: Mercer's Orthopedic Surgery. 7th Ed. Baltimore, Williams & Wilkins, 1973.
7. Pinals RS: Traumatic arthritis and allied conditions. In Arthritis and Allied Conditions. 8th Ed. Edited by JL Hollander. Philadelphia, Lea & Febiger, 1972.
8. Pinals RS, Short CL: Calcific periarthritis involving multiple sites. Arthritis Rheum 9:556–574, 1966.
9. Bridgman JF: Periarthritis of the shoulder and diabetes mellitus. Ann Rheum Dis 31:69–71, 1972.
10. Wright V, Haq AM: Periarthritis of the shoulder. II. Radiological features. Ann Rheum Dis 35:220–226, 1976.
11. Turek SL: Orthopaedics; Principles and Their Application. 3rd Ed. Philadelphia, JB Lippincott, 1977.
12. Cyriax J: Textbook of Orthopaedic Medicine. I. Diagnosis of Soft Tissue Lesions. 7th Ed. London, Bailliere Tindall, 1978.
13. Hadler NM: Industrial rheumatology; Clinical investigations into the influence of the pattern of usage on the pattern of regional musculoskeletal disease. Arthritis Rheum 20:1019–1025, 1977.
14. Neer CS, Welch RP: The shoulder in sports. Orthop Clin North Am 8:583–591, 1977.
15. Nelson CL: The painful shoulder. Postgrad Med 29:71–78, 1970.
16. McIntyre DI: Subcoracoid neurovascular entrapment. Clin Orthop 108:27–30, 1975.
17. Rathbun JB, Macnab I: Microvascular pattern of the rotator cuff. J Bone Joint Surg 52B:540–553, 1970.
18. Cannon RB, Schmid FR: Calcific periarthritis involving multiple sites in identical twins. Arthritis Rheum 16:393–396, 1973.
19. Thompson GR, Ting M, Riggs GA, et al: Calcific tendinitis and soft tissue calcification resembling gout. JAMA 203:464–472, 1968.
20. Codman EA: The Shoulder. Boston, Thomas Todd, 1934.
21. Simon WH: Soft tissue disorders of the shoulder; frozen shoulder, calcific tendinitis, and bicipital tendinitis. Orthop Clin North Am 6:521–539, 1975.
22. Schumacher HR, Smolyo AP, Tse RL, Maurer K: Arthritis associated with apatite crystals. Ann Intern Med 87:411–416, 1977.
23. McCarty DJ, Gatter RA: Recurrent acute inflammation associated with focal apatite crystal deposition. Arthritis Rheum 9:804–819, 1966.
24. Dieppe PA, Crocker P, Huskisson EC, Willoughby DA: Apatite deposition disease; A new arthropathy. Lancet 1:266–268, 1976.
25. ViGario GD, Keats TE: Localization of calcific deposits in the shoulder. Am J Roent Rad Ther and Nuc Med 108:806–811, 1970.
26. Crenshaw AH, Kilgore WE: Surgical treatment of bicipital tenosynovitis. J Bone Joint Surg 48A:1496–1502, 1966.
27. Richardson AT: The painful shoulder. Proc R Soc Med 68:731–736, 1975.
28. Hazleman BL: The painful stiff shoulder. Rheum Phys Med 11:413–421, 1972.
29. Clarke GR, Willis LA, Fish WW, Nichols PJR: Preliminary studies in measuring range of motion in normal and painful stiff shoulders. Rheumatol Rehabil 14:39–46, 1975.
30. Reeves B: Natural history of the frozen shoulder syndrome. Scand J Rheumatol 4:193–196, 1975.
31. Sheldon PJH: A retrospective survey of 102 cases of shoulder pain. Rheum Phys Med 11:422–427, 1972.
32. Wright V, Haq AM: Periarthritis of the shoulder. I. Aetiological considerations with particular reference to personality factors. Ann Rheum Dis 35:213–219, 1976.

33. Neviaser JS: Adhesive capsulitis of the shoulder; A study of the pathological findings in periarthritis of the shoulder. J Bone Joint Surg 27:211–222, 1945.
34. Brewerton DA, Hart FD, Nicholls A, et al: Ankylosing spondylitis and HL-A27. Lancet 1:904–907, 1973.
35. Bulgen D, Hazleman B, Ward M, McCallum M: Immunological studies in frozen shoulder. Ann Rheum Dis 37:135–138, 1978.
36. Steinbrocker O, Argyros TG: Frozen shoulder: Treatment by local injections of depot corticosteroids. Arch Phys Med Rehabil 55:209–213, 1974.
37. Reeves B: Arthrographic changes in frozen and post-traumatic stiff shoulders. Proc R Soc Med 59:827–830, 1966.
38. Weiser HI: Painful primary frozen shoulder mobilization under local anesthesia. Arch Phys Med Rehabil 58:406–408, 1977.
39. Moskowitz RW: Clinical Rheumatology; A problem-oriented approach. Philadelphia, Lea & Febiger, 1975.
40. Coventry MB: Recurring scapular pain. JAMA 241:942, 1979.
41. Riggins RS: The shoulder. In Musculoskeletal Disorders. Edited by RD D'Ambrosia. Philadelphia, JB Lippincott, 1977.
42. Miller LD, Stevens MD: Skeletal manifestations of polymyalgia rheumatica. JAMA 240:27–29, 1978.
43. Groves RJ, Goldner JL: Contracture of the deltoid muscle in the adult after intramuscular injections. J Bone Joint Surg 56A:817–820, 1974.

Chapter **4**

THE ELBOW

The elbow is a common site of involvement for many arthritides, including secondary osteoarthritis, rheumatoid arthritis, and gout. Elbow pain often occurs from disturbances of the regional soft tissue supporting structures. Furthermore, the clinician must keep in mind that elbow pain and dysfunction may be secondary to disorders arising in the neck, shoulder, wrist, or hand.

The two major muscle components of the forearm serving the wrist and hand include the flexor pronator group (pronator teres, flexor carpi radialis, palmaris longus, flexor carpi ulnaris, flexor digitorum sublimis) and the extensor muscle group (extensor carpi radialis longus, extensor carpi radialis brevis, extensor digitorum communis, extensor indicis proprius, extensor carpi ulnaris). The flexor pronator group arises from the medial epicondyle region of the elbow. Conversely, the extensor group joins to form the extensor communis tendon, which inserts onto the lateral epicondyle of the humerus. In addition to the well-known olecranon bursa, another bursa lies between the triceps and olecranon prominence. Also, a bursa may occur between the neck of the radius and the biceps tendon.[1]

The Examination. The history should include the quality, location, and duration of pain or disability. The physician must include in the history whether neck, shoulder, wrist, or hand position or movement aggravates the elbow problem. Numbness and tingling, in addition to pain, may suggest a local entrapment syndrome, cervical nerve root impingement, or a carpal tunnel syndrome. Aggravating factors, such as occupational repetitive movement, hobbies, sports, or other possible injury-provoking work preceding the onset of pain, should be established. Possible factors causing neuropathy (e.g., diabetes, alcoholism) should be elicited. A past history of tendinitis about the shoulder or other areas may suggest multifocal calcific tendinitis, although the elbow is an uncommon site for this.

81

Evaluation for evidence of generalized disorders, such as rheumatoid arthritis, osteoarthritis, neuropathy, gout, hyperlipidemia, and other medical conditions, should be carried out. Regional examination of the neck, shoulder, wrist, and hand may reveal disturbances at these locations, which can refer pain to the elbow.

Examination of the elbow includes muscle and neurologic examinations of the upper extremity. Palpation may demonstrate swelling of the tendon of the biceps anteriorly, swelling of the olecranon bursa, tophi, or rheumatoid nodules within the bursa. Points of tenderness at the epicondyles should be compared with the uninvolved elbow. The forearm muscles, approximately 1 to 2 inches distal to the elbow, should be palpated for cord-like induration. This may provide the examiner with evidence of a tear or adhesion within one or more of the forearm tendons.

Usually the presentation of pain at the elbow area is found to be the result of only one predominant entity. However, on occasion more than one condition may be found, such as a tennis elbow and carpal tunnel syndrome, or olecranon bursitis and tendinitis of the biceps insertion at the elbow.[2] Furthermore, these soft tissue nonarticular rheumatic disorders may be superimposed upon other arthritic disorders. Relief from these soft tissue disturbances may provide the patient with satisfactory use of the elbow, despite persistence of other rheumatic disorders.

TENNIS ELBOW

In recent years the term "tennis elbow" has been applied to several soft tissue rheumatic disorders. Similar symptoms may also result from nerve root entrapment.[3,4] Tennis elbow most accurately includes disturbances that result in pain and tenderness in the lateral epicondyle region of the elbow.[5] "Golfer's elbow" has been used to describe similar disturbances in the medial epicondyle region. The term "tennis elbow" has gained preference over "epicondylitis" or "radiohumeral bursitis," perhaps because we know little about etiology, and neither inflammation of the epicondyle nor a radiohumeral bursitis has been described.[1]

The patient with tennis elbow may present with acute, intermittent, subacute, or chronic pain during grasping or supination of the wrist. It is an occupational hazard in carpenters, gardeners, dentists, and politicians.[6] It is seen often in patients previously afflicted with shoulder tendinitis or myofascial back pain.[1] This disorder is seldom bilateral; the lateral epicondylar site is more common than the medial epicondylar site.[2,7] Tennis elbow is seldom seen in persons under the age of 40 or over the age of 60.[2,8] The patient often points to a prominent point of the lateral epicondyle as the area of maximum pain and tenderness. Often, however, the clinician can detect a cord-like, firm scar within one of the extensor tendons leading to the epicondyle. This indurated tendon generally lies approximately 2 inches distal to the epicondyle; careful palpation is needed to locate it. The pain is reproduced by having the patient extend his wrist against the examiner's resistance. Elbow motion usually is not limited by uncomplicated tennis elbow.

Etiology. A controlled pathologic study carried out by Goldie,[9] and confirmed by Nirschl,[8] revealed no evidence of a bursa on the epicondyle; rather, a subtendinous space with granulation tissue, edema, and increased vascularity was found in these patients. Fibroblast proliferation of the extensor aponeurosis was also noted,[8] and no periostitis was found.[9] The result is considered by most authors to be due to a strain or tear resulting from over-use of the forearm musculature.[1,2,5,7,10,11] More serious injury to elbow structures might present as tennis elbow, but examination for joint laxity should reveal these injuries (tear of the joint capsule or radial collateral ligament).[10] Tennis players, particularly novices, suffer tennis elbow often as a result of pressure-grip strain during backhand shots performed with a "leading elbow." The novice errs in performing a backhand shot with the elbow pointed toward the net. Also, tennis elbow is more common in loose-jointed tennis players.[11]

Laboratory and Radiographic Examination. Elbow joint roentgenographs in patients with tennis elbow rarely reveal an abnormality.[5] Unless tennis elbow is superimposed upon another inflammatory disease process, tests for inflammation are normal.

Differential Diagnosis. As mentioned, the term tennis elbow refers to pain resulting from myofascial injury, yet similar features can result from nerve entrapment, cervical nerve root impingement, or carpal tunnel syndrome. Failure to respond to local measures should raise the suspicion of these other disorders.

Management. The clinician and patient must recognize and alter aggravating activities that excessively contract the extensor muscle group. A "tennis elbow band" with velcro fastening may be helpful (Fig. 4–1). Generally, the band is 2 to 3 inches wide, and is applied across the epicondyles of the elbow just distal to the joint. It should be used during forearm work. Aggravating hand use should be avoided for at least 1 month after pain is relieved, in order to prevent recurrence.[5]

Exclude nerve entrapment syndromes, including carpal tunnel syndrome, thoracic outlet syndrome, or cervical radiculopathy.

Measures to relieve pain on the first visit depend on degree and location of tenderness elicited during the examination. If pain or tenderness is not disabling, and a well-localized point of tenderness is not found, then local corticosteroid injections should be withheld until a future visit. In such a patient, stretching exercises, protection

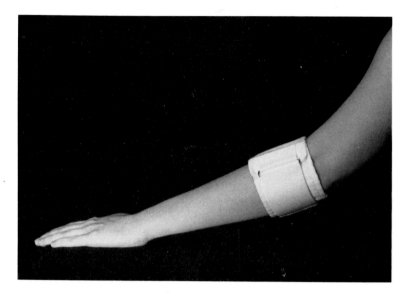

Fig. 4–1. The tennis elbow band: Although the rationale for use is uncertain, the protective influence of a tennis elbow band during arm use is helpful in most patients with tennis elbow. This is one of many available styles.

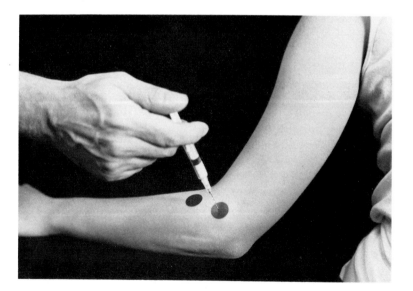

Fig. 4–2. Injection of the lateral epicondyle and the band-like trigger in the extensor tendon for the patient with tennis elbow.

from strain, and the use of local heat or ice may suffice. However, if a cord-like induration is elicited, or if symptoms are severe, local infiltration with a crystalline steroid-local anesthetic mixture with a No. 23 or No. 25 needle is usually helpful. The epicondylar region should be approached from one or more directions, so that the steroid mixture is injected into a region covering 2 cm^2 (Fig. 4–2). This is helpful in preventing local steroid atrophy. The patient should be forewarned that local pain may be worse the first day or two following injection, in which case cold applications are helpful. Oral nonsteroidal agents or analgesics are seldom necessary or effective when tennis elbow is the patient's only complaint.

Self-help physical therapy should include stretching and strengthening the forearm musculature. For lateral epicondylar tennis elbow, the extensor muscles can be stretched easily by having the patient place the arm out straight, with the hand pointed down and the back of the hand pressed gently against a wall or door. The hand and straight arm are then gently slid upward, providing tension along the extensor forearm muscles (Fig. 4–3). As the arm and hand are raised upward against the door or wall, a pulling sensation in the forearm muscles is noted. This position is held without further movement for 1 minute. As the tendons lengthen, the patient is aware that the hand can be raised higher against the door or wall before the pulling sensation is detected in the forearm musculature. Following this, the patient performs strengthening exercises by grasping a 3- to 7-pound weight. The wrist is extended and flexed slowly and gently while the hand grasps the weight, first palm down and then repeated palm up (Fig. 4–4). These exercises should be performed for 1 minute in each direction at least twice daily, and should be continued for at least 6 weeks after pain is alleviated.[2,5,6,8,11]

For the patient with tennis elbow involvement at the medial epicondyle, forearm stretching is reversed. The hand is pointed down, the palm is pressed against a door or wall, and the outstretched arm is raised slowly until a pulling sensation is perceived in the forearm flexor muscles. This position is held for 1 minute. As the muscles loosen, the arm and hand are raised to successively higher positions before the pulling sensation is perceived. If symptoms are aggravated by a particular exercise, the exercise should be modified or omitted for several weeks.

Outcome. The measures, as outlined, should provide relief without recurrence in at least 90% of patients with tennis elbow. Conservative care provided relief without recurrence in 97% of 871 patients.[2] Tennis elbow is generally a self-limiting disorder of several months' duration; in some patients, however, symptoms may last up to 12 months.[5,6,8]

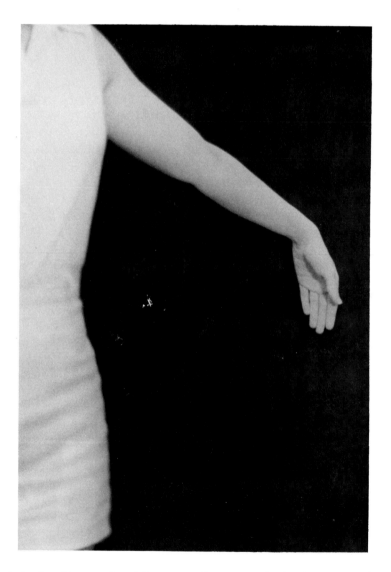

Fig. 4–3. Stretching exercise of the extensor forearm muscles for the patient with tennis elbow.

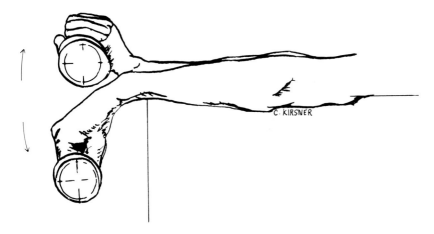

Fig. 4–4. Mobilizing and strengthening exercise for the forearm muscles in patients with tennis elbow.

In patients with continuing disability, careful neurologic investigation should be performed. Gunn reported that 42 patients with symptoms of tennis elbow had accompanying cervical radiculopathy. Of these 42 patients, 39 had relief with conservative measures directed to the neck. Electrodiagnostic tests, carefully performed, proved useful in recognizing a cervical-nerve-root cause for tennis elbow.[3] Other nerve entrapment lesions about the elbow should be considered. Tennis- or golf-related injuries may require a professional consultation for ascertaining an improper stroke.[11] An occupational therapist may be required for occupational reeducation. Local injections of corticosteroid-anesthetic mixture should generally not be required for more than a few times. Plaster immobilization is an additional therapeutic modality. Fewer than 5% of patients require surgery for chronic recurrent tennis elbow. A "lateral release" of the common origin of the radial extensors is one of the surgical procedures recommended.[12]

OLECRANON BURSITIS

The olecranon bursa occupies the posterior point of the elbow and has a synovial membrane. Inflammation or effusion of the bursa may result from gout, rheumatoid arthritis, sepsis, or trauma (Fig. 4–5). Traumatic bursitis occurs from pressure, either while seated with the elbow leaning on something, or as part of an occupational problem (e.g., carpet layers). Acute olecranon bursitis with warmth or erythema can occur in gout, pseudogout, rheumatoid arthritis, infection, or

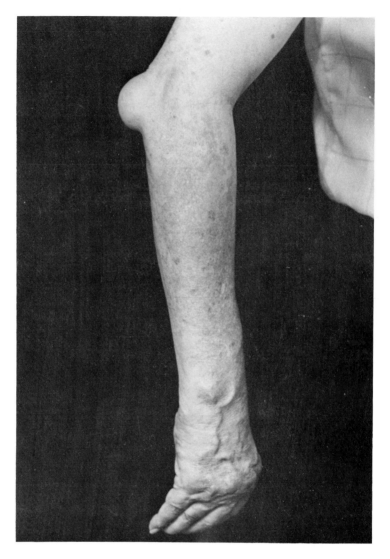

Fig. 4–5. Example of a patient with olecranon bursitis.

hemorrhage.[1,7] Whether bursitis appears acutely or subacutely in onset, septic bursitis must always be excluded. Septic bursitis may appear subacutely;[13,14] therefore, septic bursitis must be excluded by aspiration and the performance of appropriate diagnostic tests.

Laboratory and Radiographic Examination. If trauma with possible foreign body penetration is a consideration, roentgenographs with soft tissue techniques may be helpful to visualize the foreign body. Aspiration and evaluation of the bursal fluid are diagnostically helpful, and are essential if septic bursitis is even remotely suspected. Inspection of the fluid in most cases reveals a thin, watery, yellow- or brown-tinged fluid. The fluid should be examined for white blood cell count and differential, Gram stain, sugar content, and culture. A white blood cell count as low as 1400 cells/ml[3] does *not* exclude infection.[13,14] Comparison of bursal fluid sugar content to a simultaneously obtained serum sample may be helpful in cases of suspected sepsis. The majority of patients with septic bursitis have a low bursal fluid sugar level, but even this criterion is not absolute.[13] Septic bursitis may occur even in the absence of a penetrating injury. In general, the white blood cell count is less than 1000 cells/ml[3] in nonseptic bursitis fluid.[13] Crystal identification with polarizing microscopy should be performed in any patient with a history of gout, pseudogout, or recurrent olecranon bursitis.

Differential Diagnosis. Most patients with olecranon bursitis do not have a systemic disorder, yet careful palpation of the bursa for nodules can suggest the presence of rheumatoid arthritis, gout, or hyperlipidemia, before other typical features emerge. Our concern for low-grade sepsis as a cause for bursitis has been emphasized.

Management. Recognition and avoidance of aggravating pressure injury are necessary to prevent recurrence. Patients should be informed that their elbows should be kept away from the arms of chairs, or the arm rest of an automobile. In hospitalized patients, the provision of foam rubber protectors should be considered.

Following aspiration of the bursal fluid, it is our practice to instill .5 ml of a crystalline steroid-local anesthetic mixture. Obviously, if there is a high index of suspicion for sepsis, the steroid should be withheld.

Outcome. Most patients who have suffered an olecranon bursitis recognize and avoid repeated local injury. Occasionally a patient with chronic bursitis and a thickened synovial membrane requires surgical excision of the bursa.

NON-OLECRANON BURSITIS

A diagnosis of bursitis between the biceps insertion and the head of the radius may be considered in patients with pain at the elbow during wrist rotation.[1] The discomfort is milder than that of tennis elbow, and tenderness is detected over the head of the radius and accentuated during wrist rotation. Relief from a local anesthetic injection into the region of the head of the radius assists diagnosis. Exercises to stretch the lower end of the biceps are helpful.

Tendinitis and bursitis at the insertion of the triceps on the olecranon process may also cause posterior elbow pain. In this instance, there is no palpable swelling. Local anesthetic injection into the point of tenderness, with protection of this region from pressure, is usually all that is required.

TENDINITIS

Tendinitis of the distal insertion of the biceps muscle may cause pain in the antecubital fossa of the elbow with restriction of full elbow extension. Pain is dull and felt rather diffusely throughout the anterior elbow region. In all patients with elbow pain, palpation of the distal end of the biceps tendon in the antecubital space should be performed with the elbow in full extension. When biceps tendinitis is present, tenderness can be elicited along the lower ½-inch of the biceps tendon. This should be distinguished from bursitis in the area of the head of the radius. Injection of a steroid anesthetic mixture, *parallel to*, but not into the biceps tendon, provides prompt relief. Home physical therapy with gentle stretching of the biceps should be performed twice daily and continued for several weeks following relief from pain. To perform the exercise, the patient lies supine with the elbow at the edge of the bed and the arm extended beyond the bed. The patient grasps a 5-pound weight with palm upward and allows the weight to straighten the arm. The patient slowly and gently bends and straightens the elbow, allowing the weight to passively straighten the elbow each time. The arm meanwhile is supported by the bed. This is performed repetitively for 1 minute twice daily.

Tendinitis slightly distal to the elbow can occur traumatically without giving rise to tennis elbow. Careful palpation of the individual tendons during finger movement and wrist movement should allow the examiner to discern which tendon is involved. Local corticosteroid anesthetic injection and avoidance of strain should provide benefit.

NERVE ENTRAPMENT SYNDROMES

Ill-defined, diffuse, upper-forearm pain, aggravated by particular movement, should alert the clinician to the possibility of a nerve entrapment syndrome. Nerve entrapment is characterized by a positive *tourniquet test*, in which a tourniquet applied above the painful area accentuates the pain. Paresthesia may result.[4] Electrodiagnostic tests may delineate the level of entrapment (Fig. 4–6).

Radial Tunnel Syndrome

The radial nerve courses from medial to lateral around the posterior surface of the humerus, then pierces the lateral muscular septum. Compression by a contracted muscle or band may give rise to symptoms of pain and tenderness in the area of the lateral epicondyle. Of particular diagnostic value, the pain is reproduced with passive stretching or resisted extension of the middle finger. Temporary relief following anesthetic injection is diagnostically helpful. Paresthesia may or may not be present in the distribution of the superficial radial nerve. A Tinel test (tapping over the nerve), performed over the radial

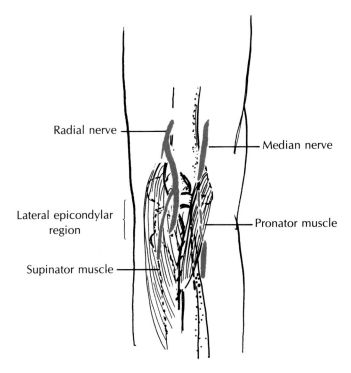

Radial nerve

Median nerve

Lateral epicondylar region

Pronator muscle

Supinator muscle

Fig. 4–6. Nerve entrapment of the elbow region: The *radial tunnel syndrome* may result from radial nerve compression in the region of the lateral epicondyle. The *pronator syndrome* results from median nerve entrapment by the pronator muscle.

head, may produce tingling along the course of the nerve. Finger-extension weakness may be noted; limitation of full extension of the elbow may also be observed.

Causes include adhesions to tissue overlying the radial head, constriction by the extensor carpi radialis brevis, or compression by the supinator muscle.[15] Nerve conduction tests may reveal slowing of impulses from the spiral groove to the medial portion of the extensor digitorum communis. In patients suspected of having radial nerve entrapment, surgical exploration and release from the overlying muscle often provide good relief.[16] The radial tunnel syndrome, as a cause for *chronic* epicondylar (tennis elbow) pain, has been refuted.[17]

Pronator Syndrome

Median nerve entrapment by the pronator muscle may result in diffuse pain in the arm and weakness of wrist pronation.[18] The pain is reproduced by resistance to pronation of the forearm and flexion of the wrist.[4] Surgical consultation for consideration of nerve release should be obtained.

Ulnar Nerve Entrapment (Cubital Tunnel Syndrome; External Compression Syndrome)

Ulnar nerve palsy may result from pressure injury to the ulnar nerve. The ulnar nerve lying behind the medial epicondyle may be palpably thickened, secondary to repeated minor trauma from pressure.[4,19,20] Paresthesia, with weakness and intrinsic atrophy in an ulnar nerve distribution, is noted. Similar symptoms may result from subluxation of the nerve, or by compression from a congenital supracondylar process of the humerus.

Carpal Tunnel Syndrome

Retrograde paresthesia into the forearm and arm may be caused by carpal tunnel syndrome. Symptoms may be reproduced by tapping over the median nerve at the wrist. (See Chapt. 5, "Carpal Tunnel Syndrome.")

REFERENCES

1. Turek SL: Orthopaedics: Principles and Their Application. 3rd Ed. Philadelphia, JB Lippincott, 1977.
2. Boyd HB, McLeod AC: Tennis elbow. J Bone Joint Surg 55:1183–1187, 1973.
3. Gunn CC, Milbrandt WE: Tennis elbow and the cervical spine. Can Med Assoc J 114:803–806, 1976.
4. Dan NG: Entrapment syndromes. Med J Aust 1:528–531, 1978.
5. Swezey RL: Arthritis: Rational Therapy and Rehabilitation. Philadelphia, WB Saunders, 1978.
6. Management of tennis elbow. In The Medical Letter, 19:33–36, 1977.
7. Pinals RA: Traumatic arthritis and allied conditions. In Arthritis and Allied Conditions. 9th Ed. Edited by DJ McCarty. Philadelphia, Lea & Febiger, 1979.
8. Nirschl RP: Tennis elbow. Primary Care 4:367–382, 1977.
9. Goldie I: Epicondylitis Lateralis Humeri, (Epicondylalgia or tennis elbow): A pathologic study. Acta Chir Scand (Suppl) 339:110–112, 1964.
10. Gardner RC: What to do about tennis elbow. Consultant 11:61–62, 1971.
11. Berhang AM, Dehner W, Fogarty C: A scientific approach to tennis elbow. Orthop Rev 4:35–41, 1975.
12. Rosen MJ, Duffy FP, Miller EH, Kremchek, EJ: Tennis elbow syndrome: Results of the "lateral release" procedure. Ohio State Med J 76:103–109, 1980.
13. Thompson GR, Manshady BM, Weiss JJ: Septic bursitis. JAMA 240:2280–2281, 1978.
14. Ho G, Tice AD, Kaplan SR: Septic bursitis in the prepatellar and olecranon bursae. Ann Intern Med 89:21–27, 1978.
15. Kopell HP, Thompson WAL: Peripheral Entrapment Neuropathies. Huntington, NY, RE Krieger Publishing, 1976.
16. Roles NC, Maudsley RH: Radial tunnel syndrome. J Bone Joint Surg 54:499–508, 1972.
17. Rossum JV, Buruma OJS, Kamphuisen HAC, Onvlee GJ: Tennis elbow—a radial tunnel syndrome? J Bone Joint Surg 60B:197–198, 1978.
18. Brown PW: Peripheral nerve lesions. In Musculoskeletal Disorders. Edited by RD D'Ambrosia. Philadelphia, JB Lippincott, 1977.
19. Wadsworth TG, Williams JR: Cubital tunnel external compression syndrome. Br Med J 1:662–666, 1973.
20. Clark CB: Cubital tunnel syndrome. JAMA 241:801–802, 1979.

Chapter 5

THE WRIST AND HAND

Pain and disability of the hand and wrist may result from local factors, or may result from systemic diseases with onset in the wrist or hand, in which case presenting symptoms may be manifest as nodular lesions or tendon and ligament problems before other systemic features are evident.

Physical Examination. The normal wrist can flex and extend approximately 80 degrees respectively from the horizontal. Ulnar wrist deviation is approximately twice the capability of radial wrist deviation (40 degrees versus approximately 20 degrees, respectively). Finger flexion should be tested by having the patient bend the distal phalanx to approximate the proximal phalanx. Flexor tendon sheath swelling, or true joint arthritis, may cause limitation of flexion of proximal interphalangeal (PIP) or distal interphalangeal (DIP) finger joints. Thumb abduction should approximate 80 to 90 degrees from a line drawn proximally along the long finger. Thumb adduction should reach to the base of the little finger. Flattening or atrophy of the thenar eminence should be noted (suggesting carpal tunnel syndrome with median nerve compression). Wasting of the interossei with "valleys" between the extensor tendons on the back of the hand may suggest ulnar nerve dysfunction. The metacarpophalangeal (MCP) collateral ligaments are tested for stability with the finger flexed to 90 degrees at the MCP joint. This tightens the collateral ligaments and allows little passive lateral finger motion (Fig. 5–1). Dorsal-volar motion of the wrist should be tested. The examiner attempts to move the patient's hand up and down within the horizontal plane of the patient's wrist. Wrist and PIP hypermobility may suggest *hypermobility syndrome* with its multiple presentations. Note the texture of the skin, presence of telangiectasia, pitting, or smoothness of the distal fingertips.

DISORDERS OF THE LOWER ARM AND WRIST

Whether from sport injury or from falling on the outstretched wrist, injury may involve tendons, ligaments, or the articular disc, or may

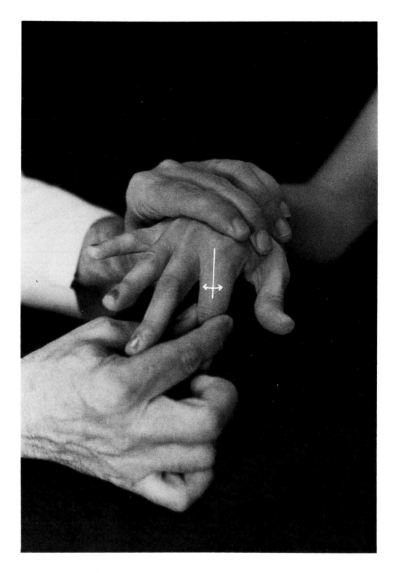

Fig. 5–1. Metacarpophalangeal (MCP) collateral ligament stability test: The finger is flexed to 90 degrees at the MCP joint in order to tighten the collateral ligament. Normally, lateral finger motion is minimal in this position.

result in joint laxity.[1,2] Acute tenosynovitis, resulting from injury or unaccustomed movement, generally involves the tendons of the lower dorsal forearm. Swelling and painful crepitus during hand extension may be detected;[2] tenderness can be elicited and internal joint derangement may be suspected.[3] In the acute stage, swelling and pain over the dorsal aspect of the wrist or over the distal radioulnar joint may occur. Clicking during hand activity may be noted. Locking does not occur. Grip strength is weakened by these injuries, and treatment requires orthopedic consultation when carpal instability is suspected.

Prominence of the distal ulna with hypermobility ("piano key" motion) may occur spontaneously, or as a result of injury or rheumatoid arthritis (Fig. 5–2). It is more prevalent in adolescents, but may follow a Colles' fracture of the wrist in others. Often, no treatment is required.[4]

If trapezium-first metacarpal joint sprain results in subluxation with limitation of pinch grasping, the region at the base of the thumb may be injected with a steroid-local anesthetic mixture, and a thumb splint provided that allows pinch grasping, yet stabilizes the carpometacarpal joint.[2] Persistent symptoms may indicate a need to consider arthroplasty.

Lastly, the pisiform-triquetral joint may be sprained, resulting in the pisiform being displaced distally. This results in pain with wrist flexion or ulnar deviation motions. The pisiform is tender to palpation in the hypothenar aspect of the palm. Reconstructive surgery may be indicated.[5]

Patients who have suffered wrist sprain and have persistent symptoms should have repeat roentgenograms, including oblique views and special scaphoid roentgenograms to detect a fracture of the

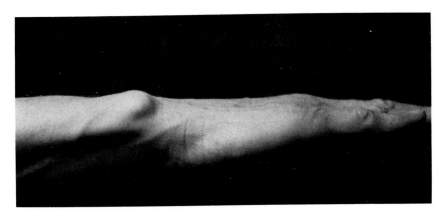

Fig. 5–2. Post-traumatic hypermobility of the distal ulna. Examination with downward pressure results in "piano key" movement of the distal ulna.

scaphoid. Also, flexion and extension wrist views help to determine instability.

SYSTEMIC DISEASES AFFECTING THE WRIST AND HAND

Systemic Rheumatic Diseases

The presenting symptom of rheumatoid arthritis is swelling of the joints of the digits, or sometimes of the flexor tendon sheaths (tenosynovitis). The patient may complain only of slight morning stiffness in the fingers and inability to fully flex the finger joints. Any patient with this complaint should have careful palpation of the flexor portion of the proximal phalanges. Swelling of the flexor tendons can be discerned as a rubbery, firm swelling when compared to the practitioner's own normal finger. Similarly, rheumatoid disease may cause flexor or extensor tendon sheath swelling in the forearm musculature, giving rise to carpal tunnel syndrome or loss of grip strength. Associated swelling of MCP and PIP joints is common. Tenosynovitis may also result from calcific tendinitis, tophaceous gout, psoriatic arthritis, Reiter's syndrome, mixed connective tissue disease, and occasionally dermatomyositis. Finger joint or tendon swelling may result from pseudogout or giant cell arteritis. The hands may be diffusely swollen in the early stage of progressive systemic sclerosis; telangiectasias, fingertip ulcers, or binding of the dorsal finger skin should suggest the diagnosis.

Clubbing of distal fingers, with or without associated periostitis or synovitis, may alert the physician to the presence of hypertrophic pulmonary osteoarthropathy and intrathoracic disease, or clubbing may be a benign inherited characteristic. The hand examination can provide clues to many systemic diseases, ranging from subacute bacterial endocarditis to hyperlipidemia; the clinician should look carefully.

Calcific Tendinitis

Calcific tendinitis may be part of recurrent multifocal attacks of tendinitis that involve the shoulder, wrist, and ankle regions. In the wrist, it may involve the lateral region with an attack of redness and swelling. Radiographic detection of periarticular calcification should alert the clinician to the disorder[6,6a] (see "Calcific Tendinitis," Chapt. 3).

HYPERMOBILITY SYNDROME

In 1967, Kirk, Ansell, and Bywaters coined the term "hypermobility syndrome."[7] Hypermobility occurs in 7% of school children and 4% of adults[7-12] (Fig. 5–3). Hypermobility may be secondary to rare diseases of the connective tissues (Marfan's syndrome, Ehlers-Danlos syn-

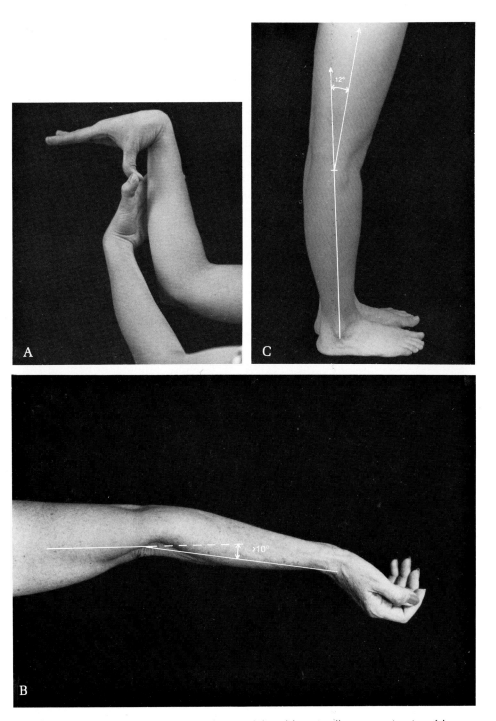

Fig. 5–3. Hypermobility syndrome: *A*, hypermobility of the wrist allows approximation of the thumb to the patient's ipsilateral forearm; *B*, hypermobility of the elbow with greater than 10 degrees of joint extension; *C*, hypermobility of the knee with greater than 10 degrees of joint extension.

drome, osteogenesis imperfecta, Achard syndrome, homocystinuria); additionally, hypermobility may result from inflammatory disorders, neurologic disease, or other metabolic disorders.[7,8] In most patients with hypermobility, the disorder is inherited as an autosomal dominant family trait,[8-10] and is benign.

The presenting complaint is often pain with use and symmetrical weakness of hand function. Hypermobility syndrome may mimic rheumatoid arthritis with a sensation of symmetric small joint swelling, morning stiffness, and fatigue. The majority of patients are children or young adults and are predominantly females. In our experience, these patients rarely perceive swelling that lasts longer than part of a day. Other features of hypermobility syndrome include genu recurvatum, lateral patellar displacement, scoliosis, and pes planus.[8-9] Hypermobility may result in premature osteoarthritis of the neck, spine, carpometacarpal joint of the thumb, or knees.[7,11,12]

Physical examination to determine the presence of hypermobility includes observation of the following: (1) passive extension of the little finger beyond 90 degrees, (2) passive apposition of the thumb to the flexor aspect of the ipsilateral forearm, (3) hyperextension of the elbows beyond 10 degrees, (4) hyperextension of the knees beyond 10 degrees, (5) ability to touch palms to floor while standing with knees extended, and (6) excessive range of passive dorsiflexion of the ankle and eversion of the foot.[7-12] Striae, a high-arched palate, eye, or cardiac abnormalities exclude the benign hypermobility syndrome.

Laboratory and Radiologic Examination. Tests for inflammation and rheumatoid factor are normal. Roentgenograms are usually normal, although in the older patient with hypermobility syndrome, they may reveal chondrocalcinosis or degenerative changes beyond that expected for age.[11]

Management. Most symptomatic patients with hypermobility are females. Perhaps this is because of greater muscle tone in males. We have found a series of graded resistance exercises helpful in alleviating symptoms. Finger extension exercises can be performed using a 2- to 3-inch wide stiff elastic band. The eight fingers are slipped into the band, sewn to fit snug. The band covers the distal ends of the fingers (Fig. 5–4). The patient repetitively extends the fingers against the elastic band, keeping the palms together.

Wrist extensor strengthening is performed against weight progressing from 1 to 7 pounds; the weight is draped across the extended fingers. The arm may rest upon a table top, and the hand is raised about an inch, then returned to a horizontal position. These exercises are performed twice daily. Exercises to strengthen extensor muscles across the knee may also be required.

Patients should be taught to avoid arm hyperextension during sleep. Since these patients can assume unusual sitting, lying, and resting

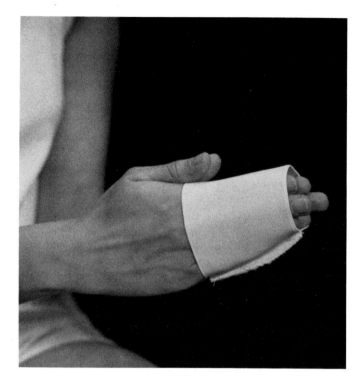

Fig. 5–4. Finger extension exercises are performed using a band made from foundation elastic. The band is sewn to fit snugly. The patient inserts eight fingers into the band and allows the band to cover the distal end of the fingers; the patient repetitively extends the fingers against the elastic band while keeping the palms together.

body positions, the physician should review each of these positions with the patient. In particular, these patients should not sit with knees tucked under or Indian style. Proper shoes should be recommended if pes planus is present. Bracing is sometimes necessary for the knees.

Outcome. In our experience, most patients, even older patients with premature osteoarthritis, respond reasonably well to a resistance-exercise program. The younger the patient, the more complete has been the response to therapy. Probably these patients should be told to avoid occupations that require prolonged repetitive hand tasks as they grow older, in the hope of preventing premature osteoarthritis.[12]

DISORDERS OF THE THUMB

DeQuervain's Tenosynovitis

Stenosing tenosynovitis of the abductor pollicis longus or the extensor pollicis brevis may result from repetitive activity or direct injury. These tendons traverse a thick fibrous sheath at the radial-styloid process. Thickening of the tendon sheath results in stenosis and inflammation. The patient notes pain during pinch grasping or thumb and wrist movement. Palpation of the tendons in the anatomic "snuff box" area may reveal swelling when compared to the uninvolved side.

The Finkelstein sign to extend the tendon and reproduce symptoms is performed by having the patient fold the thumb into her palm with the fingers of the involved hand folded over the thumb. The examiner then grasps the patient's folded hand and rotates the wrist ulnarly, gently stretching the involved tendons (Fig. 5–5). Pain is exacerbated if DeQuervain's tenosynovitis is present. In some cases, the tenosynovitis has occurred bilaterally or has been recurrent.

Treatment includes wrist protection with a splint, and one or two injections of a steroid-local anesthetic mixture into the tendon sheath, which is effective for acute relief (Fig. 5–6). Failure of this treatment may necessitate surgical release of the tendons.[5,13–15] Tasks that require repetitive thumb movement or pinch grasping should be avoided.[16]

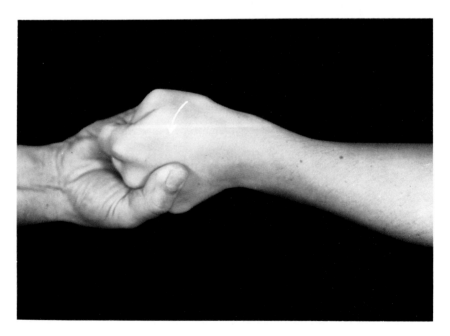

Fig. 5–5. The Finkelstein test: The examiner gently rotates the patient's wrist ulnarly (arrow) while the patient's fingers are folded over the thumb. DeQuervain's tenosynovitis can usually be distinguished from pain arising in the first carpometacarpal joint.

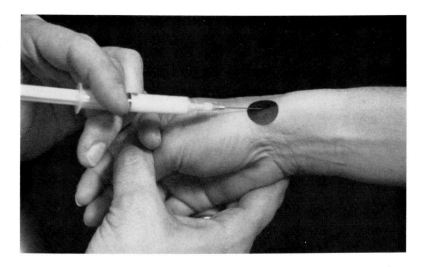

Fig. 5–6. Injection of the tendon sheath in a patient with DeQuervain's tenosynovitis.

Trigger Thumb

Stenosing tenosynovitis of the flexor pollicis longus often results in a snapping or triggering movement of the thumb. The tendon becomes compressed against a prominence of the head of the first metacarpal bone or sesamoid. Thickening of the tendon sheath is often due to repetitive movement or pressure. Trigger thumb also occurs in infants.[17] Tenderness is noted at the base of the thumb in the palmar aspect. Often, a nodule on the tendon can be palpated as it moves during thumb flexion and extension. Trigger thumb and trigger finger are frequently seen as industrial injuries.[5,13,14]

Treatment includes avoiding pressure at the base of the thumb during hand use, and injecting a steroid-local anesthetic mixture into the tendon region with a No. 25 to No. 27 gauge needle (Fig. 5–7). The tendon should then be stretched by having the patient grasp the involved thumb, and gently pull it away and back from the palm repetitively for 1 minute twice daily. If there is a recurrence, the tendon may be injected a second time, and a thumb splint provided for use during work. Failure to provide benefit after two injections should lead to consideration for surgery. Rupture of the tendon is a rare complication of repeated tendon injections.

DISORDERS OF THE PALM AND FINGERS

Trigger Finger

Fusiform swelling of the flexor sublimus tendon over a metacarpal head, accompanied by constriction of the tendon sheath, results in the

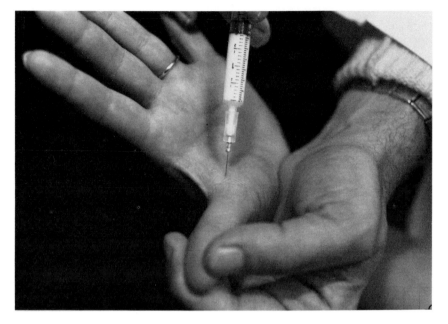

Fig. 5–7. Site for injection of a trigger thumb.

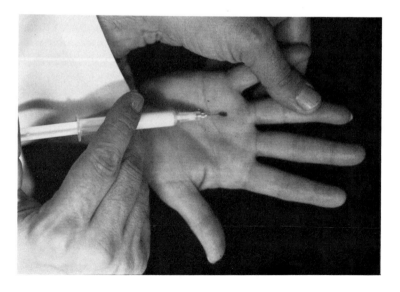

Fig. 5–8. Site for injection of a trigger finger.

locking of a finger in flexion. Often, the patient first notices locking upon arising in the morning. The bent PIP joint should be passively returned to extension; a popping sensation is perceived sometimes as the finger is straightened. Other causes of similar symptoms include: slipping of an extensor tendon, particularly in rheumatoid arthritis, a collateral ligament catching on a bony prominence on the side of a metacarpal head, traumatic splitting of the joint capsule, and an abnormal sesamoid catching on a metacarpal head.

Treatment of a trigger finger includes injection of the tendon sheath with a steroid-local anesthetic mixture (Fig. 5–8); splinting, and other joint protection measures are essential.[13-22] (See "Trigger Thumb.")

Infectious Tenosynovitis

Tuberculous tenosynovitis should be an immediate consideration if massive swelling of a single flexor tendon from the palm all the way out to the distal finger is noted. The cold swelling, with relatively little pain, should immediately be considered tuberculous until proved otherwise. Acute septic tenosynovitis may result from gonococcal, staphylococcal, and syphilitic (rare) infections.[5]

Dupuytren's Contracture

Dupuytren's contracture, which is usually painless, represents a nodular fibrosing lesion within the palmar fascia that progresses to fibrous bands, and usually radiates distally to the fourth and fifth fingers (Fig. 5–9). Ultimately the fingers are contracted by the taut bands. The flexor tendons are not intrinsically involved. Soft tissue pads over the proximal interphalangeal joints on the extensor surface (knuckle pads) may be associated findings. Nodular lesions within the plantar fascia of the feet may also develop concurrently. Dupuytren's contracture occurs in 1 to 3% of Caucasian males. Sex ratio is predominately male (10:1). The condition is probably of genetic origin (by late age, 68% of male relatives are reportedly affected), and no definite relation to occupation has been accepted by various investigators.[8,23,24] Knuckle pads may occur without palmar lesions in relatives of patients.[24] An association with diabetes was not found to be statistically significant.[25] The fasciitis histologically demonstrates fibroblastic proliferation with giant cells and vascular hyperplasia.[24a]

Differential diagnoses include congenital flexion deformity of the fourth and fifth digits (camptodactyly), traumatic scars, Volkmann's ischemic contracture, or intrinsic joint disease.[23]

Treatment of patients with minimal Dupuytren's contracture includes passively stretching the involved digits (hyperextending the digits), avoiding a tight grip by means of built-up handles (pipe insulation, cushion tape),[25a] and perhaps using a glove with padding across the palm during heavy grasping tasks. Surgery should be

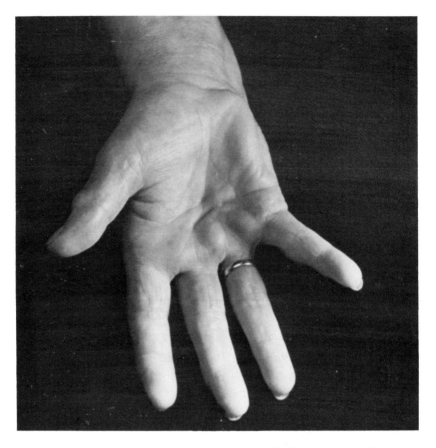

Fig. 5–9. Nodular fibrosing lesion with bands radiating distally are features of Dupuytren's contracture.

considered if functional impairment occurs, or if progressive deformity develops.[26] Unfortunately, the recurrence rate is considerable. Most patients who learn the benign nature of the contracture adapt to the disorder.

DORSAL EDEMA OF SECRETAN

Rarely, following injury to the dorsum of the hand, a peritendinous fibrosis may occur. This brawny, edematous swelling may gradually harden, and often becomes painlessly persistent. Early, consistent elevation of the affected hand may be beneficial in preventing edema.[25a] Repeated injections of a corticosteroid or excision of the fibrotic tendinous tissue have been advocated.[20]

NERVE ENTRAPMENT DISORDERS OF THE WRIST AND HAND

Carpal Tunnel Syndrome

Compression of the median nerve at the wrist may give rise to variable signs and symptoms. The most common and easily recognized symptoms are early morning numbness, tingling, or burning in the distribution of the median nerve of the hand. The patient awakes in the early morning hours, and shakes her hand, elevates it, or otherwise tries to restore sensation. At times the distress is exquisite. Symptoms may consist of sensory nerve complaints only, motor incoordination, or both. Altered motor function may predominate, in which case the patient has difficulty performing pinch grasping, writing, or holding small utensils. The symptoms generally are worse in the early morning or after prolonged use, such as knitting, working on needlepoint, or driving. Because of variable innervation, numbness, tingling, and sensory deficits may involve the entire palmar aspect of the hand, in contrast to the more typical median nerve distribution of the thumb, index, middle, and radial half of the ring fingers. Thenar flattening or atrophy are late manifestations. Raynaud's phenomenon may be seen.

Tests for nerve compression at the wrist include the Hoffman-Tinel test (Fig. 5–10) and the Phalen maneuver (Fig. 5–11). The Hoffman-Tinel test consists of a tingling sensation without pain, following

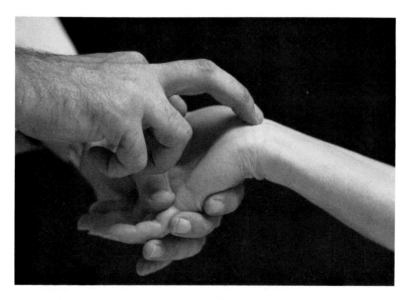

Fig. 5–10. The Hoffman-Tinel test: Tapping over a compressed nerve at the wrist reproduces pain and paresthesia, proximal or distal to the site of compression.

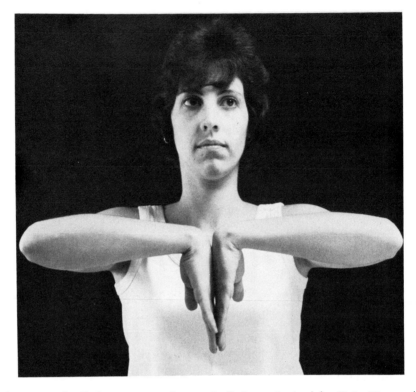

Fig. 5–11. The Phalen maneuver: Acute wrist flexion maintained for 30 to 60 seconds reproduces symptoms in patients with nerve compression in the carpal canal (the carpal tunnel syndrome).

tapping over the median nerve at the flexor surface of the wrist.[27] The Phalen maneuver is performed by having the patient approximate the back of both hands, one to the other, with fingers pointed downward, and wrists flexed maximally; this position is held for 60 seconds. A positive test reproduces numbness and tingling along the median nerve distribution.[15,28,28a] Direct compression of the median nerve may give the same findings. Electrodiagnostic testing with abnormal nerve conduction velocity is supportive of the diagnosis.[29,30] The findings include slowed conduction velocity and increased latency of evoked response potential (terminal latency of the motor impulse > 4 to 5 msec). Of patients with carpal tunnel syndrome, 10% may have normal test results.

Carpal tunnel syndrome may occur from occupations or activities that require repetitive flexor handwork such as typing or knitting,[31] or it may follow sleeping with the wrist in flexion, resting the wrists over a steering wheel, work that requires thumb rolling or kneading motion, or trauma with resulting tenosynovitis.[32] Only 3 of 658 patients with this disorder were performing heavy labor.[31] The carpal tunnel syndrome may occur secondarily to other conditions or diseases, including inflammatory connective tissue disease, secondary osteoarthritis, pregnancy, diabetes, myxedema, acromegaly, amyloid, peripheral neuropathy, or benign local tumors.[15,28,31-33a] The majority of patients with carpal tunnel syndrome do not have an underlying disease process. Rather, the disturbance results from repetitive finger motion or from forced wrist extension, such as pushing from the sides of a chair upon arising, or from development of a dense fibrotic volar-carpal ligament compressing the nerve. Pathologic findings suggest that obstruction of venous return results in increased pressure, fibrous tissue formation, and anoxia of the nerve trunk.[34]

If carpal tunnel syndrome has not resulted in atrophy of the thenar eminence, conservative treatment may suffice. These measures include 30-degree cockup wrist splinting, particularly at night,[25a] avoiding aggravating activity, and injecting a steroid-local anesthetic mixture into the carpal canal (Fig. 5–12). The injection should be placed radially to the palmaris longus tendon.[35-36] Before injection, the patient should notify the physician if the needle accentuates the numbness and tingling, since this indicates penetration of the nerve, and must be avoided. If conservative measures fail, or atrophy of the thenar eminence is detected, surgical release should be carried out. About 10% of postoperative patients unfortunately have recurrences

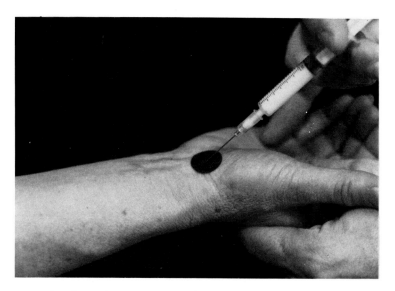

Fig. 5–12. Carpal tunnel injection: Many clinicians consider carpal tunnel injection to be diagnostic and therapeutic. The site for injection should be to the radial side of the palmaris longus tendon. The needle may be directed proximally and then distally, with aliquots of the corticosteroid-anesthetic injected in each direction.

and on occasion require repeat surgical intervention.[30] After surgery, repetitive hand use at work may still not be tolerated. Surgery does not greatly improve motor function loss, but usually aids in relieving nocturnal discomfort and in preventing further motor dysfunction.[30]

Anterior Interosseous Nerve Syndrome

Sudden loss of distal interphalangeal flexion of the thumb and distal interphalangeal flexion of the index finger may result from injury to the anterior interosseous nerve. The injury occurs during lifting, which results in strain and compression of the anterior interosseous nerve by the flexor pollicis longus and flexor carpi radialis at the neck of the radius. Occasionally, a fibrous band is found on the underside of the flexor digitorum sublimus. Electrodiagnostic tests with nerve conduction measurement assist in diagnosis. Treatment includes use of a sling, galvanic stimulation, or surgical exploration.[5]

Ulnar Nerve Entrapment at the Wrist

This disorder may result from compression through Guyon's canal, where the nerve passes deeply into the muscles of the hypothenar eminence on the ulnar side of the wrist. Such compression results in typical ulnar nerve atrophy of the interosseous muscles, and paresthesia of ulnar nerve distribution. Nerve conduction determination will assist in diagnosis. Surgical intervention for release of the nerve is usually required.[15]

NEUROVASCULAR DISORDERS OF THE WRIST AND HAND

Raynaud's Disease and Phenomenon

Sequential discoloration of the digits, progressing from pallor to cyanosis to rubor, upon exposure to cold or emotional upset may occur as a secondary *phenomenon*. Raynaud's phenomenon accompanies, or may precede, other manifestations of systemic connective tissue disease, such as progressive systemic sclerosis, systemic lupus erythematosus, rheumatoid arthritis, or mixed connective tissue disease. Raynaud's phenomenon may also result from hypothyroidism,[37] trauma or frostbite, proximal large vessel obstruction, compression within the thoracic outlet, or use of vasoconstrictive drugs.

The term Raynaud's *disease* is reserved for patients who demonstrate these manifestations, but in whom no primary underlying cause can be demonstrated after a prolonged period of time (Fig. 5–13). The diagnosis is often made only with great uncertainty, since a systemic disorder such as progressive systemic sclerosis may not appear for many years after onset of Raynaud's phenomenon. Yet 90% of patients with Raynaud's phenomenon have no apparent underlying disorder at the time of Raynaud's onset.[38] The best that the clinician can do is to

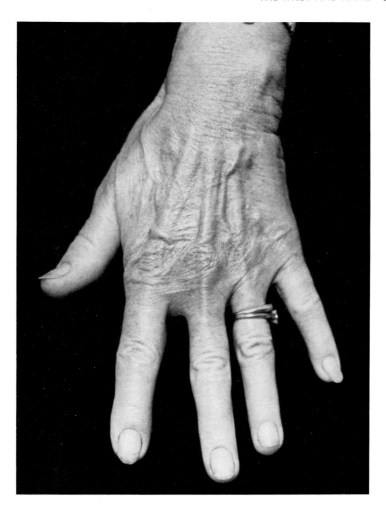

Fig. 5–13. Raynaud's disease: Despite blanching of the digits from the metacarpophalangeal joints to the fingertips for many years, this patient's hands failed to show evidence of atrophy or other features of connective tissue disease.

examine the patient carefully for subtle features of various associated disorders. The presence of distal fingertip pitting, skin telangiectasias or thickening raises concern for progressive systemic sclerosis. Physical examination of the pulses, thoracic outlet maneuvers, neurologic examination, and a general physical examination are essential.

The clinician should order rheumatoid factor test determination, antinuclear-antibody determination, serologic test for syphilis, complete blood counts, tests for sedimentation rate and cryoproteins, protein electrophoresis, urinalysis, a thyroid function test, and a chest roentgenogram.

Treatment for Raynaud's disease and phenomenon includes total body protection from cold. Cold exposure of any body part can set off the disturbance. Patients with mild symptoms need only reassurance, environmental protection from cold, and perhaps abstinence from tobacco (not of proved value). Moderate symptoms often respond to use of oral (0.25 to 0.5 mg/day) or intra-arterial (0.5 mg) reserpine. Recently, there has been concern that reserpine may induce local gangrene or breast cancer. This relationship to breast cancer has been refuted.[38a] We recommend that it be used only during the colder months. Other drugs that may be tried include prazosin (1 mg bid),[39] alpha-methyldopa (1 or 2 g/day), guanethidine (30 to 50 mg/day), phenoxybenzamine (20 to 60 mg/day), estrogen replacement,[38-42] and nitroglycerin ointment. Intravenous dextran or plasmapheresis have been used in intractable cases associated with scleroderma.[41] Stanozolol, a fibrinolytic anabolic steroid (5 mg bid) has recently been reported useful in severe cases secondary to progressive systemic sclerosis.[42] Hepatotoxicity is a limiting factor. Sympathectomy has provided relief in some patients,[38] and long-term benefit has ranged from 20 to 80% in various reports. In our experience most patients benefit with reserpine or tolazoline,[38] often used only in the colder seasons.

We have had some rewarding experience with the use of biofeedback training in patients with either Raynaud's disease or phenomenon. Some patients have raised their skin temperatures by 8 to 10 degrees for sustained periods of time.[43-44]

Erythermalgia

Redness, burning sensation, and swelling of the hands and feet after exposure to heat or after exercise suggests erythermalgia. The disorder may be primary, or secondary to a hematologic disease, diabetes, or a connective tissue disease. The attack appears to be triggered by increased skin temperature (range from 32 to 36 degrees C). Therapy includes trials of aspirin, phenoxybenzamine hydrochloride (Dibenzyline), methysergide, or sympathectomy if a treatable underlying disorder is not found.[15,40]

Acrocyanosis

Painless cyanosis, coolness, and hypoesthesia of the extremities may occur in persons with vasomotor instability, or from causes listed for Raynaud's phenomenon. When underlying disease is not found, reassurance usually suffices for therapy.[15,40]

NODULES

Pseudorheumatoid nodules (firm, rubbery, subcutaneous nodular lesions) may occur in multiple sites, particularly in the pretibial area

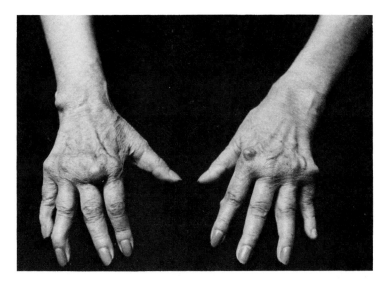

Fig. 5–14. Rheumatoid nodulosis: In patients with rheumatoid arthritis, firm nodules may erupt and persist adjacent to joints, or in the finger pulp. Similar lesions (pseudorheumatoid nodules) may occur on the extremities in the absence of rheumatoid arthritis.

and extensor finger regions, without the presence of rheumatoid arthritis. They may last for months or years, occur in both males and females but predominantly occur in children and young adults[45] (Fig. 5–14).

Giant cell tumors of tendon sheaths or pigmented villonodular tenosynovitis usually occur in women between the third and fourth decade, and are the second most common noninflammatory lesions of a tendon sheath.[46] These growths generally occur on the flexor or extensor tendons, adjacent to a proximal interphalangeal joint. Giant cell tumors of tendon sheaths also occur in the Achilles tendon, and are generally bilateral. Clinically, similar nodules are associated with hyperlipidemia or sarcoidosis; these may be pea-size, yellowish, and lobulated, and in them giant cells with lipoid foamy cytoplasm are noted microscopically.

Presenting symptoms of hemochromatosis may be nodules at the elbow and over the extensor digitorum tendons.[47] Glomus tumors occur as painful, slow-growing neurovascular tumors of an extremity; 30% arise beneath a fingernail. Pain is described as excruciating, burning, or shooting. Local contact exacerbates the pain and suggests the presence of the lesion. Surgery is necessary. An occasional patient presents with acute painful swelling in the pulp of a distal finger pad, which may be due to an infection, known as a *felon*.

Epidermoid cysts or pearls are small, hard, pearl-like cysts several

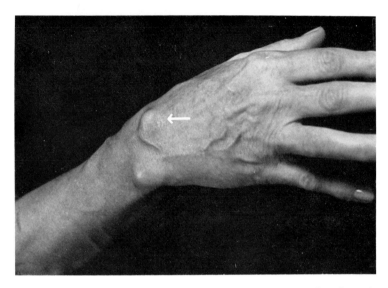

Fig. 5–15. Ganglion (arrow) on the dorsum of the wrist. Aspiration reveals a clear gelatinous fluid.

millimeters in diameter. These occur in the volar aspect of the palm, or in the web adjacent to the metacarpophalangeal joints, and generally are painless. These cysts are thought to arise from injury, when a small piece of epidermis becomes implanted in the subcutaneous tissue.[19] In most cases they disappear spontaneously.

GANGLIA

A ganglion is a cystic swelling overlying a joint or tendon sheath. It probably results as a herniation of synovial tissue from joint capsule or tendon sheath. Ganglia may be unilocular or multilocular. Inflammatory cells are not present. A soft jelly-like fluid can be aspirated from the lesion. Ganglia rarely occur after age 50, and may spontaneously regress or recur. Most commonly, a ganglion occurs at the dorsal aspect of the wrist (Fig. 5–15). Management may be one of the following: leave it alone; aspirate and inject a crystalline steroid; or surgically remove the ganglion after tracing its connection to the tendon sheath or capsule, and repair the defect.

REFERENCES

1. Linscheid RL, Dobyns JH, Beabout JW, Bryan AS: Traumatic instability of the wrist. J Bone Joint Surg 54A:1612–1632, 1972.
2. Maudsley RH: The painful wrist. Practitioner 215:42–45, 1975.
3. Posner MA: Injuries to the hand and wrist in athletes. Orthop Clin North Am 8:593–618, 1977.
4. Adams JC: Outline of Orthopaedics. London, Churchill, Livingstone, 1977.

5. Turek SL: Orthopaedics; Principles and Their Application. Philadelphia, JB Lippincott, 1977.
6. Paty JG: Flexor carpi ulnaris tendinitis. Arthritis Rheum 22:97–98, 1979.
6a. Dieppe P: Crystal deposition disease and the soft tissues. Clinics in Rheumatic Disease 5:807–822, 1979.
7. Kirk JA, Ansell BM, Bywaters EGL: The hypermobility syndrome; Musculoskeletal complaints associated with generalized joint hypermobility. Ann Rheum Dis 26:419–425, 1967.
8. James JIP, Wynne-Davies R: Genetic factors in orthopaedics. *In* Recent Advances in Orthopaedics. Edited by AG Apley. London, J & A Churchill, 1969.
9. Beighton PH, Horan ET: Dominant inheritance in familial generalized articular hypermobility. J Bone Joint Surg 52B:145–147, 1970.
10. Key JA: Hypermobility of joints as a sex linked hereditary characteristic. JAMA 88:1710–1712, 1927.
11. Bird HA, Tribe CR, Bacon PA: Joint hypermobility leading to osteoarthrosis and chondrocalcinosis. Ann Rheum Dis 37:203–211, 1978.
12. Rowatt-Brown A, Rose BS: Familial precocious polyarticular osteoarthrosis of chondrodysplastic type. N Z Med J 65:449–461, 1966.
13. Hartwell SW, Larsen RD, Posch JL: Tenosynovitis in women in industry. Cleve Clin Q 31:115–118, 1964.
14. Reed JV, Harcourt AK: Tenosynovitis. Am J Surg 62:392–396, 1943.
15. Duthie RB, Ferguson AB: Mercer's Orthopedic Surgery. 7th Ed. Baltimore, Williams & Wilkins, 1973.
16. Clark DD, Ricker JH, MacCollum MS: The efficacy of local steroid injection in the treatment of stenosing tenovaginitis. Plast Reconstr Surg 51:179–180, 1973.
17. Swezey RL, Spiegel TM: Evaluation and treatment of local musculoskeletal disorders in elderly patients. Geriatrics 34:56–75, 1979.
18. Fahey JJ, Bollinger JA: Trigger-finger in adults and children. J Bone Joint Surg 36A:1200–1218, 1954.
19. Chuinard RG: The upper extremity: Elbow, forearm, wrist and hand. *In* Musculo-skeletal Disorders. Edited by RD D'Ambrosia. Philadelphia, JB Lippincott, 1977.
20. Wolin I: The management of tenosynovitis. Surg Clin North Am 37:53–62, 1957.
21. Burton RI: The jammed finger or thumb. Contemp Orthop 1:56–81, 1979.
22. McCue FC, Baugher, H, Bourland WL, Burnet M: The 'jammed finger': How to prevent permanent disability. Consultant 19:29–38, 1979.
23. Viljanto JA: Dupuytren's contracture: A review. Semin Arthritis Rheum 3:155–176, 1973.
24. Ling RSM: The genetic factor in Dupuytren's disease. J Bone Joint Surg 45B:709–718, 1963.
24a. Gelberman RH, Amiel D, Rudolph RM et al: Dupuytren's contracture. J Bone Joint Surg 62A:425–432, 1980.
25. Bridgman JF: Periarthritis of the shoulder and diabetes mellitus. Ann Rheum Dis 31:69–71, 1972.
25a. Goodwin C, OTC: Personal communication.
26. Rodrigo JJ, Niebauer JJ, Brown RL, Doyle JR: Treatment of Dupuytren's contracture. J Bone Joint Surg 58A:380–387, 1976.
27. Sonntag VKH: Tinel's sign. N Engl J Med 291:263, 1974.
28. Pinals RS: Traumatic arthritis and allied conditions. *In* Arthritis and Allied Conditions. 9th Ed. Edited by DJ McCarty. Philadelphia, Lea & Febiger, 1979.
28a. Phalen GS: Soft tissue affections of the hand. Hosp Med 7:47–59, 1971.
29. Bendler, EM, Greenspun B, Yu J, Erdman WJ: The bilaterality of carpal tunnel syndrome. Arch Phys Med Rehabil 58:362–364, 1977.
30. Harris CM, Tanner E, Goldstein MN, Pettee DS: The surgical treatment of the carpal tunnel syndrome correlated with preoperative nerve conduction studies. J Bone Joint Surg 61A:93–98, 1979.
31. Birkbeck MQ, Beer TC: Occupation in relation to the carpal tunnel syndrome. Rheumatol Rehabil 14:218–221, 1975.
32. Kopell HP, Thompson WA: Peripheral Entrapment Neuropathies. Huntington, NY, RE Krieger, 1976.

33. Sidiq MBBS, Kirsner AB, Sheon RP: Carpal tunnel syndrome as the first manifestations of systemic lupus erythematosus. JAMA 222:1416–1417, 1972.
33a. Gerster JC, Lagier R, Boivin G, Schneider C: Carpal tunnel syndrome in chondrocalcinosis of the wrist. Arthritis Rheum 23:926–931, 1980.
34. Sunderland S: The nerve lesion in the carpal tunnel syndrome. J Neurol Neurosurg Psychiatry 39:615–626, 1976.
35. Crane RF, Hay EL: What to do when pain signals carpal tunnel syndrome. Consultant 19:81–86, 1979.
36. Moskowitz RM: Clinical Rheumatology. Philadelphia, Lea & Febiger, 1975.
37. Shagan BP, Friedman SA: Raynaud's phenomenon and thyroid deficiency. Arch Intern Med 140:832–833, 1980.
38. Halperin JL, Coffman JD: Pathophysiology of Raynaud's disease. Arch Intern Med 139:89–92, 1979.
38a. Labarthe DR, O'Fallon WM: Reserpine and breast cancer: A community based longitudinal study of 2000 hypertensive women. JAMA 243:2304–2310, 1980.
39. Waldo R: Prazosin relieves Raynaud's vasospasm. JAMA 241:1037, 1979.
40. Fairbairn JF, Juergens JL, Spittell JA: Raynaud's phenomenon and allied vasoplastic conditions. *In* Peripheral Vascular Diseases. 4th Ed. Edited by Allen–Barker–Hines. Philadelphia, WB Saunders, 1972.
41. Wong WH, Freedman RI, Rabens SF, et al: Low molecular weight dextran therapy for scleroderma: effects of dextran 40 on blood flow and capillary filtration coefficient in scleroderma. Arch Dermatol 110:419–422, 1974.
42. Jarrett PEM, Morland M, Browse NL: Treatment of Raynaud's phenomenon by fibrinolytic enhancement. Br Med J 2:523–525, 1978.
43. Emery, H, Schaller JG: Biofeedback in the management of primary and secondary Raynaud's. Abstract presented to Fortieth Annual Meeting Am Rheum Assoc, Chicago, 1976.
44. Editorial from the NIH: Biofeedback for patients with Raynaud's phenomenon. JAMA 242:509–510, 1979.
45. Williams HJ, Biddulph EC, Coleman SS, Ward JR: Isolated subcutaneous nodules (pseudorheumatoid): J Bone Joint Surg 59A:73–76, 1977.
46. Stern RE, Gauger DW: Pigmented villonodular tenosynovitis. J Bone Joint Surg 59A:560–561, 1977.
47. Bensen WG, Laksin CA, Little HA, Fam AG: Hemochromatotic arthropathy mimicking rheumatoid arthritis. Arthritis Rheum 21:844–848, 1978.

Chapter 6

THE THORACIC CAGE
AND DORSAL SPINE
REGION

Myofascial and other chest wall pain syndromes may occur as entities in and of themselves, may be secondary manifestations of other systemic disorders, or may coexist with other serious underlying diseases. Thus, a careful history and physical examination are essential. The physician may categorize the various causes for chest pain according to whether they arise from structures superior to the chest, within the chest (intrathoracic), inferior to the chest, posterior to the chest, or from structures involving the chest wall.

Chest Pain Arising from Structures Superior to the Chest. Disturbances arising in the head, neck, or thoracic outlet, such as cervical disc disease or thoracic outlet syndrome (see Chapt. 2), may give rise to referred pain that involves the chest region.[1,2,3] When chest pain results from thoracic outlet syndrome, the site of origin of the symptoms can usually be detected by characteristic manifestations involving the upper extremity (see "Thoracic Outlet Syndrome," Chapt. 2). Chest wall tenderness may also result from irritation of the cervical or vagus nerves.[1] Precordial chest pain and features of angina may be caused by cervical nerve root irritation.[4] In addition to chest wall tenderness and pain, these patients may have a positive Spurling test (see Chapt. 1) and cervical myofascial trigger points.[5] These patients improve after treatment to the neck including cervical traction.

Chest Pain of Intrathoracic Origin. A brief list of the intrathoracic origin of chest pain is seen in Table 6–1.[6]

To distinguish intrathoracic diseases causing chest pain, a careful history of the quality, duration, radiation, and precipitating causes of

Table 6–1. Sources of Chest Pain of Intrathoracic Origin

---

1. Classic Heberden's angina (arteriosclerotic heart disease)
2. Angina of pulmonary hypertension or aortic stenosis
3. Prinzmetal's angina (arteriosclerotic heart disease)
4. Acute myocardial infarction
5. Dressler's syndrome
6. Postcardiotomy syndrome
7. Pericarditis
8. Mitral prolapse
9. Dissection of the aorta
10. Diseases of the pleura
11. Pulmonary embolism
12. Pneumothorax
13. Disease of the esophagus

---

the pain must be undertaken. The pain of classic angina occurs in the retrosternal region and may radiate into the neck, left arm, and occasionally into the medial aspect of both upper arms. Angina is usually distinguishable from pain of chest wall origin by its brief duration, its aggravation by cold and exertion, and its relief with rest. Chest wall pain by contrast lasts for hours or days, occurs at rest, and may improve with general activity. Pericardial pain, which is retrosternal, is often worse while recumbent and improves by sitting up or forward, and may be accentuated by deep breathing. Complaints of chest discomfort, fatigue, dyspnea, palpitations, tachycardia, anxiety, and neurotic behavior have been described in the past under various labels, including "neurocirculatory asthenia," Da Costa's syndrome, or "effort syndrome."[7] It has been suggested that similar symptoms may be related to mitral valve prolapse (systolic click) syndrome. Although an interesting speculation, no data are available that definitively relate such symptoms to this syndrome.[8]

Pleural pain is generally located on one side of the chest, is accentuated by breathing, and is generally not aggravated by movement. A common source of pain that arises from intrathoracic structures is the esophagus, particularly for that pain emanating from a hiatus hernia with reflex esophagitis. Such pain generally radiates to the anterior chest wall, may be accompanied by tenderness of the musculature of the chest wall, and is often exacerbated by recumbency. If the examiner exerts gentle pressure to the epigastrium, this maneuver frequently reproduces pain of esophageal origin.

Chest Pain Arising from Structures Inferior to the Chest. Chest pain may result from gas entrapment syndromes, biliary tract disease, peptic or gastric ulcer, pancreatitis, and subphrenic abscess.[3] A history of bowel dysfunction, weight loss, stool changes, or dietary indiscretion should provide clues to these conditions. Gastric ulcers may be present, with marked variability in history, severity, and chronicity. We have found radiographic examination of the upper gastrointestinal tract, with careful attention for gastric ulcer, essential for diagnosis when epigastric tenderness is observed, or when patients have intractable chest wall pain.

Chest Pain Arising from Disorders Posterior to the Chest. Chest pain may arise from herpes zoster and lesions of the dorsal spine, such as osteoporosis, tumor, Scheuermann's disease, and rarely, thoracic disc disease.[2]

Chest Pain Arising from the Chest Wall Structures. Rib trauma or fracture, metastatic tumors, and other lesions evident on radiographic examination may cause pain and local tenderness. The clinician should also consider diseases of the breasts and the regional lymph nodes. However, the vast majority of patients have benign myofascial chest wall pain syndromes.[1]

MYOFASCIAL CHEST WALL SYNDROMES

Included here are subacute and chronic painful conditions of the anterior chest wall associated with tenderness of the chest wall structures (Fig. 6–1). Swelling does not occur.

The commonly described myofascial chest wall syndromes include the costosternal syndrome or costochondritis, the sternalis syndrome, xiphoidalgia, and the rib-tip syndrome. Each of these descriptive syndromes is characterized by local chest wall tenderness with accompanying pain, of severity ranging from a dull ache to a throbbing intense discomfort. In these myofascial chest wall syndromes, pain is present at rest and during chest movement, lasts up to several hours or days, and may be related to breathing. Anxiety and hyperventilation are common accompaniments.[9] The episodes are often brief and self-limited, but occasionally myofascial chest wall pain syndrome is superimposed upon true angina and causes severe disability.[10] On occasion, nitroglycerin has relieved myofascial chest wall pain unrelated to angina.[11] Although occasionally considered as one entity, *chest wall pain syndrome*,[10] most physicians prefer individual terminology, depending on points of maximum tenderness in the chest wall.[12]

Costosternal Syndrome. This term applies to conditions involving and limited to pain in the anterior part of the chest wall. The pain sometimes radiates to the whole chest and is accentuated by deep inspiration.[13] The pains are usually intermittent, last a few days, and occur intermittently for months or years. The specific feature of costosternal syndrome is the presence of tenderness and pain reproduction during palpation at one or more costosternal junctions. Ten-

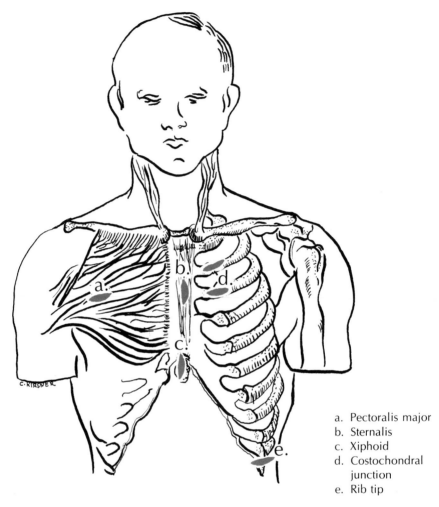

a. Pectoralis major
b. Sternalis
c. Xiphoid
d. Costochondral
   junction
e. Rib tip

Fig. 6–1. Myofascial chest wall pain: Myofascial trigger points may be found at the second or third left costochondral junction in the upper outer chest quadrant within the pectoralis major muscle, at the manubriosternal junction, at the tip of the xiphoid process, at the center of the sternum in the sternalis muscle, or on a lower rib tip.

derness may also be noted along the nearby intercostal muscles. Relief from pain by anesthetic-corticosteroid injection of the involved costochondral joint is an additional feature of the syndrome.[13]

The **Sternalis Syndrome.** The sternalis syndrome is the only myofascial disorder in which a trigger point gives rise to bilateral pain.[14] The trigger point is in the sternal synchondrosis, or in the sternalis muscle overlying the body of the sternum (Fig. 6–1). Pain is noted in the center of the chest wall, and usually the patient recognizes that the origin of the pain is in the chest wall region, rather than within the thorax. The symptoms tend to be less intermittent and the severity less frightening than those associated with the costosternal syndrome.

Xiphoidalgia. This syndrome is characterized by spontaneous pain in the anterior chest associated with distinct discomfort and tenderness of the xiphoid process of the sternum.[1] Pressure over the xiphoid reproduces the pain, which is intermittent, and often aggravated by eating a heavy meal, lifting, stooping, bending, or twisting. This pain persists for weeks or months, but tends to be self-limited without special treatment.

Rib-Tip Syndrome. This syndrome differs in that the patient presents with severe lancinating pain associated with hypermobility of the anterior end of a costal cartilage, most often the tenth rib, but occasionally involving the eighth or ninth rib.[15] The syndrome, variously called slipping rib, slipping rib cartilage syndrome, or clicking rib refers to hypermobility of a rib-tip. Digital pressure over the involved rib may reproduce a painful clicking. The slipping rib syndrome results from recurrent subluxation of a costal cartilage, and is associated with a stabbing or lancinating pain.[16] The pain is easily confused with abdominal visceral disease.[17] Injury or indirect trauma due to lifting or twisting is often the cause.[18,19] Other features of the syndrome include pain aggravated by arm abduction, audible clicking sensation in the chest wall, and relief of pain by lying down.[19]

Physical examination includes the "hooking maneuver"—the examiner's curved fingers are hooked under the ribs at the costal margin and the examiner gently pulls the rib cage anteriorly[17] (Fig. 6–2); this reproduces the snap and pain. Excision of the involved rib has been recommended, but a steroid-local anesthetic injection into the intercostal muscles adjacent to a slipping rib may be of value. In other cases, only the rib-tip of the lower ribs is tender, and the pain is self-limited. Physical examination for myofascial chest pain should include a measurement of chest expansion. Inflammatory rheumatic disease of the chest wall (e.g., ankylosing spondylitis) restricts chest expansion to 1½ inches (3 cm) or less, and may inflame the sternocostal joints.[9] Thoracic spine motion, spinal curves, and symmetry of the chest wall and the breasts should be evaluated. Careful palpation of the supraclavicular fossae and axillae for lymphadenopathy should be performed. Palpation is best performed beginning with the acromioclavicular joints, continuing to the sternoclavicular joints, and then down each of the costosternal joints. The sternal synchondrosis, the overlying sternalis muscle, and the xiphoid process should be palpated. Xiphoidalgia must be distinguished from the deeper epigastric tenderness of gastrointestinal disease. A helpful way to distinguish these is to compare the tenderness to palpation in the epigastrium while the patient performs a partial sit-up, with the severity of

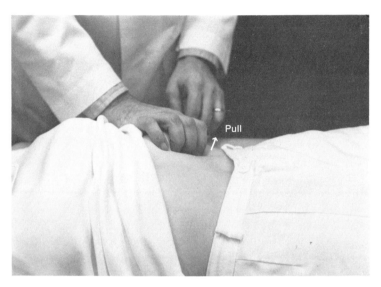

Fig. 6–2. The hooking maneuver: The examiner's curved fingers are hooked under the lower ribs, then the rib cage is gently pulled anteriorly. This reproduces a snapping sensation and pain.

discomfort during palpation while the patient is relaxed and recumbent. Xiphoidalgia and superficial lower chest wall pain are worse during the partial sit-up. Conversely, true intra-abdominal lesion tenderness is diminished during contraction of the superficial abdominal muscles, and worsens when the abdominal muscles are relaxed.

The distinguishing characteristic of myofascial chest pain is the ability to reproduce the pain state by local pressure.[10] Associated trigger points may also be found over the pectoralis muscles, the lower sternocleidomastoid area,[1] the tip of the lower costal cartilages,[15] and most commonly, the third left costochrondral joint.[20] Bilateral chest wall pain may result from a trigger point in the sternalis muscle.[14] "If local pressure applied to the anterior part of the chest wall becomes a routine procedure in the physical examination of all patients with precordial pain, a surprisingly large number of cases of costosternal syndromes will be discovered."[13]

Etiology. Inflammatory rheumatic disease can cause myofascial symptoms and must be excluded. Anxiety is common in patients with chest wall pain syndrome. However, psychologic investigations suggest that pure psychogenic chest pain is uncommon.[21] Myofascial chest wall pain syndrome usually results from "misuse" activity, similar to that which causes myofascial pain in other body regions. An attack of chest wall pain may follow prolonged sitting in a slouched position or after assuming a bent-over position.[22] The pectoral muscles may be overworked in activities that require repeated adduction of the arm across the chest (e.g., stacking logs, polishing a car). The clinician must consider household chores, job, and hobbies as possible aggravating factors. A pain-spasm-pain cycle may ensue, which is aggravated by anxiety.[23]

Laboratory and Radiographic Examination. Myofascial chest wall pain has no specific laboratory abnormalities. An erythrocyte sedimentation rate is useful to exclude tumors or other inflammatory processes. A roentgenogram of the chest and an electrocardiogram are required for most patients. Calcification of costal cartilages is commonly present, and any association to the pain is speculative.[24] An upper gastrointestinal radiographic examination is often helpful. Electrodiagnostic testing of the upper extremities, on occasion, helps delineate chest wall pain that results from cervial nerve root impingement or thoracic outlet syndrome.

Differential Diagnosis. In most cases, chest wall pain syndromes can be differentiated from other more serious disorders that were discussed earlier in this chapter.[25] In one community hospital emergency room, only 7 of 50 consecutive patients seen for chest pain had coronary artery disease.[26] Myofascial chest wall pain was the cause for chest pain in the majority of the remaining patients, and in another study was responsible for approximately 2% of all office visits.[20] The patient with *psychogenic chest wall pain* presents with atypical chest pain that bears no relation to activity, time of day, or thoracic structures. The pain is usually centered over the cardiac apex. There are no discrete trigger points that reproduce the pain. Such pain frequently accompanies anxiety and depression, has an emotional precipitant, and generally does not awaken the patient.[21]

Management. Most attacks of myofascial chest wall pain are self-limited, and the patient may require only reassurance.[1] For patients with subacute and chronic recurring myofascial chest wall pain, these six steps for management should be followed:

1. Exclude other organic disease.
2. Provide an explanation for the patient. The presence of a myofascial trigger point goes far to demonstrate to the patient that the pain does originate outside his head. The physician should briefly describe the pain-spasm-pain cycle and its aggravation by fatigue or emotion.
3. Recognize and eliminate aggravating factors. These include improper posture while sitting or working, misuse of pectoralis major muscles, and prolonged sedentary activities, such as typing.
4. Provide self-help exercises. The most helpful stretching exercise for the chest wall is the cornering exercise, or the standing push-up in a corner.[27] The patient stands facing a corner, approx-

imately 2 feet out, with each arm on an adjacent wall, fingers pointed toward the corner, and palms held to the wall at approximately shoulder height. The patient then gently presses in toward the corner until a pulling sensation is felt in the pectoral and chest wall muscles (Fig. 6–3). This position is held for 10 seconds and repeated for 1 or 2 minutes several times a day.[27] Posture correction exercises may also be necessary (see Appendix).

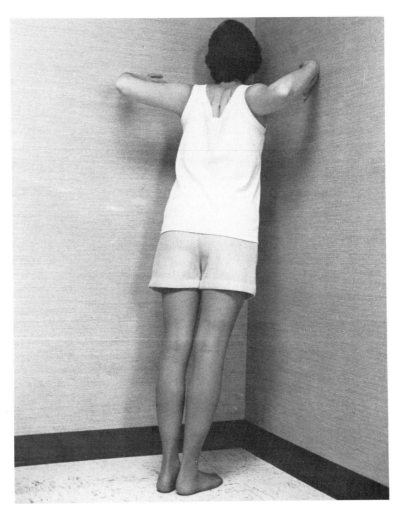

Fig. 6–3. Pectoral muscle stretching: The corner "push up" is performed with the patient standing approximately 2 feet out from the corner and both arms raised to shoulder height, hands placed on each wall, fingers pointing in toward the corner. Hands are 18 to 30 inches out from the corner to each side. The patient gently and progressively pushes into the corner until a pulling sensation is felt in the pectoral region.

5. Provide for relief from pain. Pain of myofascial chest wall trigger points may be relieved either by applying a vapocoolant spray,[1,23] or by local injection with a steroid-local anesthetic mixture (Fig. 6–4). At least two thirds of the patients obtain good results with these methods.[13]

6. Project an expected outcome. Most patients with myofascial chest wall pain who follow these management principles obtain good relief in 3 to 6 weeks. The exercises should be kept up for at least 3 weeks following relief. The patient must conscientiously avoid improper posture or repeated misuse of chest wall muscles.

When the chest wall pain syndrome and underlying arteriosclerotic heart disease coexist, careful attention to treatment of both disorders is essential. Smoking should be discontinued, since a chronic cough may cause chest wall muscle fatigue and subsequent spasm. Similarly, patients with chest wall pain superimposed upon chronic bronchitis and emphysema should stop smoking. Relaxation techniques and biofeedback training along with physical therapy are helpful. Patients with no other underlying cause for continued distress should be closely reevaluated for other causes. A trial of antidepressant medication may be rewarding. Although muscle relaxants have not proved helpful, drugs to control anxiety may be useful in an overly anxious patient. Amitriptyline and other tricyclics may be beneficial for sleep disturbances or nocturnal panic that sometimes occur in these pa-

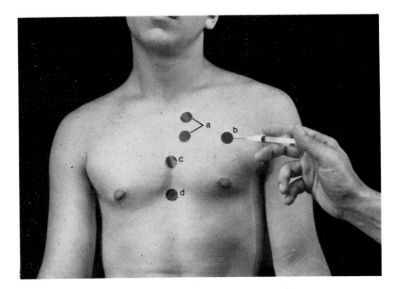

Fig. 6–4. Sites for injection: (a) second and third costochondral junctions, (b) pectoralis major muscle, (c) sternalis muscle, and (d) xiphoid process.

tients. The value of analgesic compounds is limited, but prescribing the nonsteroidal anti-inflammatory agents may be worthwhile, especially if tests of inflammation suggest the possibility of a spondyloarthritis underlying the chest pain syndrome. In some patients a therapeutic trial using a nitroglycerine compound may be rewarding. When relief does occur, it is not necessarily proof of the presence of arteriosclerotic heart disease.[10]

TIETZE'S SYNDROME

Costochondral region pain associated with *enlargement* of an upper costochondral cartilage characterizes this syndrome[9] (Fig. 6–5). Tietze's syndrome may be acute, intermittent, or chronic. The swelling is firm to bony hard, slightly elongated, or less often, round. This feature of swelling, not seen in other myofascial chest wall pain syndromes, needs emphasis. It is for this reason that Tietze's syndrome is considered separate from other chest wall pain syndromes. In approximately 80% of cases the lesion is single. Most often it occurs in the second costochondral junction, and less often in the third costochondral junction on either side.[28] The swelling is nonsuppurative, tender, and histologically reveals increased vascularity with proliferation of columns of cartilage. Cleft formation with mucoid debris is seen.[29] The etiology is unknown. Radiographic examination is usually not helpful, and tests for inflammation are generally normal. Differential diagnoses include mainly sepsis or tumors of the underlying rib, or pain from intrathoracic structures. Radiographic examina-

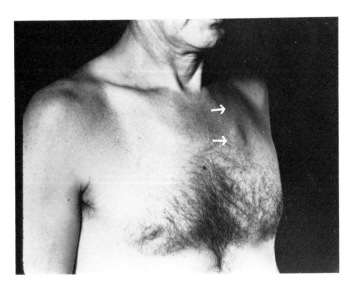

Fig. 6–5. The Tietze's syndrome lesion. Costochondral swelling is observed. (Photograph courtesy Dr. John Calabro, Worcester, Mass.)

tion may be required periodically to exclude other diseases. Although spontaneous remission generally occurs, months or years may elapse before improvement is noted. Biopsy of the rib may be required for reassurance. We have found local injections with a corticosteroid-anesthetic mixture effective. Patients with persistent symptoms may be helped by local physical therapy, including hot or cold applications, and nonsteroidal anti-inflammatory drugs.

JUVENILE KYPHOSIS (SCHEUERMANN'S DISEASE)

During puberty a child may be noted to have a slouched appearance, and may be brought to the physician for "poor posture." The child may or may not complain of discomfort. One cause of the

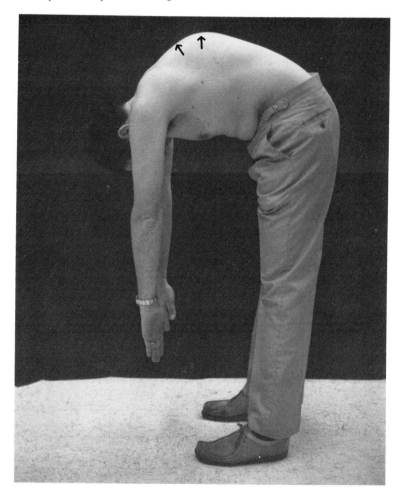

Fig. 6–6. Dorsal kyphosis may be a result of Scheuermann's disease or may be simply a postural deformity, the adult round back.

kyphosis of adolescence is an epiphysitis of the dorsal vertebrae, accompanied clinically by forward-sloping shoulders, and a round back (Fig. 6–6). Most commonly, the disease appears in the early years of the second decade of life, but may first be detected in adulthood.

The kyphosis of Scheuermann's disease is accompanied by vertebral abnormalities that can be seen on roentgenographs as vertebral end-plate irregularities, and wedging of the vertebral body.[30-34] Nonspecific kyphosis, such as adult round back, which is a postural deformity, occurs commonly in young persons, but vertebral abnormalities are not seen.[31] Juvenile kyphosis with epiphysitis (Scheuermann's disease) is accompanied by pain in up to 60% of patients, and scoliosis in 30 to 40% of patients.[31] The pain is often worse with rest and after prolonged activity, and is characterized by a dull ache in the mid-dorsal spine region between the scapulae, or diffusely in the mid-back region. This pain usually does not awaken the patient. There are no associated neurologic signs or symptoms.

Avascular necrosis of the vertebral end plate, herniation of intervertebral disc material, metabolic, endocrine, and vitamin deficiency factors have all been implicated in causation of this entity.[30] The central artery to the vertebral end plate, which usually is obliterated by the age of six, has been noted to persist in patients until age 13 in Scheuermann's disease. The persistence of this vessel beyond the normal time span is thought to lead to irregularity of the vertebral end plate.[34] In a recent investigation of the pathology of two patients with Scheuermann's disease, Bradford noted bone, cartilage and disc to be normal on histologic and electron microscopic study.[32] There was no definite evidence of avascular necrosis. However, gross examination revealed wedging and collapsing of the vertebral body with a normal disc width. Breaks in the vertebral end plate were found with protrusion of disc material into the bony spongiosum.[35] Bradford speculates that perhaps osteoporosis plays a role, although the etiology still remains unknown.[32]

No abnormalities have been noted in calcium or phosphorus values, or in tests for inflammatory processes. As noted, characteristic radiographic features include vertebral end-plate irregularity, Schmorl's nodes, and anterior wedging of the involved vertebrae[30,31] (Fig. 6–7).

Juvenile ankylosing spondylitis must be considered in the differential diagnosis of Scheuermann's disease. A history of iritis, heel pain, or synovitis of lower extremity joints in a male suggests HLA-B27 associated spondyloarthropathies. Leukemia, hemangioma of the vertebra, juvenile osteoporosis, and osteomalacia must be considered. These disorders, which may have spinal involvement, are usually readily identified by characteristic radiographic features.[33]

Management. Management includes advising parents to stop nagging the child just to "straighten up."[33] All patients should be taught

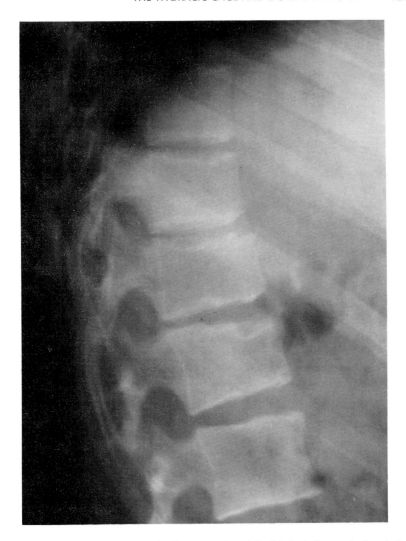

Fig. 6–7. Radiographic features of Scheuermann's epiphysitis include vertebral end-plate irregularity, herniation into the vertebral body, and anterior vertebral wedging. (Courtesy of Toledo Hospital.)

an exercise program to strengthen the extensor muscles of the dorsal spine. Hyperextension exercises should be performed at the same time as pelvic tilting. This is best performed by having the patient bend over a table flexing the hips, with the chest and abdomen in contact with the tabletop. While in this position, the patient raises the head and shoulders thus hyperextending the dorsal spine. This position is held for 10 to 30 seconds and performed for 6 to 10 repetitions twice daily. Shoulder shrugging and scapular abduction exercises may help reverse the forward inclination of the shoulders. If the kyphosis is greater than 40 degrees, a cosmetically significant deformity is noted. It is wise to refer the patient to an orthopedist who may prescribe a Milwaukee brace to improve the kyphosis and prevent the need for surgery.[30,33,36] Improvement in the kyphotic deformity is likely if treatment is begun early in the course of the disease.

OSTEOPOROSIS AND OSTEOMALACIA (OSTEOPENIA)

Osteoporosis commonly presents as back pain with segmental radiation in the distribution of the contiguous nerve roots. Sitting often aggravates the pain. The patient may be disturbed by muscle spasm during the night. Dorsal kyphosis, "dowager hump," and loss of height may be noted; T-12 and L-1 are the most common vertebrae involved.[31] Occasionally, radiographic evidence of osteoporosis and vertebral compression fracture may be observed in asymptomatic individuals.[31] Limb fracture or periodontal disease often precede the spinal complaints.[37-41]

Etiology. The etiology of osteoporosis is uncertain and complex. Many patients have a combination of both osteoporosis and osteomalacia.[42] Accordingly, the term osteopenia of bone may be preferred. Osteoporosis, characterized by loss of osteoid and mineral, is contrasted to osteomalacia, in which the primary defect is related to mineral loss alone. Factors strongly considered causative in the etiology of osteoporosis include estrogen deficiency, age, genetic factors, physical disuse, and steroid therapy.[42-47]

Laboratory and Radiographic Examination. Wedging, collapse, codfish deformity, Schmorl's nodes, vertebral end-plate irregularity and general demineralization are noted on radiographs to some degree in all patients with osteoporosis[38] (Fig. 6–8). Pseudofractures (Looser zones or Milkman's lines) (Fig. 6–9), although pathognomonic for osteomalacia, occur in less than 10% of such patients; bone biopsy is the only definite way to diagnose senescent osteomalacia.[43] Bone scans,[42] determination of serum calcium, phosphorus, alkaline phosphatase, and vitamin D levels (if available), and measures of thyroid function are useful in excluding some of the many causes of osteopenia.[43]

Primary osteoporosis must be a diagnosis of exclusion. The clinician must consider all disorders that can cause secondary osteopenia. Among the important entities to be excluded are primary or metastatic malignant disease, multiple myeloma, and causes of osteomalacia, such as malabsorption syndrome and drug-induced disease as seen in patients on long-term phenytoin (Dilantin) therapy.[31,38,43,46,48]

Management. The goals of management of osteopenia are to alleviate symptoms and arrest disease progression.[38] Although there is

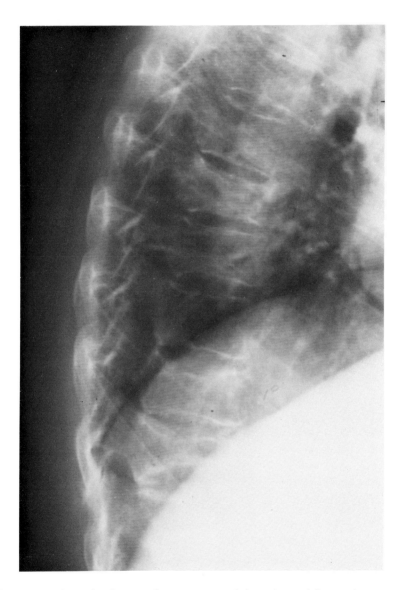

Fig. 6–8. Radiographic features of osteoporosis include wedging of the vertebra anteriorly with vertebral collapse, vertebral end-plate irregularity, and general demineralization. (Courtesy of Toledo Hospital.)

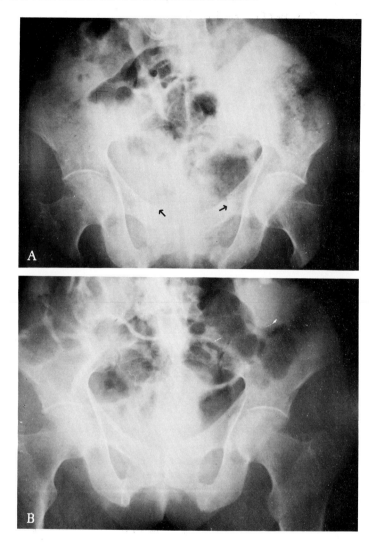

Fig. 6–9. *A,* Pseudofractures (Looser zones or Milkman's lines) are evident on the pubic rami, and, *B,* they readily disappear following treatment as seen in the follow-up roentgenograph.

only limited evidence that any presently available treatment can restore bone toward normal, dietary and physical methods of treatment may be useful. Additional therapy is aimed at preventing further loss of calcification and stimulating bone formation rather than simply symptomatic care.[38] Exercise, especially daily walks, is a recommended means of retarding progression of osteoporosis.[45] Severe pain from fractures may require bracing to allow ambulation. Prolonged bracing immobilizes the spine and can accentuate the osteoporotic process. Accordingly, bracing for pain relief should be discontinued when symptoms permit. Patients should avoid carbonated beverages at mealtime, since these retard calcium absorption. Other dietary recommendations include maintaining ideal weight and eating foods high in calcium, such as dairy products.

The use of drugs that inhibit bone resorption, such as estrogen, fluoride, and calcitonin, remains controversial and in some cases, investigational, in the treatment of osteoporosis.[41-43,47,49] A program of treatment including calcium and vitamin D ingestion may be useful for patients with repeated vertebral fractures, or with radicular segmental back pain accompanying radiographic features of osteoporosis. A baseline determination of serum and urine calcium is obtained, then 1 g of elemental calcium per day is provided as a dietary supplement, and vitamin D in doses of 50,000 units is given once or twice weekly. Dosage is later reduced depending on clinical response and results of blood and urine calcium determinations. Patients with mixed osteoporosis and osteomalacia may benefit.[38,43,50,51] This regimen is suggested for the prevention of bone loss secondary to chronic steroid use.[51] Patients on this regimen should be closely monitored with respect to serum and quantitative urinary calcium determinations to avoid hypercalcemia and renal stones.[51]

Because the benefits of potent vitamin D therapy are as yet unproved, this treatment should be reserved for patients with significant radiologic changes, distressing symptoms, vertebral fractures, or in association with prolonged high-dose steroid therapy (as a prophylactic measure). When vitamin D is used, the dose may be reduced to as little as 50,000 IU/month when clinical and radiologic improvement allow. If the patient has recurrent vertebral fractures despite use of calcium and vitamin D, the addition of estrogen and fluoride to the regimen may be considered. A new, more potent vitamin D (1-25 dihydroxy-D) may result in *worsening* of osteoporosis, since this vitamin can result in stimulation of bone *resorption*.[41] Excessive fluoride can lead to skeletal fluorosis with increased brittleness of bone or osteomalacia,[49] and has also been thought to cause plantar fasciitis (see Chapt. 11).

HERNIATED DORSAL INTERVERTEBRAL DISC

Although this disorder represents less than 1% of all patients undergoing operation for spinal disc disease,[52] a herniated dorsal intervertebral disc must be considered in the differential diagnosis of thoracic back pain. Patients with thoracic disc protrusion rarely have night pain, and there usually is no paraspinal muscle spasm. The patients do have radicular pain and sensory findings that can be intermittent or constant. Pain complaints include a dull diffuse backache. Of these patients, 50% have weakness or spasticity of the lower extremities.

Love and Schorn reviewed their experience with 61 patients in whom surgery verified thoracic disc protrusion.[52] Duration of symptoms before surgery was 1 to 2 years; gradual worsening of symptoms including pain, numbness, weakness of the lower extremities, and rarely, urinary retention or spinal shock occurred; 50% had features of bilateral spastic paralysis. Slight atrophy of the small muscles of the hand (T-1 protruded disc), or atrophy of lower extremity muscles were only seen occasionally; reflexes at the knee and ankle were often hyperactive. Positive Babinski reflexes occurred in half of the patients. Spinal fluid findings were often normal, and cerebrospinal fluid protein was elevated above 50 mg/100 ml in less than half of the patients.

Roentgenograms of the spinal column occasionally revealed calcification of the thoracic intervertebral disc, which proved to be the offending disc in every instance. Only one myelogram was normal among those studied. Computed tomography and electrodiagnostic studies were not available. Lesions found at surgery included seven instances in which the disc eroded through the anterior dura; in one case a spicule of disc material actually penetrated the spinal cord. Two cases of hematomyelia of the cord and two cases of posterior infarction of the cord at the level of the protruded disc were encountered.[52] Unfortunately, patients with a severe neurologic deficit were not improved by surgical intervention. A wide complete laminectomy of two or more vertebrae was the procedure of choice recommended by Love and Schorn.[52] Ransohoff[53] and others[54] have shown that the surgical failures resulted because of the posterior surgical approach. They recommend the anterior or anterolateral approach, which has significantly improved the outcome.

REFERENCES

1. Wehrmacher W: The painful anterior chest wall syndromes. Med Clin North Am 42:111–118, 1958.
2. Edmeads J: Pain arising from thoracic nerves, nerve roots and spinal cord. *In* Chest Pain: An integrated diagnostic approach. Edited by DL Levene. Philadelphia, Lea & Febiger, 1977.
3. Saibil FG, Edmeads J: Pain arising from extrathoracic structures. *In* Chest Pain: An integrated diagnostic approach. Edited by DL Levene. Philadelphia, Lea & Febiger, 1977.
4. Myers G, Freeman R, Scharf D, et al: Cervicoprecordial angina: Diagnosis and management. Am J Cardiol 39:287, 1977. (Abstract)
5. Nachlas W: Pseudo-angina pectoris originating in the cervical spine. JAMA 103:323–325, 1934.
6. Levene DL, Davies GM, Saibil FG: Chest pain arising from intrathoracic structures. *In* Chest Pain; An integrated diagnostic approach. Edited by DL Levene. Philadelphia, Lea & Febiger, 1977.
7. Wooley CF: Where are the diseases of yesteryear? Circulation 53:749–751, 1976.
8. Gelfand ML, Kronzon I, Decarolis P, Winer H: Mitral valve systolic click syndrome. Am Family Pract 21:135–141, 1980.
9. Pinals RS: Traumatic arthritis and allied conditions. *In* Arthritis and Allied Conditions. Edited by DJ McCarty. Philadelphia, Lea & Febiger, 1979.

10. Epstein, SE, Gerber LH, Borer JS: Chest wall syndrome: A common cause of unexplained cardiac pain. JAMA 241:2793–2797, 1979.
11. Master AM: The spectrum of anginal and noncardiac chest pain. JAMA 187:894–899, 1964.
12. Hench PK: Nonarticular rheumatism. In Rheumatic Diseases: Diagnosis and Management. Edited by WA Katz. Philadelphia, JB Lippincott, 1977.
13. Wolf E, Stern S: Costosternal syndrome. Arch Intern Med 136:189–191, 1976.
14. Pace JB: Commonly overlooked pain syndromes responsive to simple therapy. Postgrad Med 58:107–113, 1975.
15. McBeath AA, Keene JS: The rib-tip syndrome. J Bone Joint Surg 57-A:795–797, 1975.
16. Davies-Colley R: Slipping rib. Br Med J 1:432, 1922.
17. Heinz GJ, Zavala DC: Slipping rib syndrome: Diagnosis using the "hooking maneuver." JAMA 237:794–795, 1977.
18. Holmes JF: A study of the slipping rib cartilage syndrome. N Engl J Med 224:928–932, 1941.
19. Ballon HC, Spector L: Slipping rib. Can Med Assoc J 39:355–358, 1938.
20. Benson EH, Zavala DC: Importance of the costochondral syndrome in evaluation of chest pain. JAMA 156:1244–1246, 1954.
21. Billings RF: Chest pain related to emotional disorders. In Chest Pain: An integrated diagnostic approach. Edited by DL Levene. Philadelphia, Lea & Febiger, 1977.
22. Miller AJ, Texidor, TA: "Precordial catch," a neglected syndrome of precordial pain. JAMA 159:1364–1365, 1955.
23. Travell J, Rinzler SH: Pain syndromes of the chest muscles: Resemblance to effort angina and myocardial infarction, and relief by local block. Can Med Assoc J 59:333–338, 1948.
24. Lovshin L: Personal communication.
25. Greenfield S, Nadler MA, Morgan MT, Shine KI: The clinical investigation and management of chest pain in an emergency department: Quality assessment by criteria mapping. Med Care 15:898–905, 1977.
26. Mohan LA: Personal communication.
27. Swezey RL: Arthritis: Rational Therapy and Rehabilitation. Philadelphia, WB Saunders, 1978.
28. Levey GS, Calabro JJ: Tietze's syndrome: Report of two cases and review of the literature. Arthritis Rheum 5:261–269, 1962.
29. Cameron HU, Fornasier VL: Tietze's disease. J Clin Pathol 27:960–962, 1974.
30. Bradford DS, Moe JH, Winter RB: Kyphosis and postural roundback deformity in children and adolescents. Minn Med 56:114–120, 1973.
31. Benson DR: The back: Thoracic and lumbar spine. In Musculoskeletal Disorders. Edited by RD D'Ambrosia. Philadelphia, JB Lippincott, 1977.
32. Bradford DS, Moe JH: Scheuermann's juvenile kyphosis. Clin Orthop 110:45–53, 1975.
33. Winter RB, Hall JE: Kyphosis in childhood and adolescence. Spine 3:285–308, 1978.
34. Turek SL: Orthopaedics: Principles and Their Applications. Philadelphia, JB Lippincott, 1977.
35. Hilton RC, Ball J, Benn RT: Vertebral end-plate lesions (Schmorl's nodes) in the dorsolumbar spine. Ann Rheum Dis 35:127–132, 1976.
36. Levine DB: The painful low back. In Arthritis and Allied Conditions. Edited by DJ McCarty. Philadelphia, Lea & Febiger, 1979.
37. Krook, L, Whalen JP, Lesser GV, Berens DL: Experimental studies on osteoporosis. Methods Achiev Exp Pathol 7:72–108, 1975.
38. Howell DS: Metabolic bone diseases. In Arthritis and Allied Conditions. Edited by DJ McCarty. Philadelphia, Lea & Febiger, 1979.
39. Khairi MR, Johnston CC: What we know—and don't know—about bone loss in the elderly. Geriatrics 33:67–76, 1978.
40. Aaron JE, Gallagher JC, Anderson J, et al: Frequency of osteomalacia and osteoporosis in fractures of the proximal femur. Lancet 1:229–233, 1974.
41. Raisz LG: Clinical strategy in osteopenia. Hosp Pract 13:11–12, 1978.

42. Mundy GR: Differential diagnosis of osteopenia. Hosp Pract 13:65–72, 1978.
43. Avioli LV: What to do with "post-menopausal osteoporosis"? Am J Med 65:881–883, 1978.
44. Avioli LV: Management of osteomalacia. Hosp Pract 14:109–114, 1979.
45. Aloia JF, Cohn SH, Ostuni JA et al: Prevention of involutional bone loss by exercise. Ann Intern Med 89:356–358, 1978.
46. Finneson BE: Low Back Pain. Philadelphia, JB Lippincott, 1973.
47. Jowsey J, Riggs BL, Kelly PJ, Hoffman DL: Effect of combined therapy with sodium fluoride, vitamin D and calcium in osteoporosis. Am J Med 53:43–49, 1972.
48. Newcomer AD, Hodgson SF, McGill DB, Thomas PJ: Lactase deficiency: Prevalence in osteoporosis. Ann Intern Med 89:218–220, 1978.
49. Marx SJ: Restraint in use of high-dose fluorides to treat skeletal disorders. JAMA 240:1630–1631, 1978.
50. Wallach S: Management of osteoporosis. Hosp Pract 13:91–98, 1978.
51. Hahn BH, Hahn TT: Reduction of steroid osteopenia by treatment with 25 OH vitamin D and calcium. Abstract presented to Fortieth Annual Meeting Am Rheum Assoc, Chicago, 1976.
52. Love JG, Schorn VG: Thoracic-disk protrusions. JAMA 191:627–631, 1965.
53. Ransohoff J, Spencer F, Siew F, and Gage L: Transthoracic disc protrusions causing spinal cord compression. Neurosurgery 31:459–461, 1969.
54. Perot P, Munro DD: Transthoracic removal of midline thoracic disc protrusions causing spinal cord compression. Neurosurgery 31:452–458, 1969.

Chapter 7

THE LOW BACK AND PELVIS

Ever since man assumed upright posture, back pain has been an accompaniment of life. Low back pain is the most perplexing and most frequent orthopedic problem of man,[1] and is the most poorly understood. Fahrni goes so far as to suggest that "good posture" is a major cause of disc disease.[2] He prefers the Oriental stooping position and he is supported by the fact that degenerative disc disease is seen in a smaller percentage of Oriental skeletons compared to Northern European skeletons. Although degenerative joint disease may be detected within the articulations of the low back, fibrofatty nodules may be palpated in the presacral soft tissues, or a "classic sciatica" history may be obtained, no assumption can be made between these features and the cause of pain in a particular patient.[3] Sciatica is a symptom and not a disease.[1] It may result from herniation of the nucleus pulposus (ruptured disc), from extrinsic problems in the pelvis or thigh such as an entrapment neuropathy, or from a myofascial pain syndrome.[4,5] Often multiple etiologic factors are operating in an individual patient. Secondary gain, misuse injury at work or at home, or psychologic factors may predispose toward chronicity. Three times as many workdays are lost due to back pain than the number of workdays lost due to strikes![6]

Back pain is most often the result of a regional disease of the low back,[7] but may occur as part of a systemic disease. Consider systemic disease if the patient is in an older age group, has worse symptoms while lying down, has fever or other systemic complaints, or has pain localized to a point more lateral than the usual location of the myofascial trigger points.[7] A history of early morning back stiffness of gradual onset and physical findings of limitation of spinal movement in a young man would suggest inflammatory spinal disorders.[8]

135

Table 7–1. Danger Signals in Back Pain

Bladder or bowel dysfunction or impotence
Weakness of ankle dorsiflexion
Ankle clonus
Color change in the extremity
Considerable night pain
Constant and progressive symptomatology

Is the complaint of back pain a surgical emergency? Six findings that signify danger are listed in Table 7–1.

These signals should alert the clinician to consider urgent surgical consultation for such emergencies as intraspinal bleeding, infection, tumor, or massive disc herniation.[7]

Most patients have acute or subacute soft tissue injury as the predominant etiology of their back pain. The best diagnostic test may be injection of a myofascial trigger point with a local anesthetic-corticosteroid injection as a test as well as a treatment. Rapid relief of pain by this method is often more revealing than is a roentgenogram of the back.

PATHOPHYSIOLOGY OF LOW BACK PAIN

The spinal unit consists of a three-joint complex comprised of two posterior apophyseal joint articulations and the vertebral body with interposed disc.[9,10] Pathologic changes may be due to apophyseal joint synovitis or degeneration, injury or degenerative changes within the articular disc, apophyseal joint laxity, or traumatic subluxation. The result is entrapment of the nerve root as it exits through this complex. Also, stenosis of the spinal canal or additional new instability of articulating units above or below the level of involvement are also causative. Chronic low back pain resulting from these structural changes include the posterior joint syndrome (the facet syndrome), the classic herniated nucleus pulposus (ruptured disc) syndrome, and spinal stenosis.[3,9,10] "Lumbosacral strain" in many instances is misused as a wastebasket term.[3]

In 1933 Ghormley emphasized the importance of abnormalities of the posterior facet joint (zygapophyseal joint) as a cause for back pain.[10] The posterior facet joints are innervated by the posterior rami of two spinal nerve levels. Proof that these joints were capable of causing symptoms resulted from studies in which instillation of hypertonic saline into a facet joint produced low back pain, pain radiating into the trochanteric area, and pain radiating down the posterolateral thigh. Furthermore, a local anesthetic injection of the facet joint restored normality.[10]

The introduction of pressure transducers into the nucleus pulposus of humans while assuming various positions and tasks revealed complex forces occurring in the human spine.[11] Pressure in the third lumbar disc was investigated in these experiments. Measurements while the person was standing were used as a standard and the intradiscal load in other body positions was compared. Sitting increased the load by 30%, walking by 15%, coughing by 50%, jumping by 50%, bending 20 degrees forward by 85%, lifting a 20-kg weight with the knees bent by 300%, and lifting a 20-kg load with the knees straight by 500%.[12] Sitting with a backrest inclined greater than 90 degrees reduced the load on the lumbar L-3 disc by 10 to 20%.[13] Lumbar disc pressure also correlated positively to body weight.[11]

The role of abdominal and chest musculature in back support was investigated using an inflatable corset and a measuring balloon placed within the stomach. This demonstrated that 30 to 50% of lumbar disc and thoracic disc pressures could be reduced by tightening abdominal and chest muscles while performing various activities and assuming different positions.[14-16] The abdominal muscles minimize torquing and bending, and shearing stresses in the lumbar spine, thus protecting the lumbar spine.[15] Improper lifting (back bent—legs straight) can result in generating 1000 to 2000 lbs/in.^{2} of intradisc pressure. If the annulus of the lumbar disc has been previously injured the disc can rupture at 700 lbs/in.^{2}.[16] The thoracolumbar trunk may be considered a hollow chamber. If the pressure of this chamber is increased by compression of abdominal musculature, the cylinder can withstand greater stress. These studies must be considered in outlining treatment for low back pain.

Howes and Isdale examined 102 patients with backache for hypermobility.[17] Measurement included determination of spinal rotation, flexion and extension utilizing the length of the spine during these various maneuvers. In the study, 19 patients, all females, were found to be hypermobile, and only 2 of these 19 had another cause for back pain. Hypermobility as a cause of limb pain has been discussed elsewhere in this book. Whether hypermobility is a significant cause for backache requires further study.

Low back pain may bear a relationship to the lumbosacral lordotic angle (normal = 120 degrees).[1] Because a mobile spine is adjoined to the fixed sacrum, lumbosacral region strain may occur following sudden body movements. This strain occurs commonly in the female with increased lumbar lordosis, in whom L-5–S-1 disc-space narrowing is often seen. However, in other reports, pelvic lateral tilt, scoliosis, kyphosis, and lumbar lordosis did not correlate with the presence of back pain.[7] Disc degeneration, as evidenced by discography, also correlated poorly with low back pain. Rather, pain probably results only if the vertebral end plate is also fractured.[18] Although the pain appears to originate in the spinal musculature, more likely the pain is referred from ligaments or articular structures.[6] Nevertheless, once muscle spasm occurs, a complex pain-spasm-pain cycle may evolve[19] (see Chapt. 13).

Industrial physicians recognize that pre-employment radiographic examination and history are not reliable predictors of work capability. Snook et al.[20,21] developed a psychophysical method for determining ideal weights and workloads for men and women. They established a workload acceptable to the worker, based on strength and psyche. Chaffin et al.[22,23] used a rating scale for each job by measuring the workload, the distance lifted from the floor, and the distance forward from the front ankle. They also used an isometric lifting test. By rating the jobs to the strength of the individual workers, a determination was made about whether the person and the job were matched. These investigators found that three times more back injury occurred when the strength of the individual did not match the job performance, *or* if the individual had far more capability than the job required. Back pain occurred in laborers as well as in sedentary workers.

The Pain Syndromes

Because we know so little about the causes of back pain in man, we become biased in our terminology and description of the pain problems we see. In previous decades, degenerative disc disease involving the annulus fibrosus was considered the ultimate cause for most back pain. Later, herniation of the nucleus pulposus gained prominence. Today, pain of myofascial origin is considered a leading cause for back pain. The syndromes described in this chapter are presented as if they occur individually. More often, they are superimposed on other back disorders. At onset of back pain, the features may first appear to represent mechanical low back pain; later, sciatica may become evident; and finally a chronic pain state with a remarkable limitation of spinal motion may result. Thus the syndrome presentation may change with time. However, most patients with back pain have self-limited problems that the clinician can readily assist. Aggravating factors are well recognized and can be changed. Thus, the physician has an obligation not only to relieve pain, but also to prevent recurrences by providing education in back care.

Mechanical Low Back Pain

Back pain resulting from a mechanical cause should be suspected when pain is related to posture, minor trauma, or excessive use.[6] Mechanical low back pain is episodic or intermittent and is aggravated by those actions that demand more from the supporting back structures; this pain is relieved by rest and recumbency. Most patients with this type of back pain are involved in handling and lifting tasks.[24]

Often, patients with mechanical backache will describe previous "catches"—attacks that immobilize the patient in a slightly bent forward position. Such attacks are generally self-limited, last for about 4 days, and are thought to arise in the posterior articulations. Signs accompanying the pain include unilateral muscle spasm and a spinal "list" in which the patient is pulled slightly to one side. However, a list also suggests herniation of a nucleus pulposus. Flattening of the lumbar spine is similar to that seen in ankylosing spondylitis. Limb strength and reflexes remain normal.[6]

Other patients present with extremely variable symptoms, best described as a dull ache in the low back, aggravated by activity and improved with rest.[25] These patients suffer subacute episodes of worsening with radiation to one or both thighs. "Lumbosacral strain,"[1,3] "the posterior joint syndrome," or "the facet syndrome"[10] have no distinguishing features that differ from the symptoms and signs already mentioned. However, these terms do serve to point out the importance of the posterior joints, the lumbosacral ligaments, and other deep structures in the development of low back pain and spasm.

Physical examination reveals variable degrees of tenderness of the low back musculature and tightness of the hamstrings and sacrospinalis muscles (observed during straight leg raising and forward bending maneuvers). Neurologic examination is normal.

Mechanical low back pain may occur in middle age as an acute self-limited process with frequent recurrences, only to disappear in late age, or it may progress to the totally invalid "low back loser."[26] Acute low back pain accounts for approximately 2% of all office visits to physicians, with the sexes equally involved.[27] The acute painful self-limited low back attack must not be dismissed with only symptomatic care. Such attacks may be considered as "mechanical backache" when a posture or related strain is thought to be the cause.[6] The physician is then obligated to consider the patient's work position and tasks that can cause recurrences. Other conditions that may predispose to recurrent mechanical low back strain include faulty posture, structural disturbances such as spondylolisthesis and disc degeneration, all of which can be helped.[25] Specific strains or injuries are documented in only 20% of low back pain patients, and in 80%, no evident cause is elicited on careful history.[27] The presence of nerve root irritation (sciatica) bears no relation to outcome. Of ambulatory care for acute low back pain, 90% is satisfactory for pain relief, yet almost half the patients have recurrences within 4 years. No significant differences in outcome were noted in relation to sex or age.[27]

In summary, mechanical low back pain often results from a breakdown in the supporting soft tissue structures, abnormalities of the posterior apophyseal joints, or injury to spinal ligaments that assist in the maintenance of the upright spinal position. This may result from postural deficits, improper work habits, or a job or task inappropriate to the muscular control of the individual.[24] The clinical features include intermittent, subacute, or acute episodes of pain with limitation of spinal motion, sometimes related to a recent specific injurious task; physical signs include limitation of spinal motion, or listing and tightness of the hamstring and sacrospinal muscles (management is discussed later in this chapter).

Sciatica and Other Nerve Entrapment Syndromes

Sciatica, as previously mentioned, is a symptom complex that occurs as a result of many entities afflicting the low back.[4] The symptoms include pain and neuritic features such as numbness, tingling, and burning. The neuritic manifestations often occur at a location distant from the area of pain. Any activity that increases intra-abdominal or intrathoracic pressure, such as lifting, pushing, bending forward, coughing, sneezing, or the act of defecating may aggravate sciatica. This history should alert the clinician to consider an intraspinal cause. Sciatica is also aggravated during motion that hyperextends the spine. These motions generally do not aggravate the sciatica-like pain accompanying primary myofascial disease. Symptoms of sciatica that occur spontaneously during sleep strongly suggest an intraspinal pathology, such as tumor or infection. In most cases, the symptom of sciatica is an intermittent aggravation and often is layered upon chronic persistent back pain.

Herniation of the nucleus pulposus (ruptured disc) may result in pain in either the back or leg alone, or in both the back and leg, whereas sciatica that results from entrapment neuropathy often spares the back. Sciatica accompanied by pain in the anterior groin and hip suggests herniation of an L-4–5 nucleus pulposus. Patients with proven nucleus pulposus herniation usually have had episodic back pain preceding rupture. The back pain may improve when sciatica develops.[3] The intermittency of symptoms contrasts with the more chronic pain experienced by patients with intraspinal tumors. Non-disc causes of sciatica (see Table 7–2) should be suspected when physical examination has failed to demonstrate positive signs of spinal disease (reflex change, motor weakness) or if the sciatica is unrelated to activities that increase intra-abdominal or intrathoracic pressure (lifting, pushing, bending), or movements that hyperextend the spine.

Entrapment neuropathy of the sciatic nerve may occur from direct injury when sitting on a hard surface or horseback riding, with pressure occurring just below the gluteal border where the sciatic nerve lies superficially.[28] Similarly, sciatica-like pain (pseudoradiculopathy) can accompany trochanteric bursitis and other myofascial pain disorders of the pelvis. Relief may follow injection of the involved soft tissue lesion with an anesthetic-corticosteroid combination.[5,29]

Table 7–2.   Non-Disc Causes of Sciatica[3]

A. Entrapment Neuritis
  1. Obturator neuritis
    a. obturator hernia
    b. osteitis pubis
  2. Meralgia paresthetica
    a. arthritis
    b. psoas abscess
    c. traction injury
    d. obesity
    e. external pressure
  3. Lumbar spinal stenosis
  4. Spinal degenerative joint disease
  5. Ankylosing spondylitis
  6. Sacral cysts and tumors

B. Trauma
  1. Iatrogenic injections
  2. Contusion

C. Sciatic Neuritis (rare)

A rare cause of sciatica is spasm of the piriformis muscle. The piriformis muscle fills the greater sciatic foramen.[30] Pain in the buttock and point tenderness in the sciatic notch, as well as during rectal examination, strongly suggest a piriformis myofascial trigger point with secondary sciatica.[31,32] Spinal stenosis can cause piriformis spasm. When associated with spinal stenosis, symptoms are bilateral, whereas in the piriformis syndrome alone, the symptoms are unilateral. The examiner can test for this syndrome by placing his hands on the lateral aspect of the seated patient's knees, while the patient attempts to push his knees apart against the examiner's resistance. Pain and weakness of effort suggest the piriformis syndrome. Rectal palpation may disclose exquisite tenderness within the piriformis muscle in the lateral rectal wall. A local anesthetic-corticosteroid injection, carried out through the buttock over the sciatic notch, may provide relief.[31]

The sciatic nerve may rarely become trapped in the posterior thigh region with symptoms of numbness in the posterior leg, calf, and lateral foot. Pain may be noted in the posterior thigh. Entrapment is due to nerve constriction by a myofascial band running across the posterior aspect of the nerve. Electrodiagnostic testing usually establishes the zone of constriction.[33] Surgery to release the constriction is required for relief.

Another form of neurovascular entrapment is related to spinal stenosis. Stenosis may result from degenerative changes of the spine or from any cause that narrows the spinal canal (e.g., developmental and dysplastic disorders, spondylolisthesis, Paget's disease, fluorosis, and postoperative bone hypertrophy).[25,33-38] Characteristic symptoms include nerve root irritation and vascular embarrassment. Walking results in buttock pain or ache, paresthesia and loss of coordination of the lower limbs. Relief occurs after sitting, but is often followed by numbness and tingling in both lower extremities. Symptomatology may range from intermittent claudication to symptoms that mimic a herniated nucleus pulposus. Night pain occurs in the upper thigh regions. Symptoms are intermittent at first, but frequently become progressive until the patient is required to become sedentary. The patient sometimes discovers relief by bending forward, such as by leaning across a table. Physical examination reveals flattening of the lumbar curve; however, tests for nerve root irritation (straight leg raising, examination for reflexes, and determination of sensation) are often normal.[39] The back is often flexed during walking. Hyperextension of the spine during physical examination aggravates the pain and may suggest the disorder. Spinal stenosis commonly involves males from the fourth through the sixth decade of life.

Myofascial soft tissue rheumatic disorders may cause similar symptoms and should be excluded by a thorough therapeutic trial of trigger point injections and physical therapy, posture correction, and elimination of any other aggravating factors. Myelography and computed tomography are utilized in diagnosis. The risks of surgical intervention and subsequent long-term complications demand careful consideration and exclusion of all other treatable disorders before labeling a patient with the diagnosis of spinal stenosis.[9,37,40,47]

Myofascial Back Pain

Variously called fibrositis of the low back, tension myositis, or the "low back syndrome," this condition may occur as the sole cause of a painful low back or may be layered upon other disease of the low back. Myofascial back pain may involve the gluteal fascia, the iliocostalis, sacrospinalis, and other muscles, or an interspinous bursa[42] (Fig. 7-1). Pain is a constant dull aching that waxes and wanes; it is worse with working, chilling, and sitting, yet is improved with heat, walking, and bedrest. The condition may be acute or chronic, and may not have physical characteristics of spasm, listing, or limping.[1] Nevertheless, these disorders affect up to 80% of patients who come to the general practitioner with acute low back pain and in whom no other cause is evident.[27,43]

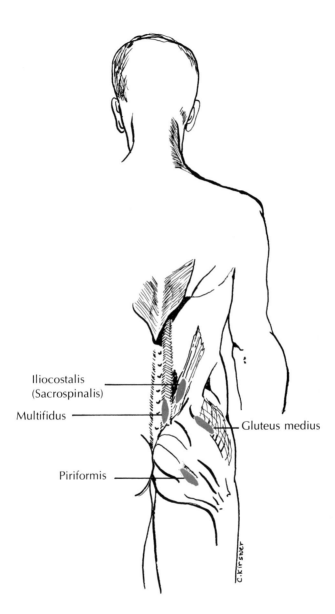

Iliocostalis
(Sacrospinalis)

Multifidus

Gluteus medius

Piriformis

Fig. 7–1. Myofascial trigger points of the low back region: Trigger points arising in the erector muscles, the gluteal fascia and the presacral fascia are common in patients with low back pain.

The subacute and chronic myofascial pain syndromes occur in the third to fifth decade of life and are rarely preceded by a single definitive injury. Repeated minor trauma of sedentary living, misuse strain,[44] or a chronic pain-spasm-pain cycle[19] are probably operational. The myofascial pain disorders certainly may be layered upon degenerative disc disease or apophyseal joint disease and may be synonymous with the "facet syndrome." By definition, these regional low back pain syndromes have a myofascial trigger point, which when palpated reproduce or accentuate the patient's pain. Episacroiliac fibrofatty nodules (lipomas) may co-exist. True sciatica is rare; if the pain has radiated to a leg, palpation of the myofascial trigger point reproduces the pain radiation. The most common sites of involvement are the origin of the sacrospinalis overlying the sacrum (multifidus triangle), the origin of the gluteus maximus adjacent to the posterior superior iliac spine, over the sacroiliac joints particularly beneath an episacroiliac nodule, or bilaterally at the origin of the gluteal fascia.[1] The patient may adopt a protective attitude of flexion during the 3 or 4 days of increased pain and spasm.[25]

The episacroiliac lipomas, as described by Ries,[45] are common soft fleshy nodules occurring over the sacroiliac joints at the insertion of the erector spinal muscles[46] (Fig. 7–2). In one study, these lipomas were found in 16% of a "normal" population (1000 persons), and of these, only 10% had back pain.[45] Their relation to pain is uncertain, although they are found in the vicinity of local pain and tenderness.[46,47] Injecting the tender lipomas and adjacent tissues with procaine and corticosteroid often provides prompt pain relief.

Psychogenic Back Pain

Psychogenic back pain and true malingering are rare, occurring in less than 2% of patients presenting with low back pain.[7] In these instances the patient's history is vague, and the patient often places emphasis on blaming others for her plight.[1] The term "compensation neurosis" is a rather ambiguous term, yet these patients often continue disabled after their claims for financial gain are settled.[1] The real question is how much are the symptoms related to anatomic disease and how much is psychologic. In such circumstances the physician must rule out organic diseases as quickly as possible, set goals for the patient, and obtain the help of a psychologist.

The patient called a "low back loser" by Sternbach[26] has the following characteristics: a history of previous physical labor and poor education; false denial of depression with a history of loss of appetite, decreased libido, poor sleep patterns, and test results two or more standard deviations above the normal mean on depression scales of the MMPI (Minnesota Multiphasic Psychologic Inventory Assessment); and a life style of invalidism. The patient perceives herself

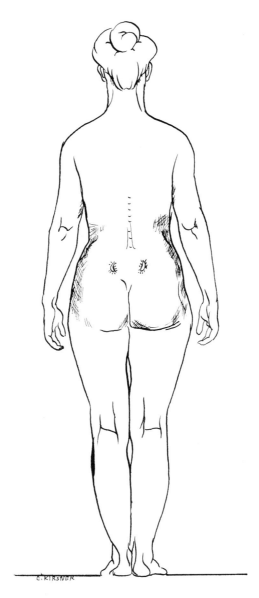

Fig. 7–2. Episacroiliac lipomas: These fleshy fibrofatty nodules commonly occur over the sacroiliac joints at the insertion of the erector muscles.

more ill than rheumatoid arthritis patients on the Cornell Medical Index scale. These patients are home-bound and their illness perception is as hard to break as chronic alcoholism. During history taking, these patients are likely to "play games" with the clinician and frustrate the diagnostic evaluation. Psychologic assessment of patients begins with the first physician encounter, which should include the patient's social, occupational, and marital history.

The psychodynamics of chronic back pain have received considerable investigation. Prospective studies have revealed no relation between a psychologic profile and future outcome or disability.[48] Positive answers to two questions at the outset of a treatment program are good predictors of a bad outcome: (1) "Has your appetite decreased recently?" or (2) "Has your sexual interest diminished?"[49] Although the MMPI has not been a reliable predictor of the results of surgery, the MMPI may be a useful warning device in undertaking treatment of patients with chronic back pain.[49,50]

MacNab described the "racehorse syndrome," which applied to tense, hard-working, hyper-reactive persons who tend to hyperextend their spines, and the "razor's edge syndrome," which signified persons on the razor's edge of emotional stability who present outlandish appearances and complaints.[51] Persons suffering from anxiety may confuse "hurting" with "harming."[51] Careful examination, followed by reassurance, is necessary for care.

HISTORY AND PHYSICAL EXAMINATION

In taking a history of a patient with low back pain the clinician must consider the age of the patient, history of previous back pain, aggravating factors in home or job performance, the presence of litigation or other secondary gain factors, and the general demeanor of the patient.[50] Pain localization is important, as is the distance and direction of the pain radiation. The pain history is often better evidence for localization than is sensory nerve testing.[50] The clinician should elicit which activities reproduce the pain, which aggravate the pain, and which alleviate the pain. Has there been a decrease in the level of work activity to a more sedentary life, with resultant loss of muscle tone?

The symptom of stiffness should be considered separately from pain. Stiffness that begins insidiously and occurs during the night or early morning hours may suggest inflammatory diseases of the spine (e.g., ankylosing spondylitis).[8] A history of aching, numbness, and tingling radiating posteriorly or posterolaterally into the lower extremity below the knee (sciatica), or pain and burning that radiate anteriorly into the groin or anterior hip region, is often present in herniated disc disease. Aggravation by coughing, sneezing, or straining at defecation also suggests intraspinal disease. Certain symptoms may suggest a diagnosis or location of disease origin: night pain is often a result of intraspinal tumors or disease within abdominal or retroperitoneal structures; chills or fever suggest septic causes of back pain; changes in bowel and sexual function or urination suggest lesions of the cauda equina; and claudication followed by numbness and tingling suggests spinal stenosis. Spinal stenosis often causes the patient to stop walking because of aching in the buttock and calf regions; then upon resting, numbness and tingling may occur in one or both lower extremities. Relief in these patients may occur with bending forward, such as leaning over a table.[41]

Physical examination begins with observation of the appearance of the patient while sitting, rising, standing, walking, and bending. Observing the patient undressing can be helpful. Structural abnormalities can only be demonstrated with the patient completely disrobed. Pes planus should be noted. Mobility can be observed as the patient bends over. Can the patient touch the palms to the floor with legs straight? This is an important clue to hypermobility. Scoliosis, when evident, should be described as occurring to the right or left, depending on the convexity direction of the curve.[25] Using a tape measure the examiner measures the chest circumference at the breast line, after expiration and again after inspiration. A difference of two or more inches is normal.[52] Restriction of chest expanse may suggest ankylosing spondylitis or other inflammatory disease of the spine or rib cage. The spinal curvatures are examined with forward flexion, extension, and lateral flexion (Fig. 7–3). The examiner notes rigidity, spasm, pain, or listing of the body to one side. Symmetric loss of spinal motion may occur in degenerative disease of the posterior joints and ankylosing spondylitis, whereas asymmetric loss of movement suggests disc disease; this is not a hard-and-fast rule.[6,25] With the patient bent over a table, myofascial trigger points are palpated, and pain reproduction is sought[53] (Fig. 7–4).

While the patient is bent over the examining table with knees flexed, firm percussion in the center and to each side of the lumbar vertebrae may reproduce sciatica[25] (Fig. 7–5). In our experience, a positive percussion test is as good an indicator of lumbar disc disease as a positive straight-leg-raising maneuver (Fig. 7–6) or a reflex change. Tenderness in the sciatic notch in patients with sciatica is often due to herniated nucleus pulposus (ruptured disc), but may also occur in the piriformis or other myofascial syndromes.

While the patient is supine on the examining table (lying on his back), the examination continues with careful palpation of the abdomen. Auscultation for bruits over the abdominal, iliac, and femoral vessels is performed. Examination of range of hip movement, and straight-leg-raising (Lasègue's sign), with comparison of the opposite side, is carried out (Fig. 7–6). Most commonly, straight-leg-raising is

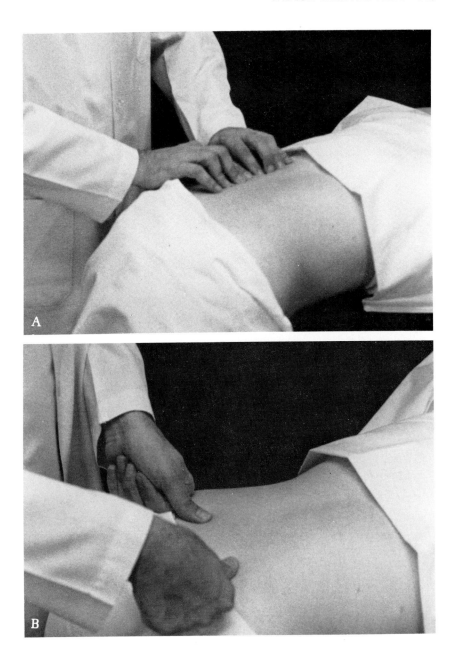

Fig. 7–4. Physical examination for myofascial trigger points is best performed with the patient lying across an examining table with knees bent. This relaxes the hamstrings and allows careful palpation for the tendon trigger points that reproduce the pain: A, erector muscles, and, B, presacral fascia, gluteal fascia, and episacroiliac nodules.

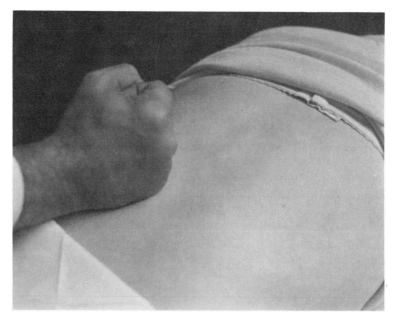

Fig. 7–5. Firm spinal percussion should be performed over each vertebra in the midline and to the symptomatic side as well as the side opposite. A positive test occurs with pain reproduction in the symptomatic hip or limb. A positive test is highly suggestive of herniated nucleus pulposus (ruptured disc).

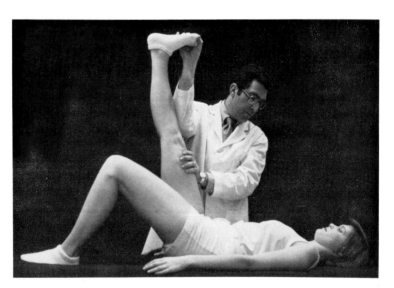

Fig. 7–6. The straight-leg-raising maneuver (Lasègue's sign): After gradually raising the straight leg to the maximum tolerated position, the foot is then drawn to a 90 degree angle. Paresthesias are accentuated if the sciatic nerve has been irritated. Tightness of the hamstrings may result in a false position straight-leg-raising maneuver.

limited by tightness of the hamstring muscles rather than by sciatic nerve irritation, and is poorly correlated with the presence or absence of herniated disc disease. Shortening of the hamstring muscle itself is a frequent cause of low back pain.[1]

The classic features of herniated nucleus pulposus with sciatica are pain in the buttock, characterized by aching, and nonburning pain radiating into the posterior thigh and calf, or into the posterolateral thigh and lateral foreleg. Paresthesia may be noted all the way to the heel, or within a zone of the lateral foreleg. The pain distribution rarely extends down the entire nerve trunk, but when the S-1 nerve root is compressed, the pain often radiates into the posterior gluteal fold and down the posterior thigh into the calf and heel. Maneuvers that stretch the nerve trunk include straight-leg-raising (Lasègue's sign), and the reversed straight-leg-raising test.[6] The straight-leg-raising test is usually performed with the patient lying flat on his back with the uninvolved knee bent 45 degrees, and that foot resting on the table. The involved leg is raised straight up, while the ankle is kept at 90 degrees of flexion (Fig. 7–6). Generally, if hamstrings are not tight, straight-leg-raising can reach 90 degrees of upright vertical position.[41] When this test is positive, pain and tingling are reproduced; this test is nonspecific, and any type of irritation of the sciatic nerve may cause a positive result. Dorsiflexion of the foot increases the pain during the straight-leg-raising maneuver. Reversed straight-leg-raising is performed while the patient is lying on his stomach with his legs raised backwards, one at a time. Pain over the involved nerve root may be reproduced regardless of which leg is posteriorly raised.[41]

Range of hip movement should always be performed to exclude muscle spasm referred from intrinsic hip disease (Fig. 8–1). Special maneuvers to increase intraspinal pressure, using jugular compression (Naffziger's test), may prove useful in some patients. Sensory deficits to pinprick testing may not be as valuable as the patient's description of pain pattern and radiation. When the L-5 nerve root is compressed, pain radiates into the posterolateral hip, and numbness and tingling may be noted in a lateral zone of the foreleg.[50] Impingement of the L-3–4 nerve roots is associated with depression of the knee jerk; impingement of the first sacral nerve root is associated with depression of the ankle jerk, and impingement of the L-5 nerve root may be associated with depression of the posterior tibial tendon reflex.[25] The pain is often complicated by reflex muscle spasm, which results in pain during rest and flattening of the lumbar spine. Trigger points may be present, and atrophy is usually not evident. The physical examination is not complete until strength has been determined in the lower extremities. Gait abnormalities should be noted. Inability of the patient to walk on her toes and heels provides evidence of weakness in the gastrocnemius or tibialis anterior muscle groups, respectively.

Foot and toe dorsiflexion testing against the examiner's resistance picks up more subtle weakness of involved muscle groups. Limb length measurement should be performed. Rectal and pelvic examinations are carried out to complete the examination.

A careful history and physical examination may suggest more than one condition causing low back pain; however, in most cases only one condition predominates. Often myofascial trigger points with accompanying muscle spasm are aggravating degenerative disease of apophyseal joints or other structural disorders.

Laboratory and Radiographic Examination

Tests of inflammation, particularly erythrocyte sedimentation rate, should be utilized to aid in excluding underlying tumor or inflammation, such as ankylosing spondylitis or diverticulitis. Urinalysis, blood counts, serum acid and alkaline phosphatase, serum protein electrophoresis, HLA B27 determination, and other tests should be performed as appropriate.

Exclusion of tumor, sepsis, effects of trauma, or congenital abnormalities are some reasons for performing radiographic examination of the spine. Radiographic examination of the lumbar spine for basic assessment should include anteroposterior (AP) and lateral views of the lumbosacral spine, and a true AP view of the pelvis. Additional views that may be helpful in certain circumstances include sacroiliac joint films, and left and right oblique views of the spine. Spurs and other evidence of degenerative changes of the articular structures are so prevalent[54,55] that the clinician should interpret the relationship of radiologic findings to symptoms with caution.[7]

Osteoarthritis with marginal vertebral and apophyseal joint spurs is likely to be significant if the neuroforamina are encroached upon. Osteoarthritis, if severe, does result in limitation of spinal motion.[1] Most patients with proved herniation of the nucleus pulposus have normal roentgenograms.[1] Congenital deformities of the low lumbar and lumbosacral spinal areas are seen in up to 30% of radiographic surveys.[1] Changes in the neural arch, abnormality of the transverse process of the fifth lumbar vertebra, with or without sacralization, or a spina bifida occulta often are unrelated to symptoms.[13] Rarely, after trauma, symptoms may occur in relation to such structural changes in younger individuals. Roentgenographic examination may also reveal squaring of the vertebral bodies, erosion, sclerosis characteristic of ankylosing spondylitis, and other spondyloarthritides.[6] Spinal roentgenographic examination reveals the occasional abscess, with soft tissue swelling adjacent to an involved disc and its adjacent vertebra. Specialized radiographic techniques include tomograms and computed tomography for determining the size of the spinal canal and for identifying tumors. Less expensive techniques include routine and pulsed-echo ultrasound, if available.[56]

An exciting new factor in consideration of back disability is the determination of HLA B27. This test should be considered for patients under age 40 with spinal distress that has an insidious onset, a duration greater than three months, is accompanied by morning stiffness, and is improved with exercise.[8] In such individuals, particularly in the absence of radiographic abnormalities, a B27 determination may support a working diagnosis of spondyloarthritis.[7] A chemical battery of tests should be obtained in patients with persistent back pain and disability. Cushing's syndrome, Paget's disease, tumor, hematologic disorders with marrow encroachment, and osteomalacia are some of the systemic disorders that chemical and blood count determinations might reveal. A urinalysis should be part of the back examination. A Westergren sedimentation rate is an inexpensive and excellent screening test for the presence of tumors, infection, and inflammatory diseases of the spine.

An EMG may be falsely normal if performed too early after onset of symptoms. This test cannot detect nerve compression until demyelination has occurred. Later it may help confirm nerve root compression. Electromyography and nerve conduction studies may be helpful in patients with atypical sciatica, nerve root entrapment syndromes, peripheral neuropathy, and herniated nucleus pulposus. If danger signals of spinal cord compression are present, do not wait for an electrodiagnostic determination; get surgical consultation promptly. Elective contrast myelography is reserved for patients with atypical pain, or for localization of the site of pathology, preceding operative intervention. Discography is still a controversial diagnostic procedure.[3]

Most patients have acute or subacute soft tissue injury as the predominant etiology of their back pain. The *best test* may be injecting a myofascial trigger point with a local anesthetic-corticosteroid, as a test as well as a treatment. Rapid relief of pain by this method may be more revealing than a roentgenogram of the back.

Differential Diagnosis

In addition to what we have discussed, the following points are stressed again. Systemic infections cause few local findings on back examination, and local tenderness is rarely significant. Weight loss, fever, and elevation of the erythrocyte sedimentation rate should raise suspicion for an infectious origin of low back pain. Fractures, congenital spinal deformities, spondylolysis, spondylolisthesis, the spondylarthritides, Paget's disease, osteitis condensans ilii, osteoporosis, osteomalacia, tumors, and infections are disorders that are suggested by clinical and radiographic examination. Intraspinal neoplasms, including ependymoma, neurofibroma, or metastatic tumors, usually cause constant pain without relief when the patient is recumbent. Benign bone tumors, such as giant cell tumors, hemangioma, and osteoma, are rare. Don't forget herpes zoster as a cause for unilateral back pain. Back pain may be referred from the hip, and physical examination should detect the limitation of hip motion. Hip pain often limits the patient's ability to cross the leg while putting on a stocking.[25,57]

Many disorders can cause *referred pain* in the back. Peptic ulcer disease produces pain localized near the midline of the lower thoracic region, kidney disease causes flank pain with radiation into the groin, and neurofibromatosis (with café-au-lait spots) may cause sciatica-like pain that radiates into the legs.[41] Pelvic disease and aortic aneurysms may first cause low back pain. Renal colic (stone) often refers pain into the testicle, in addition to producing back distress. Retroperitoneal fibrosis may raise the erythrocyte sedimentation rate, and prostatitis or pyelonephritis may cause a dull persistent ill-defined back pain.

Management

Treatment for back pain varies with acuteness, mode of onset, duration, and etiology. The earlier a comprehensive evaluation and treatment are introduced, the greater the likelihood that the individual can return to an improved state of function, regardless of the site or severity of injury.[58] Spontaneous improvement occurs in many back disorders. Conversely, psychogenic and compensation factors are known to prolong disability. Psychopathology may be more complex in the back-injured individual than in the extremity-injured individual, yet even in these persons, the outcome tends not to be influenced by the psychopathology.

Aggravating factors that may cause recurrences should be sought. Beals suggests that we inquire whether the patient has a fear of returning to a former job, or has vocational dissatisfaction for any reason.[58] Other recognizable aggravating factors to be determined include lifting, stooping, bending, prolonged sitting, stair climbing, use of high-heeled shoes, and strains resulting from occupational sources or new hobbies.[3] Nachemson has stressed consideration for the strain involved in lifting with the knees straight instead of flexed, and the back flexed instead of straight.[13] (In nearly all cases of gluteal fasciitis a history of lifting with straight knees can be obtained.)

Proper sitting and sleeping positions should be provided. Keegan has performed a roentgenographic study for the determination of proper posture and sitting.[59] No sitting position was found to achieve vertebral alignment comparable to erect standing. However, the best results that could be obtained occurred when the trunk-thigh angle was 105 degrees or greater. Thus, the upright portion of the chair should be tilted slightly backward from the vertical position, the seat should be convex, and support for the lumbar region should be present across the back of the chair. Sitting forward or backward from this position increases lumbar flexion and thereby increases lumbar disc compression. The height of the chair should allow frequent changes in position, the distance of eye level to a work surface should be approximately 16 inches (eye glasses are set for this distance). There should be an open space beneath the seat of the chair to allow knee flexion beyond 90 degrees.[59] The patient's feet should be able to touch the floor or footrest.

Proper resting position for patients with back pain should reduce lumbar lordosis. Such a position is provided by the semi-Fowler position (Fig. 7–7). This position is achieved by having the patient lie on her back with a thin pillow under her head, with the thighs and legs elevated on cushions, pillows, or blankets.[1,13,60] Use of a bed pan actually *increases* lumbar lordosis and disc pressure, and is more aggravating than allowing the patient to use a bedside commode.[3,6] Proper bed rest as the *only treatment* of low back pain resulted in good pain relief in patients so treated and followed for 8 years. In this group, only 9% subsequently came to surgery, and only 44% required any other medical treatment.[61]

Use of pelvic traction is often subjectively beneficial. Because enormous forces are necessary to distract the lumbar spine, the traction serves the purpose of providing rest. It may have a placebo effect. We place the patient in a semi-Fowler position (head of mattress elevated 45 degrees, foot of mattress elevated 15 to 25 degrees). This places the low back into a more convex position; 15 to 30 pounds of traction are applied as much of the time as is tolerated. If the treatment program provides relief, the duration in traction during

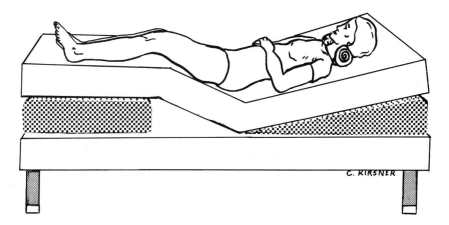

Fig. 7–7. The semi-Fowler bed position: A helpful resting position for patients with back pain.

daytime is progressively shortened. Traction, however, should never be the only treatment of back pain.[62]

The use of corsets is controversial. The corset may be utilized for the patient who is unwilling to remain in bed; however, there are no controlled data on their use.[7] If a corset is used, it should provide abdominal compression and be utilized only briefly. The patient should learn to depend on stronger abdominal muscle tone for back support.[1,3,25,50,53] In general, fewer than 5% of patients with back disease follow through on wearing the corset after purchase.[63] A back brace differs from a corset in having horizontal rigid elements, producing more restriction of spinal motion. A brace is utilized predominantly for patients with osteoporosis and vertebral compression fractures, or for post-traumatic vertebral fractures.[3] Patients with chronic or repeated pain occurrences should be referred for a back protection program provided by a physical or occupational therapist.

Therapeutic exercise is the cornerstone of management of the painful low back. Although their value in controlled studies is unproved, exercises nevertheless remain an extremely important and useful part of management in the experience of most physicians.[7] Exercises that specifically strengthen the abdominal muscles are of reasonably established value.[64] Also, good quadriceps power allows the legs to assist in lifting. The most sensible exercises are those that provide some back protection. These include exercises that develop

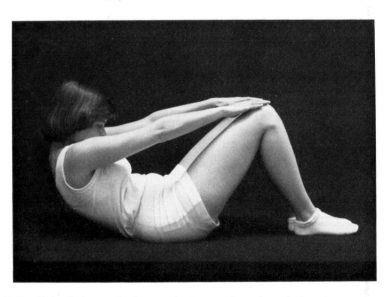

Fig. 7–8. Abdominal strengthening exercise is properly performed when the knees are kept bent and the patient does not sit up fully. Rather, the patient raises the trunk approximately 6 inches from the table. This contracts the superficial abdominal muscles without bringing the psoas muscle into play.

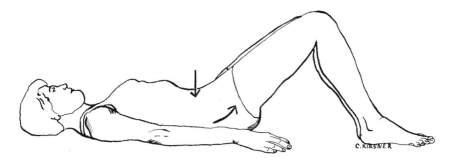

Fig. 7–9. Pelvic tilt exercise: To correct the lumbar lordosis, the abdominal muscles and gluteal muscles are contracted, and the lumbar spine is flattened.

abdominal strength (Fig. 7–8), provide posture correction (Figs. 1–6 and 7–8) and pelvic tilting[7,50,65,66] (Fig. 7–9). The Williams flexion exercises have proved useful in over 30 years of experience, yet theoretically these exercises increase disc pressure.[7] The knee-chest exercises are helpful, whether performed while lying on the back or sitting (Figs. 7–10, 7–11). Tight hamstring muscles and Achilles tendons can accentuate lumbar lordosis and should be stretched[3] (Fig. 7–12). General torso-stretching is an excellent warm-up maneuver (Fig. 7–13). As the patient achieves increased abdominal strength, she should reinforce conscientious continued voluntary contraction of the abdominal muscles throughout daily activities.[64,66] A "trapeze" exercise that is helpful for some patients is performed by gripping a chinning bar overhead. Knees are drawn up from below, and the weight of the pelvis stretches the low spine region; a chinning bar is available at athletic supply stores (Fig. 7–14).

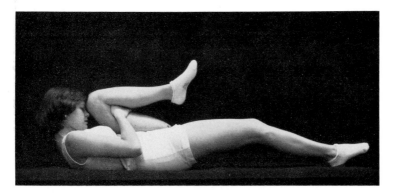

Fig. 7–10. The knee-chest exercise: Stretching of the low back muscles and fascia is obtained through these mobilizing exercises. One and then both knees are drawn toward the chest, the sacrum is lifted up, and the patient should perceive a pulling sensation in the low back tissues.

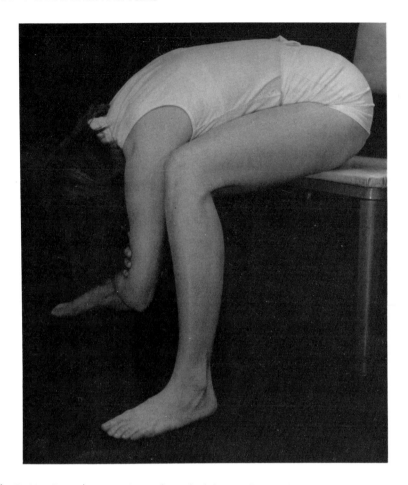

Fig. 7–11. Knee-chest exercise performed while seated on a chair: If standard knee-chest exercise (Fig. 7–10) does not provide a pulling sensation in the low back (perhaps due to hypermobility of the hip), the exercise should be attempted while the patient is seated as shown above.

Satisfactory results may also require proper resting position with the knees flexed, while lying on the back, with the thighs elevated with pillows; exercises to correct posture and strengthen the abdomen; recognition and correction of improper habits of sitting, lying, lifting; and, when necessary, use of vocational rehabilitation measures.

Myofascial trigger point injection has also proved itself over the course of time. Steindler,[67] in 1938, advocated the use of local anesthetic injections of trigger points within the soft tissue of the low back, and claimed lasting relief in the vast majority of patients with

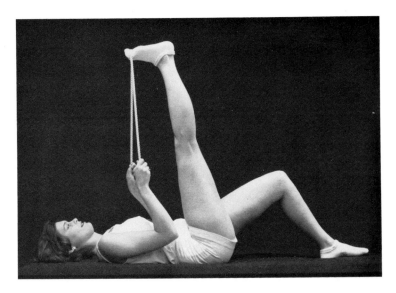

Fig. 7–12. Straight leg stretching: Tightness in the hamstring muscles, gastrocnemius, soleus, and Achilles tendon may be stretched progressively using a 4-ft length of rope looped across the ball of the foot. The extremity is pulled gradually toward the maximum tolerated upright position and held for 1 min during which further stretching may be accomplished.

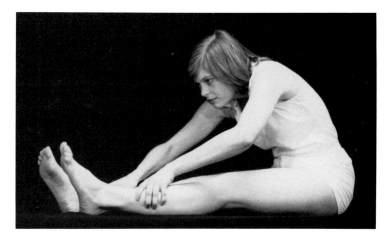

Fig. 7–13. Trunk stretching exercise: An excellent warm-up exercise to stretch posterior trunk and leg muscles before performing sport activities or more selective exercises.

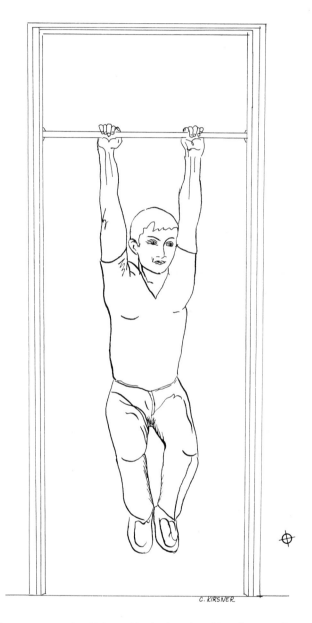

C. KIRSNER

Fig. 7–14. The trapeze exercise: Using a chinning bar placed in a doorway, the patient grasps the bar overhead and draws the knees up. The weight of the lower body stretches the musculature and soft tissues about the lumbar spine region. The patient should spend a minute or two repetitively holding this position as long as grasping permits.

low back pain. He emphasized the importance of using the needle as a probe; contact of the needle with the trigger point must reproduce the patient's pain before injection. We have found local corticosteroid-anesthetic injections helpful in providing lasting benefit (Fig. 7–15). The corticosteroid-anesthetic should be a long-acting preparation. Injection into a painful trigger point is no different than injection for bursitis or tendinitis.[63] The trigger point injection provides pain relief, which allows the patient to pursue corrective exercises and to return to normal function quickly.[1,3,10,29,50,53,63,67,68] The patient with low back pain associated with episacroiliac lipoma may have substantial and lasting pain relief by an injection of the lipoma and adjacent tissue.[45,47]

Oral medication has a limited role in the treatment of back pain,[63] yet the use of muscle relaxants at night has had some advocates.[69] There is a growing recognition of the value of mood altering drugs, such as amitriptyline, in providing improvement.[50,63,70,71] Use of tricyclic antidepressants for nocturnal sedation as well as depression has been helpful for most patients with *chronic* back pain. These agents should be started slowly, and may be given every 2 hours for 2 or 3 doses each evening (e.g., 8 PM, 10 PM, midnight). This regimen decreases the side effects, including morning hangover and daytime dry mouth. Nonsteroidal anti-inflammatory agents may be helpful in some patients with chronic myofascial back pain, especially those

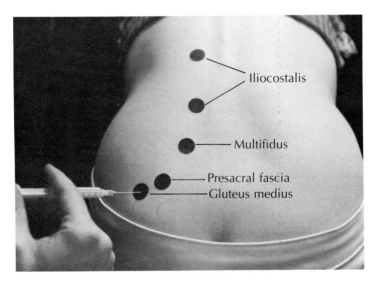

Fig. 7–15. Myofascial trigger point injection: Using the needle as a probe, the points of tenderness are located. Following skin penetration, aliquots of a corticosteroid-local anesthetic mixture are injected. Needle length varies with the size of the patient and ranges from a 1½-in. No. 22 needle to a 4-in. No. 20 spinal needle. Often both sides require injection at the same time, but we seldom exceed a volume of 5 ml.

with associated degenerative arthritis of the posterior apophyseal joints. Benefit is related to analgesic or anti-inflammatory effects. *There is no place for long-term oral corticosteroids in any myofascial disease of the low back.*

Outcome and Additional Suggestions

Most causes for low back pain are poorly understood at this time, and exacerbation and remissions of symptoms are the rule. Return to the previous accepted level of function represents a "satisfactory outcome." This, of course, is modified by age and other health situations.[63,72] Outcome often depends on the motivation of the patient and good communication between all involved parties (employer, insurer, physician, attorney, patient, and the patient's family).[63]

The importance of a comprehensive program was reported by Reed and Harvey in 1964.[72] In this study, medical, psychologic, sociologic, and vocational evaluations were performed on 185 persons, all of whom were on welfare although previously employed. Of these, only 69 patients were felt likely to be employable full-time; 31 of these 69 welfare recipients did become fully employed; in addition, 16 became part-time employees. Interestingly, 33 other patients left the evaluation program prematurely because they had obtained full-time employment. Only 4 were felt to be malingering. In another series of 100 chronic low back pain patients, 80% were reportedly improved; however, of those previously working, only 3 actually returned to work.[63] Yet in most series, less than 2% of patients with back pain are malingering. These 2 reports, a decade apart, offer conflicting return-to-work results. The later report had the poorer result. Is this a result of greater financial support of illness in the more recent decade?

In another study, ambulatory care provided relief in 90% of patients at follow-up.[27] Over the 4-year period of evaluation, surgery was unnecessary for any patient, yet 44% did have recurrences. In those patients with established disc disease, 74% had recurrences of pain, and sciatica alone was not of prognostic value.[27]

Subacute and chronic back pain often respond to a comprehensive treatment program, and the methods outlined are available to any practitioner. Additional new measures receiving attention include transcutaneous nerve stimulation, implantable stimulators, acupuncture, spinal manipulation, biofeedback training, and special inpatient "pain center" therapy. The most commonly used of these treatments, transcutaneous nerve stimulators, are expensive little black boxes with electrodes applied to the skin over various trigger points or nerve trunk pathways. Objective reduction in pain sensitivity has been reported.[26,73] Long noted that use of electric eels for medical purposes was common among the ancients.[74] Implanted electrical nerve stimulating devices have hazards, including scarring, nerve deficits, and the possible complications from the laminectomy necessary for implantation. Acupuncture (recommended by Osler 50 years ago!)[7] has come and gone in the treatment of low back pain in this country. When the acupuncture therapist provided *no suggestion* of benefit to the patient, only 4% of the patients had lasting relief.[75]

Manipulation of the spine has been utilized for nearly a century, and a major segment of the patient population with chronic back pain utilizes this treatment. Finneson details seven types of manipulation that include thrusting, hyperextension, rotation, torsion, and pelvic rock;[3] in general, rotational and mobilizing types are also used.[76-78] Doran and Newell reported the results of osteopathic manipulation versus standard medical care in 456 patients with painful limitation of spinal movement, unassociated with overt disc herniation or vertebral lesions.[78] After 3 months, nearly all patients in both therapeutic groups improved, so that no conclusions could be drawn. Analgesics were of little help. Almost all of the patients were back to work, but 44% still had pain interfering with their work regardless of the treatment modality. Similarly, studies comparing outcome from manipulation versus routine medical care gave results that were comparable.[77,79] Current orthopedic literature is accepting manipulation as a valid treatment.[1,3,63,80]

Indications for surgical intervention for low back pain have altered considerably in the last decade. Selection for surgery and a successful outcome are based upon a definite diagnosis that can be helped by a specific surgical therapy (e.g., laminectomy, fusion, abscess drainage). Probably fewer than 5% of patients with herniated nucleus pulposus require surgical intervention. Surgical results parallel the size of defect seen on myelograms (i.e., the larger the defect, the greater the chance for a good outcome). The severity of a patient's pain is a poor indicator for surgical outcome. Surprisingly, surgical outcome has not correlated well with psychopathology as evidenced by personality inventory determination.[81] However, there was a correlation of outcome with the patient being a recipient of workman's compensation.[81] Resumption of normal activity postoperatively was 16 days when no secondary gain was present, compared to 36 days if secondary gain was evident. Also, surgical failures were twice as common in those having secondary gain.[82]

Caudal or epidural blocks and posterior rhizotomy are specialized, potentially hazardous procedures used rarely in unresponsive cases of sciatica,[37,83] and should be considered experimental undertakings.[84]

Chronic back pain is seldom due to a single structural disorder. More often social and psychologic factors equally contribute to "injury." We discussed Sternbach's description of the "low back loser" (p. 144). Treatment requires that the patient must want to recover. The patient must have goals that she wishes to achieve.[26]

Pain centers are utilizing multiple treatment modalities in an inpatient setting. The eight points of treatment listed by Gottlieb are:[85] biofeedback relaxation, self-control techniques to handle stress and anxiety, patient-regulated medication, case conferences, physical therapy education, vocational rehabilitation, patient education, and a therapeutic milieu.

A comprehensive back therapy program requires active patient participation. Structural causes for pain, if present, are treated with anesthetic blocks or corticosteroid-anesthetic blocks and injections. In one such program,[86] patients participate in daily activities under the direction of a psychologist, a physical therapist, an occupational therapist, a recreational therapist, and a physician. The patient has an appointment list and must keep the appointments or does not obtain a weekend pass. Should the patient fail on the initial program, she then enters "operant conditioning" in an inpatient facility for 4 to 6 weeks of therapy. This "operant unit" has a "performance and reward" concept. Each bed is connected to a monitor that records the duration of time the patient is up and about. Activity quotas are provided each patient. A psychologist is in charge of such a unit. The patient does obtain positive reinforcement support for demonstrating improvement. Such improvement includes decreased dependency on drugs other than psychotropic agents. Discharge goals are set by the patient in group therapy sessions. Patients, also in group therapy, learn to recognize manipulative factors of chronic pain complaints and their effect on interpersonal relationships. A ten-month follow-up revealed that 70% of the patients had increased their activity or were working. However, most of these patients still regard themselves as failures, and require rewards for the smallest improvements.[86] It should be obvious to the physician that a pain center must provide a multifaceted program. "Center" programs that provide only one or two modalities, such as biofeedback training or acupuncture, do not suffice and can only delay comprehensive care.

Most patients with low back pain require supportive and preventive therapy. They usually do not have a complex esoteric disease. A treatment regimen, readily provided in an outpatient setting, includes (1) recognition and modification of aggravating factors through the use of vocational guidance personnel or an occupational therapist, (2) physical therapy and exercise to restore proper soft tissue support for the spine, (3) relief from pain with mild analgesics, or with local soft tissue injections using an anesthetic-corticosteroid mixture, (4) proper instructions in rest, with or without a corset or traction, and (5) possible use of mood altering drugs for nocturnal sedation and for altering pain perception. Even the patient with chronic, longstanding back pain can be helped in most instances by the personal physician.

PAIN SYNDROMES OF THE PELVIS

Osteitis Condensans Ilii

For a long time this entity has been erroneously considered a radiographic curiosity detected in asymptomatic persons. Sclerosing densities occur on the iliac side of the pelvis. This is usually readily distinguishable from radiographic features of ankylosing spondylitis in which the lesion involves both the sacrum and ilium. Blaschke, however, reviewed 109 patients with the finding of osteitis condensans ilii and discovered that a third suffered from sciatica, two thirds of them had a diffuse fibrositis syndrome, and nearly half the patients had elevation of the erythrocyte sedimentation rate.[87] The symptoms often are self-limited and may respond to nonsteroidal anti-inflammatory agents. HLA B27 typing is reported positive in 25% of these patients.[88]

Osteitis Pubis

Inflammation on each side of the periosteal bone of the symphysis pubis is detectable clinically by local direct point tenderness, and radiographically by erosion, sclerosis, and widening of the symphysis pubis (Fig. 7–16). This disorder may result from regional spread of sepsis following surgery of the prostrate or bladder, or herniorrhaphy. However, it often occurs insidiously without any known provoking cause. The vast majority of patients are females in the third to fourth

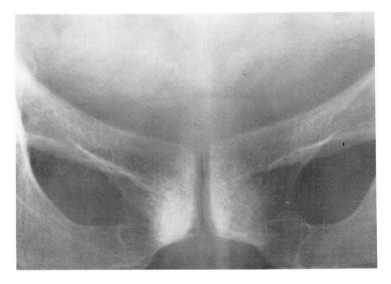

Fig. 7–16. Radiographic features of osteitis pubis include erosion, sclerosis, and widening of the symphysis pubis.

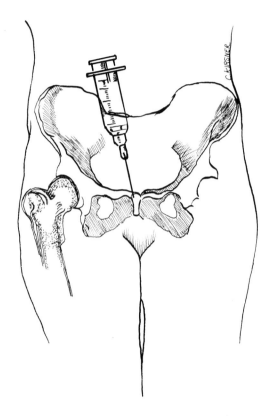

Fig. 7–17. Injection for osteitis pubis: After proper preparation a 1½-in. No. 22 or No. 23 needle is used as a probe. The corticosteroid-local anesthetic mixture is injected at the proximal symphysis pubis region along the bony surface. Strict aseptic technique is essential.

decades of life. The presentation consists of pain in the low anterior pelvis with radiation into the adductor muscles of both thighs. The patient may assume a duck-waddling gait. Local tenderness with reproduction or accentuation of pain by pressure over the symphysis pubis is diagnostic. Tenderness may occur before radiographic changes are evident. Later, the radiographic features of bone rarefaction and erosion with separation of the symphysis pubis and subsequent new bone repair are revealed.[89]

Osteitis pubis may be secondary to ankylosing spondylitis, chondrocalcinosis,[90,91] or polymyalgia rheumatica.[92] Often the condition is self-limited, and symptomatic benefit may be obtained from use of nonsteroidal anti-inflammatory agents,[93] or local corticosteroid injections into the tender regions of the symphysis pubis (Fig. 7–17), if sepsis has been excluded. Use of a sacral belt to stabilize the pelvis has also provided symptomatic benefit. Obviously, radiographic progression suggests osteomyelitis, and surgical consultation should then be obtained.[89]

Coccygodynia

This disorder may occur secondary to low back disorders with referred pain to the coccyx region; from visceral, rectal, or genitourinary disturbances with regional muscle spasm; from local myofascial injury with point tenderness at the sacrococcygeal joint; or from local inflammatory or post-traumatic lesions involving the coccyx and its ligamentous attachments.[25,94,95] An L-4 herniation of the nucleus pulposus may result in pain in the coccyx region. Percussion over the L-4 often reproduces such pain. Local treatment measures include injection with a local anesthetic-corticosteroid into soft tissue at the level of vertebra, if a spinal percussion test is positive. Local myofascial injury with point tenderness at the sacrococcygeal joint may be benefited by a local anesthetic-corticosteroid injection directly into the tender area. Use of a thick, soft, foam rubber cushion with a hole cut out of the center provides additional comfort. The cushion may prevent a pain-spasm-pain cycle. Surgical resection of a radiographically normal coccyx has not been necessary. Persistent pain raises suspicion for an L-4 ruptured disc.

Aching discomfort in the rectum, pelvis, coccyx, or low back with radiation to the legs and pain during defecation or during sexual intercourse may result from presumed spasm of the piriformis, levator ani, and coccygeus muscles.[95] The symptoms are often aggravated by sitting longer than 30 minutes and are relieved by lying down. Anxiety and fatigue are other aggravations. Tenderness upon rectal examination with reproduction or accentuation of pain occurs when the gloved examining finger palpates the involved muscle. Neurologic examination is normal and there are no radicular features. Rectal massage of the muscles in the lateral rectal walls surrounding the coccyx (the piriformis, the levator ani, and the coccygeus) performed 4 to 6 times over a 10 day period is recommended. The massage is carried out with a gentle stroking of the lateral and posterior rectal walls within reach of the examiner's fingers. The underlying muscles are massaged continually with gradual increased pressure. Relief occurs in approximately two thirds of patients.[94,95] Careful assessment for underlying disc disease is important in those who fail to benefit. We have tried the tricyclic anti-depressants without benefit in these patients.

REFERENCES

1. Duthie, RB, Ferguson AB: Mercer's Orthopedic Surgery. 7th Ed. Baltimore, Williams & Wilkins, 1973.
2. Fahrni WH: Conservative treatment of lumbar disc degeneration: Our primary responsibility. Orthop Clin North Am 6:93–103, 1975.
3. Finneson BE: Low Back Pain. Philadelphia, JB Lippincott, 1973.

4. King JS, Lagger R: Sciatica viewed as a referred pain syndrome. Surg Neurol 5:46–50, 1976.
5. Swezey RL: Pseudo-radiculopathy in subacute trochanteric bursitis of the subgluteus maximus bursa. Arch Phys Med Rehabil 57:387–390, 1976.
6. Matthews JA: Backache. Br Med J 1:432–434, 1977.
7. Quinet RJ, Hadler NM: Diagnosis and treatment of backache. Semin Arthritis Rheum 8:261–287, 1979.
8. Calin A: Back pain: Mechanical or inflammatory? Am Fam Pract 20:97–100, 1979.
9. Kirkaldy-Willis WH: Five common back disorders: How to diagnose and treat them. Geriatrics 33:32–41, 1978.
10. Mooney V, Robertson J: The facet syndrome. Clin Orthop 115:149–156, 1976.
11. Nachemson A, Morris JM: Lumbar discometry: Lumbar intradiscal pressure measurements in vivo. Lancet 1:1140–1142, 1963.
12. Nachemson A, Morris JM: In vivo measurements of intradiscal pressure: Discometry, a method for the determination of pressure in the lower lumbar discs. J Bone Joint Surg 46A:1077–1092, 1964.
13. Nachemson A: Towards a better understanding of low-back pain: A review of the mechanics of the lumbar disc. Rheumatol Rehabil 14:129–143, 1975.
14. Morris JM, Lucas DB, Bressler B: Role of the trunk in stability of the spine. J Bone Joint Surg 43A:327–351, 1961.
15. Farfan HF: Muscular mechanism of the lumbar spine and the position of power and efficiency. Orthop Clin North Am 6:135–144, 1975.
16. Bartelink DL: The role of abdominal pressure in relieving the pressure on the lumbar intervertebral discs. J Bone Joint Surg 39B:718–725, 1957.
17. Howes RG, Isdale IC: The loose back: An unrecognized syndrome. Rheum Phys Med 11:72–77, 1971.
18. Hirsch C: The mechanical response in normal and degenerated lumbar discs. J Bone Joint Surg 38A:242–243, 1956.
19. Bonica JJ: Management of myofascial pain syndromes in general practice. JAMA 164:732–738, 1957.
20. Snook SH, Irvine CH, Bass SF: Maximum weights and work loads acceptable to male industrial workers: A study of lifting, lowering, pushing, pulling, carrying, and walking tasks. Am Ind Hyg Assoc J 31:579–586, 1970.
21. Snook SH, Ciriello VM: Maximum weights and work loads acceptable to female workers. J Occ Med 16:527–534, 1974.
22. Chaffin DB, Park KS: A longitudinal study of low-back pain as associated with occupational weight lifting factors. Am Ind Hyg Assoc J 34:513–525, 1973.
23. Chaffin DB: Human strength capability and low-back pain. J Occ Med 16:248–254, 1974.
24. Hadler NM: Industrial rheumatology: Clinical investigations into the influence of the pattern of usage on the pattern of regional musculoskeletal disease. Arthritis Rheum 20: 1019–1025, 1977.
25. Levine DB: The painful low back. In Arthritis and Allied Conditions. 9th Ed. Edited by DJ McCarty. Philadelphia, Lea & Febiger, 1979.
26. Sternbach RA, Murphy RW, Akeson WH, Wolf SR: Chronic low-back pain: The "low-back loser." Postgrad Med 53:135–138, 1973.
27. Dillane JB, Fry J, Kalton G: Acute back syndrome—a study from general practice. Br Med J 2:82–84, 1966.
28. Gelmers HJ: Entrapment of the sciatic nerve. Acta Neurochir 33:103–106, 1976.
29. Breneman JC: The herniated disc syndrome. J Occ Med 11:475–479, 1969.
30. Retzlaff EW, Berry AB, Haight AS, et al: The piriformis muscle syndrome. J Am Osteopath Assoc 73:799–807, 1974.
31. Pace JB, Nagle D: Piriform syndrome. West J Med 124:435–439, 1976.
32. Brown BR: Diagnosis and therapy of common myofascial pain syndromes. JAMA 239:646–648, 1978.
33. Banerjee T, Hall CD: Sciatic entrapment neuropathy. J Neurosurg 45:216–217, 1976.
34. Kestler OC: Posterior lumbar fusions, spinal stenosis, and arachnoiditis. An overview. Contemp Orthop 1:43–53, 1979.

35. Shenkin HA, Hash CJ: Spondylolisthesis after multiple bilateral laminectomies and facetectomies for lumbar spondylosis. J Neurosurg 50:45–47, 1979.
36. Choudhury AR, Taylor JC: Occult lumbar spinal stenosis. J Neurol Neurosurg Psychiatry 40:506–510, 1977.
37. Wiltse LL: Common problems of the lumbar spine: Degenerative spondylolisthesis and spinal stenosis. JCE Orthop 7:17–30, 1979.
38. Wilson ES, Brill RF: Spinal stenosis: The narrow lumbar spinal canal syndrome. Clin Orthop 122:244–248, 1977.
39. Keim HA: Awareness that spinal nerve entrapment syndromes really exist is most important step in treatment. Orthop Rev 7:79–86, 1978.
40. Verbiest H: A radicular syndrome from developmental narrowing of the lumbar vertebral canal. J Bone Joint Surg 36B:230–237, 1954.
41. Benson DR: The back: Thoracic and lumbar spine. In Musculoskeletal Disorders: Regional Examination and Differential Diagnosis. Edited by RD D'Ambrosia. Philadelphia, JB Lippincott, 1977.
42. Bywaters EGL: Tendinitis and bursitis. Clin Rheum Dis 5:883–927, 1979.
43. Sarno JE: Therapeutic exercise for back pain. In Therapeutic Exercise. 3rd Ed. Edited by JV Basmajian. Baltimore, Williams & Wilkins, 1978.
44. Fowler WM, Taylor RG: Differential diagnosis of muscle diseases. In Musculoskeletal Disorders: Regional Examination and Differential Diagnosis. Edited by RD D'Ambrosia. Philadelphia, JB Lippincott, 1977.
45. Ries E: Episacroiliac lipoma. Am J Obstet Gynecol 34:490–494, 1937.
46. Pace JB, Hening C: Episacroiliac lipoma. Am Fam Physician 6:70–73, 1972.
47. Singewald ML: Sacroiliac lipomata—an often unrecognized cause of low back pain. Johns Hopkins Med J 118:492–498, 1966.
48. Crown S: Psychological aspects of low back pain. Rheumatol Rehabil 17:114–122, 1978.
49. Forrest AJ, Wolkind SN: Masked depression in men with low back pain. Rheumatol Rehabil 13:148–153, 1974.
50. Pheasant HC: The problem back. Curr Pract Orthop Surg 7:89–115, 1977.
51. MacNab I: Backache. Baltimore, Williams & Wilkins, 1977.
52. Brown MD: Diagnosis of pain syndromes of the spine. Orthop Clin North Am 6:233–248, 1975.
53. Russek AS: Biomechanical and physiological basis for ambulatory treatment of low back pain. Orthop Rev 5:21–31, 1976.
54. Lawrence JS, Bremner JM, Bier F: Osteoarthrosis: Prevalence in the population and relationship between symptoms and x-ray changes. Ann Rheum Dis 25:1–24, 1966.
55. Lawrence JS: Disc degeneration: Its frequency and relationship to symptoms. Ann Rheum Dis 28:121–138, 1969.
56. Porter RW, Wicks M, Ottewell D: Measurement of the spinal canal by diagnostic ultra-sound. J Bone Joint Surg 60B:481–484, 1978.
57. Terry AF, DeYoung R: Hip disease mimicking low back disorders. Orthop Rev 8:95–104, 1979.
58. Beals RK, Hickman NW: Industrial injuries of the back and extremities. J Bone Joint Surg 54A:1593–1611, 1972.
59. Keegan JJ: Alterations of the lumbar curve related to posture and seating. J Bone Joint Surg 35A:589–603, 1953.
60. Kraus H: Clinical Treatment of Back and Neck Pain. New York, McGraw-Hill, 1970.
61. Pearce J, Moll JMH: Conservative treatment and natural history of acute lumbar disc lesions. J Neurol Neurosurg Psychiatry 30:13–17, 1967.
62. Mathews JA, Hickling J: Lumbar traction: A double-blind controlled study for sciatica. Rheumatol Rehabil 14:222–225, 1975.
63. Mooney V, Cairns D: Management in the patient with chronic low back pain. Orthop Clin North Am 9:543–557, 1978.
64. Nachemson A: Physiotherapy for low back pain patients: A critical look. Scand J Rehabil Med 1:85–90, 1969.
65. Kendall PH, Jenkins JM: Exercises for backache: A double-blind controlled trial. Physiotherapy 54:154–157, 1968.

66. Kendall PH, Jenkins JM: Lumbar isometric flexion exercises. Physiotherapy *54*:158–163, 1968.

67. Steindler A, Luck JV: Differential diagnosis of pain low in the back: Allocation of the source of pain by the procaine hydrochloride method. JAMA *110*:106–113, 1938.

68. Dilke TFW, Burry HC, Grahame R: Extradural corticosteroid injection in management of lumbar nerve root compression. Br Med J *2*:635–637, 1973.

69. Hindle TH III: Comparison of carisoprodol, butabarbital, and placebo in treatment of the low back syndrome. Cal Med *117*:7–11, 1972.

70. Beaumont G: The use of psychotropic drugs in other painful conditions. J Int Med Res *4*: [Suppl (2)]56–57, 1976.

71. deJong RH: Central pain mechanisms. JAMA *239*:2784, 1978.

72. Reed JW, Harvey JC: Rehabilitating the chronically ill: A method for evaluating the functional capacity of ambulatory patients. Geriatrics *19*:87–103, 1964.

73. Ignelzi RJ, Sternbach RA, Callaghan M: Somato-sensory changes during transcutaneous electrical analgesia. *In* Advances in Pain Research and Therapy. Vol I. Edited by JJ Bonica, DG Albe-Fessard. New York, Raven Press, 1976.

74. Long DM: Use of peripheral and spinal cord stimulation in the relief of chronic pain. *In* Advances in Pain Research and Therapy. Vol I. Edited by JJ Bonica, DG Albe-Fessard. New York, Raven Press, 1976.

75. Murphy TM: Subjective and objective follow-up assessment of acupuncture therapy without suggestion in 100 chronic pain patients. *In* Advances in Pain Research and Therapy. Vol I. Edited by JJ Bonica, DG Albe-Fessard. New York, Raven Press, 1976.

76. Maigne R: Orthopedic Medicine: A New Approach to Vertebral Manipulations. Springfield, IL, Charles C Thomas, 1972.

77. Glover JR, Morris JG, Khosla T: Back pain: A randomized clinical trial of rotational manipulation of the trunk. Br J Ind Med *31*:59–64, 1974.

78. Doran DML, Newell DJ: Manipulation in treatment of low back pain: A multicentre study. Br Med J *2*:161–164, 1975.

79. Kane RL, Leymaster C, Olsen D, et al: Manipulating the patient: A comparison of the effectiveness of physician and chiropractic care. Lancet *1*:1333–1336, 1974.

80. Firman GJ, Goldstein MS: The future of chiropractic: A psychosocial view. N Engl J Med *293*:639–642, 1975.

81. Waring EM, Weisz GM, Bailey SI: Predictive factors in the treatment of low back pain by surgical intervention. *In* Advances in Pain Research and Therapy. Vol I. Edited by JJ Bonica, DG Albe-Fessard. New York, Raven Press, 1976.

82. Finneson BE: Modulating effect of secondary gain on the low back pain syndrome. *In* Advances in Pain Research and Therapy. Vol I. Edited by JJ Bonica, DG Albe-Fessard. New York, Raven Press, 1976.

83. Stanton-Hicks M: Therapeutic caudal or epidural block for lower back or sciatic pain. JAMA *243*:369–370, 1980.

84. Tarlov E: Therapeutic caudal or epidural block for lower back or sciatic pain. JAMA *243*:369, 1980.

85. Gottlieb H, Strite LC, Koller R, et al: Comprehensive rehabilitation of patients having chronic low back pain. Arch Phys Med Rehabil *58*:101–108, 1977.

86. Cairns D, Thomas L, Mooney V, Pace JB: A comprehensive treatment approach to chronic low back pain. Pain *2*:301–308, 1976.

87. Blaschke JA: Clinical characteristics of osteitis condensans ilii. Abstract. Paper presented to VI Pan-American Congress on Rheumatic Diseases, June 16–21, 1974.

88. Singal DP, deBosset P, Gordon DA, et al: HLA antigens in osteitis condensans ilii and ankylosing spondylitis. J Rheumatol [Suppl (3)] *4*:105–108, 1977.

89. Samellas W, Finkelstein P: Osteitis pubis: Its surgical treatment. J Urol *87*:(4)553–555, 1962.

90. Scott DL, Eastmond CJ, Wright V: A comparative radiological study of the pubic symphysis in rheumatic disorders. Ann Rheum Dis *38*:529–534, 1979.

91. Pinals RS: Traumatic arthritis and allied conditions. *In* Arthritis and Allied Conditions. 9th Ed. Edited by DJ McCarty. Philadelphia, Lea & Febiger, 1979.

92. O'Duffy JD: Increasing evidence suggests polymyalgia rheumatica is not a muscle disease. Wellcome Trends in Rheumatology 1:1–2, 1979.
93. Barnes WC, Malament M: Osteitis pubis. Surg Gynecol Obstet 117:277–284, 1963.
94. Thiele GH: Coccygodynia and pain in the superior gluteal region and down the back of the thigh: Causation by tonic spasm of the levator ani, coccygeus, and piriformis muscles and relief by massage of these muscles. JAMA 109:1271–1275, 1941.
95. Sinaki M, Merritt, JL, Stillwell GK: Tension myalgia of the pelvic floor. Mayo Clin Proc 52:717–722, 1977.

Chapter 8

THE PELVIS AND THIGH REGION

Pain in this region may be referred from disorders arising in the low back, abdomen, peripheral nerves, retroperitoneal region (with irritation of the psoas muscle), within the hip joint, or may result from lesions in the soft tissue of the hip region. Patients with intrinsic hip disease usually have the associated complaint of limitation of movement. For example, the most specific complaint is a loss of the ability to rotate the leg into abduction when putting on a slipper or stocking in the morning. In essence, the patient is performing the Patrick or "Fabere test." The *Fabere test* is comprised of the abbreviations for four maneuvers: *F*lexion, *Ab*duction, *E*xternal *R*otation and *E*xtension.[1] As mentioned previously, night pain often is the result of inflammation of myofascial structures, bursitis, or tumor. If a patient with known hip disease does suffer night pain, the clinician should be alert to a coexisting extra-articular treatable soft tissue cause for the pain, although severe intra-articular disease can also cause night pain. Numbness, tingling, stabbing, and sciatica-like pain may be of myofascial origin rather than disc disease, or the symptoms may result from an entrapment neuropathy. Entrapment neuropathies are characterized by intermittency of symptoms, lancinating pain, and aggravation by a particular motion.

The fascia lata and its component, the iliotibial tract, are important soft tissue structures, the involvement of which is capable of causing frustrating chronic leg pain.[2] The fascia lata is a thickened deep fascia of the lateral thigh. Superiorly the fascia lata attaches to the anterior superior iliac spine, the inguinal ligament, the body of the pubic bone, the ischial tuberosity, the sacrotuberous ligament, the sacrum, and the iliac crest. The iliotibial tract is a conjoint aponeurosis of the fascia lata and the gluteus maximus muscle. The iliotibial tract inserts on the

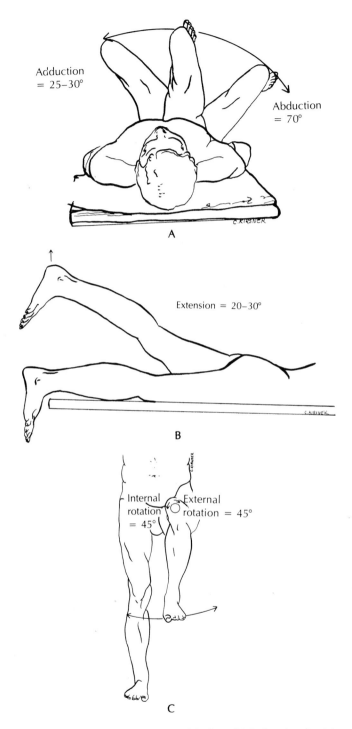

Fig. 8–1. Examination for range of movement of the hip. This ball-and-socket joint provides, A, adduction, abduction, and flexion; B, extension; C, internal and external rotation. These illustrations demonstrate some of the methods for the determination of these movements.

173

anterolateral aspect of the tibia.[1] If contracted, it exerts a pull upon the hip resulting in flexion and abduction; it can also cause the "snapping hip syndrome." Knowledge of the location of the superficial and deep trochanteric bursae, the iliopectineal bursa, and the origin and points of potential injury or entrapment of the various superficial peripheral nerves of this region allow the examiner to palpate for trigger points and to reproduce the pain that results from disturbances of these soft tissue structures.

Physical Examination. The following degrees of hip movement are considered normal: Flexion–120 to 135 degrees; abduction in extension–35 to 40 degrees; abduction in flexion–70 to 75 degrees; adduction (crossing leg)–25 to 30 degrees; internal rotation in extension or flexion–45 degrees; external rotation in extension or flexion–45 degrees; and hip extension–20 to 30 degrees[3] (Fig. 8–1).

The examiner should measure leg lengths, after determining the patient's ability to fully straighten the knees. With the leg drawn straight and the patient lying flat on her back, the true leg length can be measured from the anterior-superior iliac spine to the medial malleolus of each ankle. Normal individuals may have as much as 1-cm discrepancy without symptoms. "Apparent" limb length disparity is determined by measuring the distance from the umbilicus to each medial malleolus.[3]

Special Maneuvers or Other Tests. The *Trendelenburg* test is important for the detection of involvement of the hip stabilizers (gluteus medius, gluteus minimus). The examination consists of having the patient stand with her back to the examiner; two points are marked on each of the posterior iliac spines; then the patient stands on one foot and raises the other; the side supporting the body's weight is the side being tested. If the pelvis falls on the side *not* bearing weight the test is positive and suggests muscle disease affecting the abductors or the stabilizers of the hip, congenital dislocation of the hip, coxa vara, Legg-Calvé-Perthes disease, or abnormalities in the proximal femoral epiphysis.[3]

The *Fabere test* (also called Patrick's test) is a physical examination maneuver that requires placing the foot of the involved extremity on the opposite knee. The examiner then presses the knee and thigh downward and pain results if intrinsic hip disease is present (Fig. 8–2).

Erichsen's sign: The examiner provides compression across the iliac bones; if pain occurs, the test is suggestive for sacroiliac joint inflammation.

Ober's test (for contracture of the iliotibial band): The patient lies with the affected side up and the opposite side down; the uppermost leg (symptomatic side) is drawn backward at the hip (with hyperextension of the hip) and then bent at the knee (Fig. 8–3). The Ober test

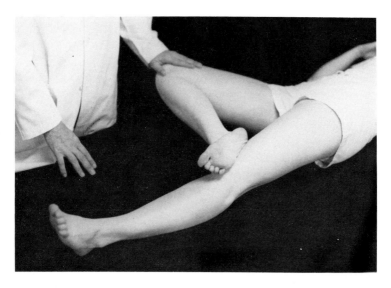

Fig. 8–2. The Patrick or Fabere test: If pain results when the examiner presses the knee and thigh downward, then intrinsic hip disease should be suspected.

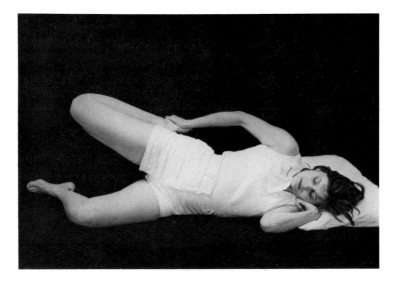

Fig. 8–3. The Ober test: This test is useful for determining the presence of a contracture of the iliotibial band or tightness in the hip flexor musculature.

is positive if, after letting go of the involved thigh, the knee does not drop to the table. Failure of the leg to fall suggests a contracture of the iliotibial band. The Ober test (Fig. 8–3) also reproduces pain resulting from hip flexor muscle contractures.[3]

Differential Diagnosis. The conditions described in this chapter are regional local disorders. However, pain in the region can also arise from systemic or multifocal disease, such as herniation of a lumbar disc, Paget's disease, migratory osteolysis, inflammatory rheumatic diseases, panniculitis, occult sepsis, or neoplastic disorders.[4–7] Patients with persistent pain in this region require appropriate laboratory and radiographic examinations. Radiographic examination should include the spine and both hips for appropriate evaluation. An erythrocyte sedimentation rate, a complete blood count, urinalysis, rectal examination, and stool examinations for occult blood are essential in patients with any persistent pelvic or hip region pain. A careful vaginal pelvic examination should be performed by the clinician experienced in this examination. The pelvic ligaments are uncommon sites of origin for low pelvic pain in females, and the degree of tenderness is a subjective determination.

MYOFASCIAL PAIN SYNDROMES

Snapping Hip

An actual dislocation of the hip is painful, whereas the snapping hip is a painless annoying noise.[8] The snapping hip often results from a

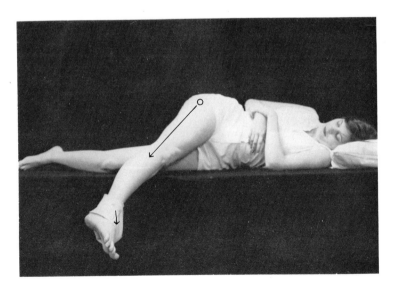

Fig. 8–4. Exercise or method of examination for taut iliotibial band or fascia lata fasciitis.

taut iliotibial band slipping over the greater tuberosity.[1,3] Treatment consists of stretching the iliotibial band for a few moments twice daily (Fig. 8–4). Usually within a period of weeks the snapping diminishes.

Fascia Lata Fasciitis

Symptoms may result from inflammation or tightness of the fascia lata due to overuse or disuse. The patient may describe vague discomfort upon arising in the morning and after prolonged walking. Initially, symptoms may be relieved by walking, only to be aggravated by further prolonged walking. The discomfort is a dull ache over the low back and lateral hip and thigh region radiating down the lateral thigh to the lateral knee region. Physical examination requires positioning the patient on the examining table with the involved hip uppermost. The straight leg is then drawn over the edge of the table

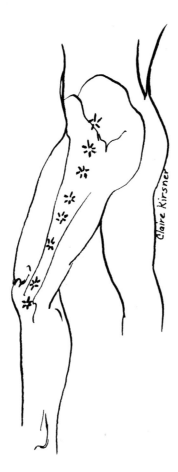

Fig. 8–5. Sites of tenderness or adhesions along the fascia lata.

and pressure is placed upon the ankle (Fig. 8–4). The weighted straight leg is drawing the fascia lata taut. In a slender individual we have seen dimpling along the fascia resulting from adhesions (Fig. 8–5). The dimpling or tenderness to palpation may be detected in the region of the trochanteric bursa, 2 inches below the trochanteric bursa, and then along the crevice palpable between the anterior and posterior muscle compartments of the lateral thigh. These areas should be marked for later injection. Tenderness should be sought as high as the gluteus medius and as low as 2 or 3 inches below the fibular head. Treatment consists of injecting local anesthetic-corticosteroid mixture into the involved symptomatic locations. The fascia should be stretched by having the patient assume the same position as described for the examination. The patient lies on the edge of a bed with a weight (ranging from 3 to 10 pounds depending on tolerance) applied to the ankle. The patient should flex the hip to a degree that allows a pulling sensation to be felt along the lateral compartment of the thigh[2] (Fig. 8–4).

BURSITIS

Of the 18 or more bursae described in the hip region, the most important are the trochanteric, iliopectineal, and ischiogluteal bursae.

Trochanteric Bursitis

The trochanteric bursa lies between the tendon of the gluteus maximus and the posterolateral prominence of the greater trochanter.[1,3,9] A more superficial bursa directly over the greater trochanter may also become inflamed and tender. Characteristic night pain of bursitis may be added to that secondary to osteoarthritis of the hip. Point tenderness over the trochanteric bursa with pain reproduction is strong evidence for the presence of bursitis. This point of tenderness usually lies approximately an inch posterior and superior to the greater trochanter, and is located about 3 inches deep to the skin. Obesity, compression injury, or other minor local trauma may be aggravating factors. The act of arising from a position of lumbar spine flexion (back bent forward), while the knees are kept straight requires a lever action of the glutei and is perhaps the most common cause for gluteal strain, which in turn may predispose to trochanteric bursitis. Such patients must learn to bend their knees before bending their backs. Treatment consists of injecting the trochanteric bursa with a local anesthetic-corticosteroid agent (Fig. 8–6), sleeping with a small pillow under the involved buttock to keep the body weight shifted off of the bursa, and stretching the gluteal muscles utilizing knee chest exercises (Fig. 7–10).

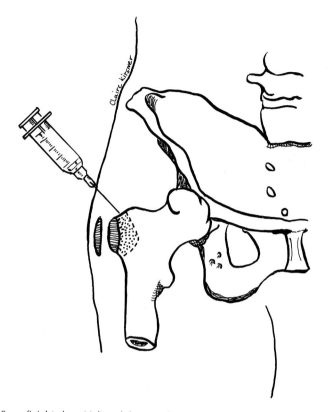

Fig. 8–6. Superficial (adventitial) and deep trochanteric bursitis: After localizing the points of maximum tenderness by deep palpation, a 1½- to 4-in. needle is used as a probe; the points of maximum tenderness are determined, and aliquots of a corticosteroid-local anesthetic are injected into each site.

Iliopectineal and Iliopsoas Bursitis

The iliopectineal bursa lies between the iliopsoas muscle and the iliopectineal eminence. Posteriorly it lies lateral to the femoral vessels and overlies the capsule of the hip. The iliopsoas bursa lies medially in Scarpa's triangle. Bursitis in the anterior hip region (rare in our experience) causes pain in the anterior pelvis, groin, and thigh region.[1,3] The iliopectineal bursa often communicates with the hip joint; bursitis may result from intrinsic joint disease.[1] Careful injection of the bursa with a corticosteroid-local anesthetic mixture probably is best performed by a rheumatologist or orthopedist. Persistence may indicate surgical intervention and excision of the bursa.

Ischial (Ischiogluteal) Bursitis

"Weaver's bottom" or "tailor's bottom" represents pain in a bursa overlying the ischial prominence, and irritation of the sciatic nerve may coexist.[10] The patient often has exquisite pain when sitting or lying. Such patients often are given floor exercises to do and find them painful. Point tenderness with pain reproduction is suggestive. Occasionally we have seen similar pain accompany silent prostatitis in males, in association with ankylosing spondylitis, or in Reiter's syndrome. Rectal examination for prostate irritation should be considered in patients with atypical symptoms. Ankylosing spondylitis or other spondyloarthritides should be excluded. Local anesthetic-corticosteroid injection and use of a 3-inch foam rubber cut-out cushion as described for "coccygodynia" is helpful.[1] When injecting the bursa, warn the patient to call out if neuritic pain occurs, since the sciatic nerve is nearby and should *not* be injected.[10]

ENTRAPMENT NEUROPATHIES

Symptoms of intermittent numbness, tingling, and a sensation of swelling suggest an entrapment neuropathy.

Abdominal Cutaneous Nerve

The patient is often a teenage girl who notes a dull burning pain with sharp exacerbations. The pain radiates transversely across the lower abdomen to the mid-line, and often the patient can localize the origin of pain with one finger.[11,12] The abdominal cutaneous nerves arise from the thoracoabdominal nerve trunks and divide into anterior, lateral, and posterior branches. The nerves pass through a tough fibrous ring in the abdominal wall. Traction of the nerve against this ring may result in a burst of pain. In some patients the nerve is overstretched and angulated as a result of spinal, rib, or other skeletal structures. Symptoms may also result from abdominal distention, but often no apparent cause is found.[11,12] The nerve is easily put under tension and angulated within the abdominal wall's fibrous ring. Most cases involve the anterior cutaneous branch at the rectus margin. Examination with careful palpation of the rectus abdominis usually localizes and reproduces the pain at the fibrous ring. Local anesthestic injection of the region is both diagnostic and therapeutic.[11]

Obturator Nerve

Often following a pelvic fracture, osteitis pubis, or development of an obturator hernia, the patient notes pain and paresthesia in the groin that travels down the inner aspect of the thigh; these symptoms are aggravated during passive or active hip motion.[13] Local nerve block is necessary to establish the diagnosis.

Meralgia Paresthetica

Entrapment of the lateral femoral cutaneous nerve is a frequent entrapment neuropathy of the thigh region. Intermittent paresthesia, hypesthesia, or hyperesthesia over the upper anterolateral thigh occur (Fig. 8–7). The entrapment occurs at the anterior superior iliac spine where the nerve passes through the lateral end of the inguinal ligament or adjacent iliacus fascia.[13,14] The nerve also perforates the sartorius muscle and exits through a canal in the fascia lata.[15] Trauma, a pelvic tilt resulting from a short limb, prolonged sitting with crossed legs, or increased abdominal girth with bulging fat may be causative.

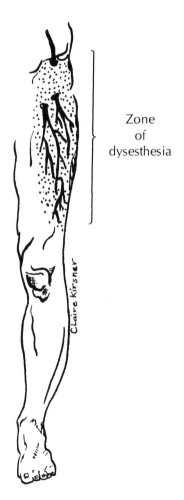

Zone
of
dysesthesia

Fig. 8–7. Entrapment of the lateral femoral cutaneous nerve (meralgia paresthetica): The nerve is frequently impinged at the anterosuperior iliac spine; dysesthesias are noted over the upper anterior lateral thigh.

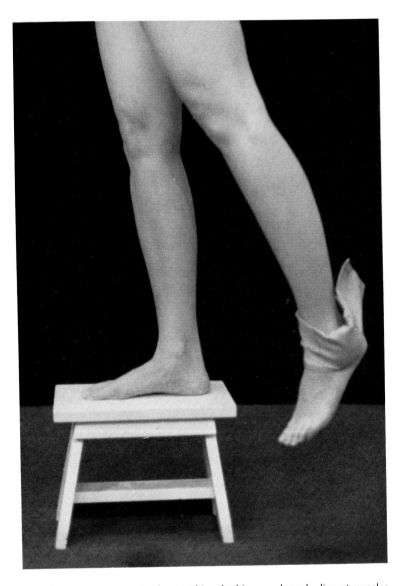

Fig. 8–8. Pendulum exercise for stretching the hip capsule and adjacent muscles.

Pregnancy, rapid weight gain, and constriction from a corset, belt, or seatbelt are other common causes.[16] Treatment includes local infiltration with anesthetic-corticosteroid agents into the site of nerve exit at the inguinal ligament and into the region of dysesthesia. Also helpful are avoiding contact pressure in the region of the inguinal ligament, loss of weight, and if necessary, use of a heel-lift for a short limb.[13]

Sciatic Pseudoradiculopathy

A pseudoradiculopathy may result from trochanteric bursitis; relief of the sciatica-like pain occurs following injection of the trochanteric bursa.[17] Sometimes hip capsule stretching is of additional help (Fig. 8–8). In addition, the sciatic nerve may be involved in disease entities beyond the pelvis. Constricting myofascial bands in the posterior thigh have been described.[18]

No single entity stands out as a cause for low pelvic, hip, and thigh region pain. We have presented a potpourri of disorders seen frequently as causes for treatable discomfort in the hip and thigh. Management obviously depends on careful assessment. The relief provided by treatment often establishes the diagnosis. However, failure to recognize an aggravating factor often results in recurrence. The six points of management described previously apply to this body region as well.

REFERENCES

1. Turek SL: Orthopaedics; Principles and Their Application. 3rd Ed. Philadelphia, JB Lippincott, 1977.
2. Lowman EW: Connective tissue diseases. In Handbook of Physical Medicine and Rehabilitation. 2nd Ed. Edited by FH Kruzen. Philadelphia, WB Saunders, 1971.
3. D'Ambrosia RD: The hip. In Musculoskeletal Disorders. Philadelphia, JB Lippincott, 1977.
4. Benson R, Fowler PD: Treatment of Weber-Christian disease. Br Med J 2:615–616, 1964.
5. Pinals RS: Traumatic arthritis and allied conditions. In Arthritis and Allied Conditions. 9th Ed. Edited by DJ McCarty. Philadelphia, Lea & Febiger, 1979.
6. Swezey RL: Transient osteoporosis of the hip, foot, and knee. Arthritis Rheum 13:858–868, 1970.
7. Duncan H, Frame B, Frost HM, Arnstein AR: Migratory osteolysis of the lower extremities. Ann Intern Med 66:1165–1173, 1967.
8. Carter C, Wilkinson J: Persistent joint laxity and congenital dislocation of the hip. J Bone Joint Surg 42B:40–45, 1964.
9. Swezey RL, Spiegel TM: Evaluation and treatment of local musculoskeletal disorders in elderly patients. Geriatrics 34:56–75, 1979.
10. Swartout R, Compere EL: Ischio-gluteal bursitis. JAMA 227:551–552, 1974.
11. DeValera E, Raftery H: Lower abdominal and pelvic pain in women. In Advances in Pain Research and Therapy. Vol 1. Edited by JJ Bonica, D Albe-Fessard. New York, Raven Press, 1976.
12. Applegate WV: Abdominal cutaneous nerve entrapment syndrome. Am Fam Physician 8:132–133, 1973.
13. Kopell HP, Thompson WA: Peripheral Entrapment Neuropathies. Huntington, NY, RE Krieger, 1976.

Chapter 9

THE KNEE

The knee performs a complex series of gliding, sliding, rotating, and bending functions.[1] Knee movement includes the "screw home" mechanism; specifically, as the knee extends or straightens from the bent position, the tibia rotates externally and the femur rotates internally. This rotation mechanism requires joint stability, particularly while running. Although the functions of the menisci are not completely understood, they act both as shock absorbers and as stabilizers to help rotational stability.[1] At least a dozen bursae are situated in the knee region; several of them communicate with the joint itself (Fig. 9–1).

History. The physician who deals with disabling problems of knee pain must consider the age of the patient, any preceding injury, and the pain pattern. In addition, the mode of onset, the localization of pain, and any associated phenomena of locking, clicking, catching, buckling, swelling, or loss of motion should be noted.[2,3]

Intermittent "giving way" (buckling) or locking, followed by a period of recovery, may result from a torn meniscus, intra-articular loose bodies, cruciate ligament inadequacy, patellofemoral instability, hypertrophy of the infrapatellar fat pad, or intra-articular tumors of the knee. These disorders collectively are termed "internal derangements of the knee."[4] Early recognition of an internal derangement of the knee, followed by appropriate therapy, may relieve symptoms and prevent secondary osteoarthritis. Warmth and swelling in association with a persistent locked knee are signs of serious internal derangement; surgical consultation is often required.

Asking the patient to point to the area of maximum pain, or having the patient indicate whether the pain is anterior, posterior, medial, or lateral assists the clinician in diagnosis. Pain at the medial joint line is seen with injury to the medial collateral ligament, disease of the medial joint compartment, anserine bursitis, or an internal derange-

185

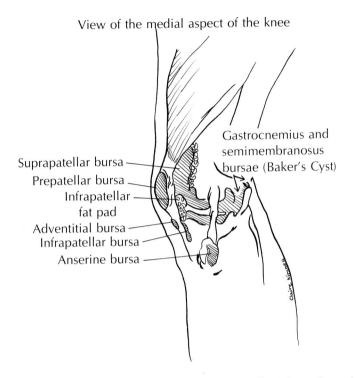

View of the medial aspect of the knee

Suprapatellar bursa
Prepatellar bursa
Infrapatellar
fat pad
Adventitial bursa
Infrapatellar bursa
Anserine bursa

Gastrocnemius and
semimembranosus
bursae (Baker's Cyst)

Fig. 9–1. Bursa of the knee region: The suprapatellar, prepatellar, infrapatellar, and adventitial bursae lie anteriorly; the anserine bursa and the sartorius bursa (not shown) are located on the medial aspect; posteriorly, the large popliteal (Baker's cyst) may originate from the gastrocnemius or semimembranosus bursa.

ment. Pain posterior to the knee joint may result from a shortened hamstring, a popliteal cyst, or tendinitis. Pain at the lateral aspect of the knee joint may represent bursitis adjacent to the head of the fibula, arthritis, or internal derangement of the lateral compartment of the knee. Pain anterior to the knee is strongly suggestive of patellofemoral disturbances or derangements of the quadriceps mechanism. Although pain location is helpful, referred pain may be present and confuse the diagnosis. Burning, throbbing, or other neuritic-like symptoms may result from reflex sympathetic dystrophy in the knee region,[5] or from a prepatellar neuralgia.[6]

Physical Examination. A careful examination includes evaluation of the appearance of the extremity when the patient is lying, rising, standing, and walking. Some specific physical examination maneuvers that assist in determining the integrity of the internal knee structures are described. A more comprehensive discussion and description of post-traumatic knee problems is beyond the scope of this book, and the interested reader may find the article by Hughston of value.[7]

While the patient is standing with feet slightly apart and parallel (pointing directly forward), the clinician may note congenital abnormalities, including genu recurvatum (excessive backward joint mobility), patella alta (a high-riding patella), or abnormal patellar alignment, when viewed in relation to the tibial tubercle. From the frontal view, the patellae each may point away from the midline, denoting lateral patellar subluxation ("grasshopper eye patellae"); this often occurs in association with chondromalacia patellae.[2,8]

Genu valgum* (knockknee) may also predispose to lateral patellar dislocation or displacement. Displacement may be observed as the seated patient straightens the knee and the patella moves outward instead of straight upward. Prepatellar bursitis, synovitis with suprapatellar fullness, or a Baker's cyst may be apparent by observation while the patient is standing. Pes planus (flatfootedness) may give rise to knee region discomfort and should be noted. The patient should be observed while rising from a seated position without the use of hands for assistance; this is a simple test for the integrity of the quadriceps extensor mechanism, but may also suggest knee disorders located in the patellofemoral region, or primary muscle disease. Inspection and palpation of the knee may reveal a relatively painless chronic granular cellulitis in the patellar region, as seen in coal miners (the beat knee).[10] Chronic prepatellar bursal thickening occurs in relation to certain occupations, such as carpet laying (Fig. 9–2).

The joint capsule is supported on each side by complex medial and lateral collateral ligament systems,[7,11] and inadequacy of these structures may result in excessive sideway motion. Cruciate ligament insufficiency is associated with excessive anteroposterior motion. If there is any suggestion of instability, stress testing is important to help define the problem. Post-traumatic ligamentous instability that is not treated may lead to quadriceps atrophy, which complicates the clinical presentation.

Stress testing includes the collateral ligament stress test for excessive medial or lateral movement, and the "drawer tests" for anteroposterior instability. The collateral ligament stress tests are performed by the examiner first grasping the involved leg with the knee in full extension (Fig. 9–3); the test is then repeated with the knee flexed 30 degrees. The examiner attempts to deviate the foreleg away from the midline inwardly and outwardly (varus, valgus respectively). Performing the maneuver with the knee extended tests the integrity of both the posterior cruciate and collateral ligaments; repeating the stress

---

*The terms varus, or valgus, through common usage, imply inward or outward deviation respectively. Recent discussions in the literature have emphasized that these commonly used terms are inaccurate.[9] Accordingly, it is usually best to add additional descriptions when defining changes related to these anatomic deviations.

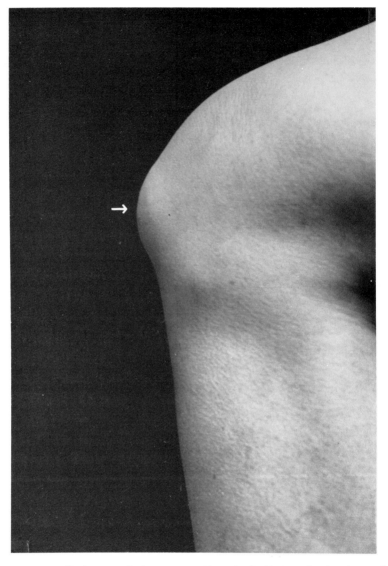

Fig. 9–2. Prepatellar bursitis: The bursitis is visible and palpable superficial to the patella.

test with the knee bent tests the collateral ligaments alone. The examiner observes for opening or widening of the medial or lateral joint compartment. Stress tests may be misleading if reflex spasm from pain prevents relaxation during the examination.

The anterior drawer sign is performed with the patient supine, the hip flexed 45 degrees, and the patient's head supported on a pillow; otherwise, should the patient arise to look forward, the hamstring

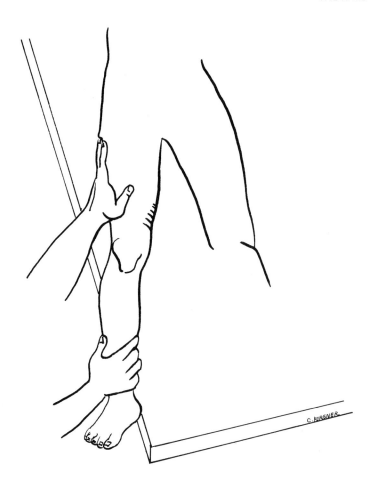

Fig. 9–3. The valgus stress test: When the examiner attempts to deviate the knee into a valgus position with the knee extended, the integrity of both the posterior cruciate and the medial collateral ligaments is tested; repeating the test with the knee bent tests the collateral ligament alone.

muscles may become tense. The involved knee is flexed approximately 80 to 90 degrees, and the foot is stabilized by the examiner sitting on it. The hamstrings should be relaxed. The tibia is gently pulled and pushed straight in and out, anterior and posterior, back and forth. The maneuver should be performed separately with the foot in the straight-forward or neutral position, then with the foot rotated internally, and lastly with the foot rotated externally. Both legs should be compared. Excessive anterior motion supports a diagnosis of insufficiency of the anterior cruciate ligament or of the medial portion of the joint capsule. Instability may be graded from 1 to 3+; greater than 5 mm of excess motion equals 1+ instability; greater than 10 mm equals 3+ instability.[7]

The posterior drawer sign is determined passively by observing whether the tibia is displaced posteriorly while the patient is resting in the same position as described for the anterior drawer sign. The examiner then grasps the tibia and attempts to displace it further posteriorly. A positive posterior drawer sign detects insufficiency of the posterior cruciate ligament.[12]

The McMurray sign and the Apley grinding maneuver may help distinguish a torn meniscus from other causes of internal knee derangement. The McMurray test is performed by acutely flexing the symptomatic knee, so that the heel of the involved extremity approximates the buttock. The examiner then grasps the ankle and straightens the tibia, while rotating the tibia medially and then laterally. A palpable or auditory click represents a positive test.[2,11,13] The Apley grinding maneuver is performed with the patient prone (on the stomach); the knee is flexed 80 to 90 degrees. The examiner then presses down upon the foot and foreleg while rotating them. Pain, clicking, or locking are noted if the Apley grinding maneuver is positive.[2] This usually indicates a derangement of the meniscus or articular surface rather than the ligament complex.

Sometimes a patient provides a history of the knee "giving way" but stress tests reveal only slight or no abnormal motion. In such patients a diagnosis of hypermobility syndrome with disuse quadriceps weakness should be considered; signs of hypermobility elsewhere in the musculoskeletal system should be sought.[1,11,14,15] Similar symptoms may result from patellofemoral disturbances (see "Disturbances of the Patella," this chapter).

Loose bodies (joint mice) may cause symptoms similar to that of a torn meniscus with sensations of locking, grating, giving way, and swelling of the knee. The loose body may represent a chondral or osteochondral fragment, meniscus material,[4] or a sequestered fragment from an osteochondritis dissecans lesion.[16] Radiographic evidence may not be apparent if the fragment is of cartilaginous origin or is hidden in the posterior compartment. Occasionally, a loose body may be the first sign of synovial chondromatosis. Periodic giving way or locking, without apparent injury, strongly suggests the presence of a loose body.

QUADRICEPS MECHANISM DERANGEMENT

Quadriceps Muscle and Tendon Disruption

In young athletes the extensor quadriceps mechanism consists of strong tendons so that rupture generally involves the muscle mass. In older persons rupture usually occurs at the tendinous portion.[11] The injury generally occurs during forced knee joint flexion with a contracted quadriceps. Swelling occurs above the patella and the patient notes various degrees of loss of extension activity of the knee joint. With complete rupture at any age, immediate surgical repair is recommended. Occasionally a partial muscle rupture occurs with less severe trauma. In such patients, acute pain, swelling, and hemorrhage occur, but knee extension is possible. These patients are treated by immobilization in extension, followed by gentle physical therapy and exercise.[11]

Disuse Atrophy

This is one of the most common disorders leading to knee joint instability. It occurs secondary to other knee joint disturbances,

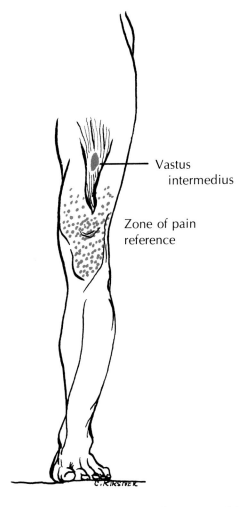

Vastus
intermedius

Zone of pain
reference

Fig. 9–4. A myofascial trigger point in the region of the insertion of the vastus intermedius may cause pain in the anterior lower leg and knee region.

including rheumatoid arthritis and osteoarthritis. Often disuse quadriceps atrophy results from the chronic use of hands to assist in the act of rising from the seated position. Middle-aged and elderly persons should be advised to use their thighs, not their hands when rising from a chair. This prophylactic advice may prevent a significant number of chronic painful knee joint disabilities. Often a trivial self-limited knee joint disturbance becomes a major disability because of disuse quadriceps atrophy or myofascial pain (Fig. 9–4). Resistant quadriceps exercise may be performed by patients at any age in the comfort of their home, and does not require frequent physical therapy supervision (Fig. 9–5). Hip stretching is helpful in patients with a taut vastus intermedius (Fig. 9–6).

Acute Calcific Quadriceps Tendinitis

Pain in the region of the suprapatellar pouch may be associated with calcification in the region of the quadriceps tendon, particularly at the superior pole of the patella (anterosuperior patellar whiskers). These radiographic findings may be seen in patients without symptoms; when associated with chronic knee pain, such patients frequently have evidence of degenerative joint disease.[17] Accordingly, the calcification may be an asymptomatic coincidental finding. The possibility that calcific quadriceps tendinitis is related to calcific tendinitis in other joint areas as a general metabolic disturbance has been suggested.[17]

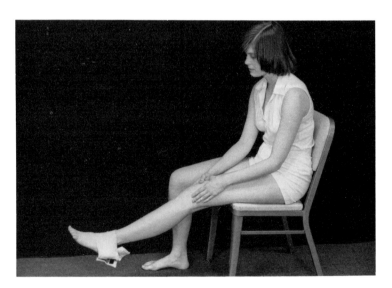

Fig. 9–5. Resistance quadriceps exercise: Utilizing weights ranging from 10 to 30 or more pounds, the arc of movement must be determined for each patient depending on comfort and tolerance. Often the patient notes an arc that achieves maximum results.

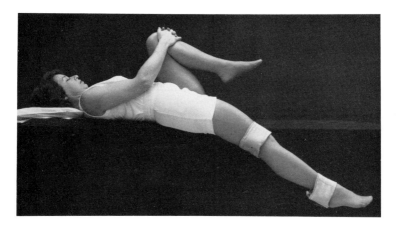

Fig. 9–6. Stretching the hip flexors and quadriceps mechanism for patients with myofascial knee region pain.

DISTURBANCES OF THE PATELLA

Patellar region pain results from a number of complex problems; most of them respond well to nonsurgical treatment. These disorders include the patellofemoral pain syndrome, infrapatellar fat pad disturbances, infrapatellar tendinitis and bursitis, prepatellar bursitis, and prepatellar neuralgia. Patellar dysfunction may also result from contracture or insufficiency of the quadriceps mechanism, the hypermobility syndrome, or contracture of the iliotibial band. The disorders described often are symptomatic only because of injury or misuse, and although mild structural disturbances may coexist, symptoms respond to treatment with restoration of stability to the limb.

The Patellofemoral Pain Syndrome. This syndrome is characterized by pain and crepitation in the region of the patella during activities that require knee flexion under load conditions, such as stair climbing. Joint swelling may be seen; symptoms are often intermittent.[18] Primary idiopathic adolescent chondromalacia, post-traumatic adolescent chondromalacia, "patellofemoral syndrome of adolescents and young adults," and "adult chondromalacia with secondary degenerative joint disease" are various terms for a group of disorders with similar symptoms. Underlying etiologic disturbances include malalignment of the quadriceps with lateral displacement of the patella,[4] an abnormal medial patellar facet,[19] the patella alta, and the hypermobility syndrome. Chondromalacia of the patella is a prominent associated finding. The exact relationship of patellofemoral crepitation to the presence of pain is debatable.[4,18,19]

In one study of "normal" students, more than half had patellofemoral crepitation unrelated to the presence or absence of patellar pain.[18] The "cinema sign" describes patellofemoral pain following prolonged sitting with knees in flexion, relieved by subsequent knee extension.[11]

Physical findings suggestive of the patellofemoral pain syndrome include reproduction of pain when the examiner presses the patella against the femur during knee motion, or detecting tenderness over the medial articulating surface of the patella. Patellofemoral crepitation during knee flexion and extension is usually palpable.[19] Pain may be reproduced by patellofemoral compression with the knee flexed or straight as the patella is pushed from side to side (Perkin's test).[2,11] The examiner must avoid squeezing the synovium during the examination. The young adult or teenager with patellofemoral pain should be observed for lateral patellar displacement (dislocation or subluxation) during knee flexion and extension.

Lateral displacement of the patella can be detected by having the patient seated, and the examiner's index finger and thumb positioned upon the lateral and medial upper borders of the patient's patella. The examiner observes and palpates for lateral patellar displacement as the flexed knee is extended; this finding is commonly seen in patients with hypermobility syndrome. "Grasshopper eye patellae" is a term in which the patellae point outward from the midline, suggesting the appearance of grasshopper's eyes when viewed from the front.[2] This correlates with lateral patellar subluxation and chondromalacia.

Hoffa's Disease. This syndrome refers to hypertrophy of the infrapatellar fat pad in young persons after mild injury. The infrapatellar fat pad may then become impinged between the femur and tibia when the flexed knee is suddenly extended. Pain is localized and occurs during weight-bearing knee activity. Symptoms simulate internal knee derangements, but locking does not occur. Physical examination reveals swelling on either side of the infrapatellar ligament, and quadriceps atrophy may be seen.[13] Hypertrophy of the infrapatellar fat pad may be recurrent as a premenstrual syndrome.

Infrapatellar Tendinitis. This disorder is common in persons with lateral patellar displacement or malrotations of the tibia or fibula.[1] Infrapatellar pain or crepitation may result from jumping in athletic endeavors (Jumper's knee).[2] Infrapatellar bursitis causes similar discomfort in the infrapatellar region.

Traumatic Prepatellar Neuralgia.[6] This type of neuralgia follows trauma to the anterior patella and may be preceded by transient prepatellar swelling. After a few weeks, exquisite tenderness occurs over the medial outer border of the patella at the site of emergence of the neurovascular bundle; even slight stroking is exquisitely painful. Treatment with a local anesthetic or corticosteroid injection into the point of maximum tenderness is usually helpful.[6,11]

Etiology. These patellofemoral disturbances are often associated with conditions that result in a change in the angle of pull of the patellar tendon. Such disturbances include malrotation of the tibia or femur, alteration of the quadriceps muscle, abnormal position of the iliotibial band, or malformation in the posterior surface of the patellae or femoral condyles. Symptoms may also result from chronic trauma, such as repeated scrubbing of floors on hands and knees. Hypermobility syndrome has been noted as a predisposing disorder. Degenerative pathologic findings of cartilage softening and fissuring are frequently noted; there is often a lack of correlation between pathologic findings and symptoms.

Laboratory and Radiographic Findings. Inflammatory connective tissue disease is rarely associated with these patellar disturbances. Therefore, tests of inflammation are normal. Radiographic examination should include the tangential patellofemoral roentgenographic techniques (skyline, Hughston views) that best demonstrate the patellar facets and lateral patellar deviation.[4]

Differential Diagnosis. Anterior knee pain in the absence of locking strongly suggests the patellofemoral pain syndromes, but may also occur from a tight hamstring. In the latter instance, straight leg raising to the point of maximum tolerance may reproduce the anterior knee distress.

Management. Conservative measures that are helpful include aspirin or other nonsteroidal anti-inflammatory agents for pain, restriction of competitive activities or overuse, weight reduction for obese patients, and resistance quadriceps strengthening exercises.[8] Bracing with an elastic support and a lateral felt pad may also be tried. A trial of isometric quadriceps strengthening exercises with maximum resistance is essential. The leg should be almost in full extension as the quadriceps exercise is performed.

Disturbances of the infrapatellar fat pad, infrapatellar ligament, and the infrapatellar bursa usually respond to rest followed by graded resistance quadriceps exercise; relief usually requires many weeks of therapy. Injecting the infrapatellar fat pad with a local anesthetic-corticosteroid is rarely needed. If necessary, the injection is administered from a lateral approach; the needle should rest well beneath the tendon (Fig. 9–7). The tendon must not be penetrated as future tendon rupture may occur. These patients rarely require more than one injection. *Athletes or persons who must kneel repeatedly should not be given a local corticosteroid injection.*[20] Management also requires recognition and prevention of aggravating factors, such as improper kneeling, working on the hands and knees excessively, and prolonged sitting.

Outcome and Additional Suggestions. Adolescents with patellofemoral pain syndrome (chondromalacia patellae) frequently have spontaneous improvement without residual disturbance.[1,11,18,19] As

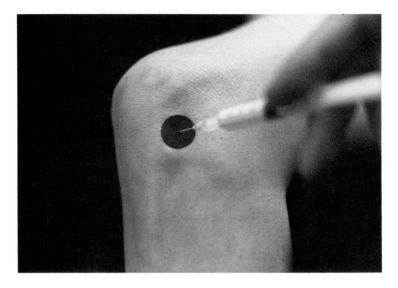

Fig. 9–7. Injection for disturbances of the infrapatellar region must be performed with the needle well beneath the infrapatellar tendon. Furthermore, patients receiving such an injection must be warned to limit stressful activities for several weeks in order to avoid tendon disruption.

mentioned, the key to managing patellar disturbances is to maintain a strong quadriceps mechanism with normal alignment.

In patients in whom symptoms are resistant to conservative programs, surgical intervention may be indicated. Surgery may have to be directed toward the underlying basic abnormality, such as patella alta or recurrent subluxation with hypermobility. Other corrections may have to be directed toward more general problems, such as genu valgum or tibial torsion. Surgery may have to be directed as well toward any chondromalacia present. Therapeutic procedures for the latter include patellar shaving, drilling, and rarely, patellectomy. When chondromalacia patellae is associated with lateral patellar displacement or dislocation, the future development of osteoarthritis may be prevented or retarded by surgical repair.[11,21]

Although surgery may be indicated at times, quadriceps setting exercises and associated conservative management measures often result in pain relief in patients with patellofemoral pain syndrome. We strongly encourage an intensive trial of conservative therapeutic modalities for all patients with this entity.

BURSITIS ABOUT THE KNEE

At least 12 bursae regularly occur in the knee region: the suprapatellar, prepatellar, infrapatellar, and an adventitious cutaneous bursa lie in the anterior knee region; the gastrocnemius and semimembranosus bursae are located in the posterior region and often give rise to a popliteal (Baker's) cyst; the sartorius and anserine bursae lie medially; three bursae lie adjacent to the fibular collateral ligament[22] and the popliteus tendon in the lateral region of the knee.[11,13,23-25] Not to be forgotten is the "no name-no fame" bursa of Stuttle,[26] located at the front edge of the anterior fibers of the medial (tibial) collateral ligament.

Bursitis is characterized by pain, which is aggravated by motion and which at times is worse at night. Point tenderness is present over the involved bursa; active motion may or may not be limited. Inspection may immediately reveal a swollen prepatellar bursa. *Prepatellar* bursitis may be a chronic condition secondary to certain occupations, such as coal mining, farming, or activities performed by overconscientious housewives.[25] The "no name-no fame" bursa may be palpable during knee flexion when the examiner feels a small tender rounded nodule jumping onto the leading edge of the medial collateral ligament.[26] Another bursa, the adventitious cutaneous bursa, may be palpable as a swelling over the tibial tuberosity.[13] Popliteal bursitis is discussed under the commonly used term "Baker's cyst" in this chapter.

Anserine bursitis should be suspected when pain occurs in the medial knee region. It is often bilateral, and may accompany panniculitis in obese postmenopausal females.[24] Osteoarthritis often is present and may predispose to bursitis. Pain originating in the medial collateral ligament may also coexist. Pain of both anserine bursitis and medial collateral ligament disease is worse with activity. Pain at night is more characteristic of anserine bursitis.

Etiology. Bursitis about the knee often occurs in females. Pes planus may be a predisposing cause for bursitis in the medial knee region.[26] The suprapatellar bursa and the posterior bursae often communicate with the knee joint. Swelling of these "pouches" often reflects synovial swelling due to inflammatory arthritis or internal derangement of the true knee joint; the most common cause is rheumatoid arthritis.[13] None of the bursae in the medial or lateral knee regions communicate with the synovial cavity; therefore, inflammatory joint disease rarely is related to inflammation of these bursae.[24] Women with large fat panniculi overlying the medial knee joint may present with pain that is worse at night; this nocturnal pain should alert the physician to the presence of an anserine bursitis deep to the panniculus. Whether pressure from the panniculus is significant in the cause of anserine bursitis is unknown. Following treatment, the bursitis seldom recurs despite the continued presence of the panniculus.

Laboratory and Radiographic Examination. Prepatellar bursitis, though usually secondary to pressure phenomenon, may also result from infection. Aspiration of prepatellar bursa fluid for white cell count and differential, gram stain, sugar, culture and sensitivity determination, and crystal identification are diagnostically indicated. In acute knee bursitis of local origin, tests for systemic inflammation are normal. Radiographic examination is seldom abnormal but may reveal osteoarthritis consistent with age. Calcific tendinitis and bursal calcification may rarely be seen. Chondrocalcinosis with pseudogout syndrome may occur in elderly patients with bursitis, but the findings are likely coincidental.

Differential Diagnosis. Diagnosing acute bursitis is seldom a problem. Swelling in the region of the bursa may also result from tumors of the bursae, including osteochondromatosis, villonodular synovitis, xanthomatosis, and synovioma.[11]

A patient with osteonecrosis of the femur may present with medial compartment knee pain that is constant (day and night). Radiographic features may be normal. Radionuclide imaging with strontium 85 or technetium 99 reveals a localized increased area of uptake in the involved femoral condyle.[27]

Management. Nonseptic bursitis about the knee responds readily to reduction in local pressure and local corticosteroid-anesthetic injections[24] (Fig. 9–8). Patients with bursitis in the medial aspect of the knee should sleep with a small cushion placed between the thighs so that the opposite knee does not rest upon the medial aspect of the involved knee. Use of kneeling pads is important for miners and other persons whose occupations expose them to prepatellar bursitis. Septic bursitis requires the use of parenteral antibiotics and immobilization. Aspiration and open drainage may be required. Recurrence of infection should lead to consideration of total bursal excision during the quiescent phase of the disease.

Outcome and Additional Suggestions. Chronic bursitis about the knee is rarely encountered; it is limited mostly to the prepatellar bursa.[25] Gout, rheumatoid arthritis, and villonodular synovitis are differential diagnostic entities that should be considered in patients with bursitis. As noted, surgical excision may be indicated in chronic bursitis.[25]

POPLITEAL CYST (BAKER'S CYST)

Swelling in the posterior aspect of the knee (in the popliteal fossa) may occur in children and adults. In children, the cyst is usually congenital and usually disappears spontaneously after a prolonged period of observation; surgery is rarely indicated.[28] In adults, a Baker's cyst is usually secondary to underlying disease of the knee joint, such as internal derangements, osteoarthritis, or rheumatoid arthritis. The patient frequently presents with aching discomfort in the popliteal region, leg, and calf. The discomfort is aggravated by walking, and

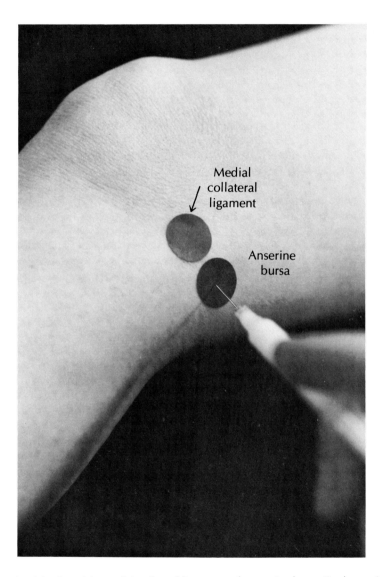

Medial
collateral
ligament

Anserine
bursa

Fig. 9–8. Injection of the medial collateral ligament or the anserine bursa: Tenderness in the medial region of the knee may result from one or both structures, and with the needle used as a probe, points of maximum tenderness should be injected. A 1½-inch No. 22 or No. 23 needle is appropriate.

often relieved by rest. Frequently the patient reports the presence of an egg-shaped mass behind the knee (Fig. 9–9).

When a Baker's cyst is suspected but not certain after physical examination, have the patient perform the hamstring stretching exercise using a 4-foot length of rope to pull the leg up in the air (Fig. 9–10); this results in a more readily palpable cyst. Needle aspiration of the Baker's cyst reveals fluid ranging from jelly-like consistency or cholesterol-laden fluid to acute inflammatory fluid, depending on the presence of underlying inflammatory disease in the knee joint. A large-bore (15 gauge) needle may be needed for aspiration.

Occasionally a Baker's cyst ruptures acutely before the physician has been consulted. This may occur with any activity, but is especially common during repetitive squatting movements, such as taking inventory or redoing the stock in a store. Patients with a *ruptured Baker's cyst* present with features suggestive of thrombophlebitis. They may have minimal or no synovitis in the knee, the cyst is often no longer palpable, and swelling, heat, and diffuse tenderness of the calf and posterior foreleg is evident.

A Homan's sign, suggestive of phlebitis, may be positive. At this point it is apparent that the diagnosis may be uncertain, and the differential between a ruptured popliteal cyst and acute phlebitis is an

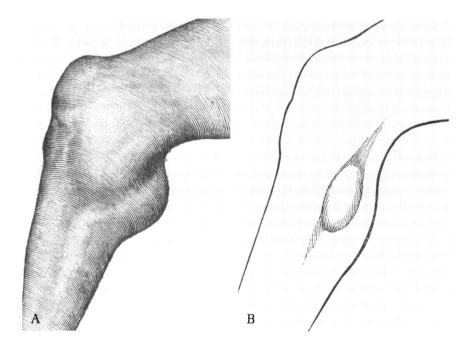

Fig. 9–9. Popliteal (Baker's cyst) bursitis. Reprinted from the original report by W.M. Baker. Saint Bartholomew's Hospital Reports, London, 1877.

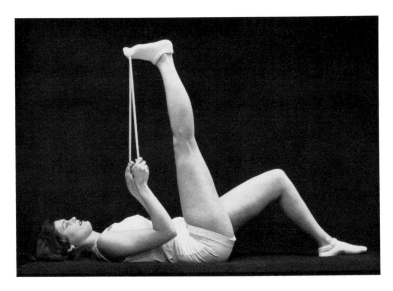

Fig. 9–10. Hamstring and posterior leg muscle stretching may be helpful by providing a more readily palpable popliteal bursa. Hamstring stretching exercise is useful for treatment of posterior myofascial pain disorders of the posterior knee region.

important consideration. In those patients in whom the diagnosis is unclear, venography should be performed to exclude phlebitis to clarify this important question. Contrast pneumoarthrograms reveal evidence of rupture with extravasation of dye into the calf. Although this study is diagnostically confirmatory, it is not always essential if clinical findings are characteristic.

In patients in whom the diagnosis of ruptured cyst has been made, management consists of treatment with bed rest, heat, and elevation. Introduction of local steroids into the joint that has an effusion may be helpful. Nonsteroidal anti-inflammatory agents may also be of assistance. After symptoms have begun to show significant improvement, ambulation can slowly be increased. Patients sometimes demonstrate evidence of both popliteal cyst formation, with or without rupture, and thrombophlebitis. This combined process results when prolonged pressure from the cyst has led to venous stasis.

Management of an uncomplicated Baker's cyst includes aspiration of the contents of the cyst (and of the knee if synovitis is present), and instillation of a corticosteroid-anesthetic mixture into the cyst and joint cavity. A mild pressure bandage applied to the posterior popliteal region is helpful, as are isometric quadriceps exercises. Weightbearing should be minimized for several days or weeks.

The need for surgical excision of the cyst depends on recurrences and the presence of primary disease within the knee joint. Cyst excision without therapy directed to the primary knee disease is usually associated with cyst recurrence. This results from fluid transmission through the one-way valve, which exists in the communication between the knee and cyst. The fluid accumulates in the bursa and is unable to go back into the knee. The bursa gradually descends into the calf; it may rupture and produce further local inflammation. Proper care of the underlying knee joint arthritis or internal derangement is essential.

MISCELLANEOUS DISORDERS OF THE KNEE

Popliteal Region Tendinitis

Tenosynovitis of the popliteal tendon or hamstring may cause pain in the posterior or posterolateral aspect of the knee. Tenderness to palpation with the knee at 90 degrees may be found,[2] and straight leg raising to maximum tolerance can accentuate the tenderness. Palpation during straight leg raising reveals marked tightness in the involved muscles.[29] Corticosteroid-anesthetic injections into points of tenderness often provide prompt relief. Hamstring stretching exercises performed twice daily are helpful.

Pellegrini Stieda Syndrome

Following knee strain, an occasional patient notes progressively worsening symptoms, and knee joint *flexion* becomes restricted. Presumably a soft tissue injury in the region of the medial tibial collateral ligament is followed by *calcification* in this area with permanent obstruction to knee joint motion.[11] Similar medial joint calcification has been reported in the ankle and elbow joint regions.[13] If present, synovitis is usually transient. Palpable indurated swelling in the soft tissues about the femoral condyle, restriction of knee joint flexion, and evidence of calcification on roentgenographic films of the knee joint are noted. Adult males are most commonly affected. The calcification appears 3 to 4 weeks following injury, and has the appearance of a narrow elongated amorphous shadow adjacent to the medial aspect of the femoral condyle (Fig. 9–11). Similar calcification may be seen without symptoms.[11] Pain gradually disappears over a period of months or years. Surgical excision of the bony mass may be considered if symptoms persist.

Iliotibial Band Friction Syndrome

The iliotibial band is a thickened part of the fascia lata that inserts over the lateral tibial condyle. Patients with this syndrome present with pain in the region of the lateral knee joint following vigorous running or hiking. These patients develop a painful limp and experi-

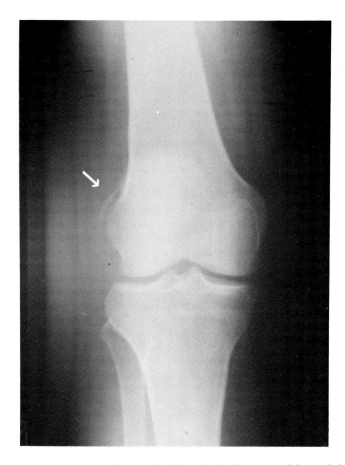

Fig. 9–11. Pellegrini Stieda syndrome of calcification in the region of the medial or lateral tibial collateral ligament. This narrow elongated amorphous shadow adjacent to the femoral condyle may occur in patients with or without symptoms. (Courtesy of Toledo Hospital.)

ence point tenderness over the lateral femoral condyle. Friction is thought to provoke the inflammation. Pain is accentuated by having the patients support all of their weight on the affected leg with the knee bent 30 to 40 degrees. Furthermore, a palpable "creak" during flexion and extension of the knee is noted; this has the consistency of rubbing over a wet balloon.[30] Synovial effusion or excessive lateral joint motion does *not* occur. Nonsteroidal anti-inflammatory drugs and joint rest are helpful. Local corticosteroid injection into the point of insertion may be attempted, if necessary.

Knee problems in runners are often secondary to abnormal foot positions, flatfeet, or high arches. Stretching exercises, proper shoes, and if necessary, an orthotic insert consisting of leather with a molded plastic insert is usually beneficial.[31]

The Plica Syndrome

Folds, pleats, bands, or shelves of synovium are normally present in the knee joint; the term "plica" is used to describe these synovial remnants.[32] The most common remnant is the medial suprapatellar plica originating beneath the quadriceps tendon and extending to the medial wall of the joint. Also common is the infrapatellar plica, which is attached to the intercondylar notch and runs distally to the infrapatellar fat pad. Knee joint pain and effusion often follow a blunt or twisting trauma. Additional features, similar to internal derangement, include a sensation of giving way. During physical examination a palpable snap may occur. Definitive diagnosis is based on demonstrating the plica(e) by arthroscopy or pneumoarthrography. Conservative treatment with hamstring stretching, rest, heat, and anti-inflammatory agents is helpful in some patients; in others the plica can be released during arthroscopy, but the majority require arthrotomy and partial synovectomy.[32]

REFERENCES

1. Grossman RB, Nicholas JA: Common disorders of the knee. Orthop Clin North Am 8:619–640, 1977.
2. James SL: The knee. *In* Musculoskeletal Disorders. Edited by RD D'Ambrosia. Philadelphia, JB Lippincott, 1977.
3. Burry HC: The painful knee. Practitioner *215*:46–54, 1975.
4. Johnson RP, Brewer BJ: Internal derangement of the knee. Arthritis and Allied Conditions. 9th Ed. Edited by DJ McCarty. Philadelphia, Lea & Febiger, 1979.
5. Kim HJ, Kozin F, Johnson RP, Hines R: Reflex sympathetic dystrophy syndrome of the knee following meniscectomy. Arthritis Rheum 22:177–181, 1979.
6. Gordon GC: Traumatic prepatellar neuralgia. J Bone Joint Surg *34B*:41–44, 1952.
7. Hughston JC, Andrews JR, Cross MJ, Moschi A: Classification of knee ligament instabilities. J Bone Joint Surg *58A*:159–172, 1976.
8. Dehaven KE, Dolan WA, Mayer PJ: Chondromalacia patellae and the painful knee. Am Fam Physician *21*:117–124, 1980.
9. Houston CS, Swischuk LE: Varus and valgus—no wonder they are confused. N Engl J Med *302*:471–472, 1980.
10. Sharrard WJ: Aetiology and pathology of beat knee. Br J Ind Med *20*:24–31, 1963.
11. Turek SL: Orthopaedics: Principles and Their Application. 3rd Ed. Philadelphia, JB Lippincott, 1977.
12. Kennedy JC, Roth JH, Walker DM: Posterior cruciate ligament injuries. Orthop Digest *7*:19–31, 1979.
13. Duthie RB, Ferguson AB: Mercer's Orthopedic Surgery. 7th Ed. Baltimore, Williams & Wilkins, 1973.
14. Kirk JA, Ansell BM, Bywaters EGL: The hypermobility syndrome; Musculoskeletal complaints associated with generalized joint hypermobility. Ann Rheum Dis *26*:419–425, 1967.
15. Howorth MB: General relaxation of the ligaments. Clin Orthop *30*:133–143, 1963.
16. Zeman SC, Nielsen MW: Osteochondritis dissecans of the knee. Orthop Rev *7*:101–112, 1978.
17. Trujeque L, Spohn P, Bankhurst A, et al: Patellar whiskers and acute calcific quadriceps tendinitis in a general hospital population. Arthritis Rheum *20*:1409–1412, 1977.
18. Abernethy PJ, Townsend PR, Rose RM, Radin EL: Is chondromalacia patellae a separate clinical entity? J Bone Joint Surg *60B*:205–210, 1978.

19. Goodfellow J, Hungerford DS, Woods C: Patello-femoral joint mechanics and pathology. J Bone Joint Surg 58B:291–299, 1976.
20. Ismail AM, Balakrishnan R, Rajakumar MK: Rupture of patellar ligament after steroid infiltration. J Bone Joint Surg 51B:503–505, 1969.
21. Grana WA, O'Donoghue DH: Patellar-tendon transfer by the slot-block method for recurrent subluxation and dislocation of the patella. J Bone Joint Surg 59A:736–741, 1977.
22. Hendryson IE: Bursitis in the region of the fibular collateral ligament. J Bone Joint Surg 28:446–450, 1946.
23. Moschcowitz E: Bursitis of sartorius bursa: an undescribed malady simulating chronic arthritis. JAMA 109:1362–1364, 1937.
24. Brookler MI, Mongan WS: Relief for the pain of anserina bursitis in the arthritic knee. Cal Med 119:8–10, 1973.
25. Quale JB, Robinson MP: An operation for chronic prepatellar bursitis. J Bone Joint Surg 58B:504–506, 1976.
26. Stuttle FL: The no-name and no-fame bursa. Clin Orthop 15:197–199, 1959.
27. Lotke PA, Ecker ML, Alavi A: Painful knees in older patients. J Bone Joint Surg 59A:617–621, 1977.
28. Dinham JM: Popliteal cysts in children. J Bone Joint Surg 57B:69–71, 1975.
29. Halperin N, Axer A: Semimembranous tenosynovitis. Orthop Rev 9:72–75, 1980.
30. Renne JW: The iliotibial band friction syndrome. J Bone Joint Surg 57A:1110–1111, 1975.
31. Lutter LD: Foot related knee problems, presented to Am Orthopaedic Foot Society, San Francisco. Orthop Rev 8:123–126, 1979.
32. Hardaker WT, Whipple TL, Bassett FH: Diagnosis and treatment of the plica syndrome of the knee. J Bone Joint Surg 62A:221–225, 1980.

Chapter 10

THE FORELEG REGION

Overuse from running, jogging, or other conditioning activities often results in pain syndromes of the lower extremities. Other disorders of diverse or unknown etiology are presented in this chapter with suggestions for safe and empiric therapy.

SHIN SPLINTS

"Shin splints syndrome" is loosely used jargon that has been applied to a symptom complex of pain and discomfort in the lower leg after repetitive overuse, such as in running, jogging, or walking. Discomfort emanates from the lower half of the posteromedial border of the tibia, the anterior tibial compartment, the tibia itself, or the interosseous membrane region of the foreleg. The symptoms are a dull ache followed by a gradually worsening pain, which is at first relieved by rest, and later becomes continuous. Accompanying foreleg pain, numbness or loss of sensation over the fourth toe may be noted. The pain and discomfort in the leg are associated with repetitive running, particularly on a hard surface, or with forcible, excessive use of foot flexors. Usually the pain is confined to the anterior portion of the leg, but the site of involvement may be more diffuse. Tenderness can usually be elicited over symptomatic sites.[1] Stress fractures, tears of musculotendinous structures, or definite ischemic compartment syndromes are important alternate diagnostic considerations.[2,3]

Etiology. Shin splints syndrome often is related to overuse of underdeveloped, untrained muscles, particularly the posterior tibial muscle.[1,2] Small tears at the origin of the muscle or herniation of the muscle through fascia are thought to occur.[3] The lesion may be located at the origin, belly, or musculotendinous junction of the involved muscles.[2]

Differential Diagnosis. If pain is out of proportion to the clinical findings, an intermittent or complete ischemic compartment syndrome should be excluded. A compartment syndrome results from any increased tissue pressure within an anatomic space that compromises the circulation to the compartment.[4-6] It requires a constricting envelope (a constricting fascia or cast) and an increased volume (blood, swelling). Ischemic compartment syndromes that must be distinguished from shin splints include those due to involvement in the anterior tibial compartment.[7] Symptoms related to these ischemic syndromes often begin 10 to 12 hours after unaccustomed exercise, or in association with serious trauma; aching pain in the compartment region is noted. Increased pain in the anterior compartment following passive flexion of the toes is an early sign. Pain, pallor, and pulseless paralysis are late hallmarks of the serious ischemic post-traumatic compartment syndromes. Elevated compartment pressure is a confirmatory diagnostic finding. In addition to ischemic compartment syndrome, fracture and vascular claudication must also be considered in the differential diagnosis of severe shin splints syndrome.[4,7,8]

Management. Stretching followed by strengthening exercises directed to the musculature of the involved site of the leg are helpful. Use of proper footgear is important; runners should avoid running on hard surfaces.

Outcome and Additional Suggestions. Brief rest usually allows the pain to subside, at which time activity may be resumed. Recurrent or persistent pain requires exclusion of a true compartment syndrome or a stress fracture.[7] The latter may be difficult to distinguish from shin splints; bone scans, positive in the presence of stress fracture, are diagnostically helpful.[1,9,9a]

OTHER LEG PAIN AND DYSFUNCTION

Patients may suffer from a partial rupture of one of the calf muscles. Symptoms commonly are due to a tear of the plantaris muscle, but may also result from a partial rupture of any of the other muscles of the popliteal and calf region. The term "tennis leg" has been given to this symptom complex. The patient often perceives a "snap" followed by a sudden burning in the calf; the leg gives way and the patient finds himself on the ground. Examination reveals pain aggravated by passive dorsiflexion of the ankle. Treatment of the partial tear is protective with the use of adhesive strapping to immobilize the ankle in plantarflexion and to limit weight bearing; the use of heat, massage, and gentle exercise are helpful. Limited activity for 3 to 4 weeks is usually needed.[10]

Spontaneous *rupture* of the *posterior tibial tendon* results in pain, tenderness, and swelling behind and below the medial malleolus with loss of foot stability. Often a tenosynovitis characterized by slight swelling behind and beneath the medial malleolus has been present for some time. Lower leg pain after walking is noted.[10]

Osgood Schlatter Disease

Usually seen in boys during periods of rapid growth, patients with this disease present with pain, tenderness, and soft tissue swelling about the tibial tubercle just below the patella. Pain occurs when climbing stairs, kneeling, or kicking in association with quadriceps muscle contraction. The discomfort and swelling usually cease before or by age 18.

The etiology is thought to be traumatic and may result from avulsion of the tibial tubercle during adolescence.[8] Radiographic findings may include fragmentation of the tibial tubercle, soft tissue swelling, avulsion of an ossification center,[8] or avascular necrosis. On the other hand, radiographic study often reveals normal findings.

Treatment includes the use of a cylinder cast for several weeks, avoidance of contact sports, and maintenance of quadriceps strength with cautious use of isometric exercise (10 to 20 pounds, depending on age and size of the patient). The end result is a prominent tubercle that is usually painless. Excision of the fragments is rarely necessary.

Growing Pains

The term "growing pains" attributed to Deschamp in the early 19th century[11] is in fact a misnomer, because the most common age of occurrence is *not* at the time of rapid growth. These pains usually occur around age 8 and disappear by age 12.[12] The discomfort is described as an intermittent annoying pain or ache usually localized to the muscles of the legs and thighs, associated with a feeling of restlessness. These pains do not occur in joint areas and are often bilateral;[11] they often awaken the child from sleep and may be relieved by movement such as walking about the room. A hot tub bath, leg elevation, and leg massage are additional helpful measures. The discomfort is accentuated by running or other strenuous play activities.

Naish and Apley, in a study of British school children, noted leg pain in 5% of the children.[12] Patients identified in the study had a history of nonarticular pain of at least 3 months' duration, and severe enough to cause some limitation of activity. The sexes were equally involved. Except for two children who were found to have tuberculosis, and one child who developed osteochondritis of the knee, the remainder had a confirmed diagnosis of benign leg pain after 1 to 3 years of observation. A family history of rheumatic pain was found in over half the children with growing pains, compared to 10% in a control group. A child with only nocturnal pain often had relatives with only nocturnal pain, whereas children with diurnal pain had a strong family history of diurnal pain. Although no acceptable cause for these pain disturbances has been recognized,[11] a relation to exertion, fatigue, mechanical factors, and structural deficits such as pes planus or scoliosis has been noted.[12]

The differential diagnosis of recurrent pain in the lower limbs in children and adolescents includes trauma, occult infection, avascular necrosis of bone, vascular disturbances, congenital structural disorders, tumors, connective tissue diseases, and the soft tissue rheumatic pain disorders. Workup might include an erythrocyte sedimentation rate, complete blood count, and roentgenogram of the limb and chest if clinically indicated.[11,12] Benign causes of leg pain are usually bilateral, whereas most of the serious disorders with leg pain are unilateral.

Treatment for children with these benign leg pains is empiric. If the leg muscles are tight, gentle hamstring muscle stretching exercises may be beneficial. These should also be done as a warmup before competitive sports. When myofascial trigger points have been found, a vapocoolant spray has been found to be helpful. Improvement with these measures aids in diagnosis of a soft tissue rheumatic pain disorder.[13] Most children seem to improve by age 12.

Infrequently the clinician sees a child or adolescent with leg pain without any distinguishing features; psychogenic factors may have to be considered.[12,14] The clinician should then look for the following:

1. Death of a parent or separation from a significant other person.
2. Marital discord between parents.
3. Family pathology or similar complaints of pain in parents or siblings.
4. Difficulty in school with academic subjects, teachers, or peers.

When an emotionally charged situation has been discovered, therapeutic intervention must focus on the psychosocial disorder as well as on its resulting symptoms. With removal of the emotionally charged situation, the pain or dysfunction state often improves.[14]

Night Cramps

Cramps that involve the legs and feet are probably more common than physicians realize. Effective treatment may be a problem. Patients often do not mention the complaint unless asked. Inappropriate use of folk medicines and snake venom for this and other pain syndromes serves only to emphasize our failure to understand and treat this syndrome adequately.

Benign nocturnal leg and foot aches and cramps may be related to exertion, and often awaken the patient. These patients usually have normal peripheral pulses on examination and no evidence of significant vascular disease. Symptoms have to be differentiated from pain of intermittent claudication, which occurs during limb use and is relieved by rest. Although common in childhood and in the elderly, night cramps occur in all decades of life. Patients with the complaint of nocturnal leg and foot pain and cramp should be carefully examined for structural disorders, including flat feet, genu recurvatum, hypermobility syndrome, and inappropriate leg position during sedentary activity. Patients who sit for prolonged periods or who tuck a leg up under themselves may be predisposed to night cramp.

A history of working on a concrete floor, or having moved to a home built on a cement slab foundation (even with floor coverings) may correlate with the occurrence of leg cramps. Wearing thick crepe-soled shoes is often helpful in such situations. Symptoms frequently recur in clusters. Quinine given at bedtime may be helpful in preventing recurrences. This agent is administered daily at bedtime until the patient has been free of night cramps for several days. Therapy is then discontinued and reinstituted when a new cluster of cramps recurs. In patients allergic to this agent, or who fail to respond, a trial of diphenhydramine (Benadryl) may be of value. Other medications recommended for night cramps include vitamin E,[15] meprobamate, and other simple muscle relaxants.[15-17]

If a structural disorder or muscle contraction is found, muscle stretching or strengthening exercises, and use of long-countered shoes and other proper footgear may be of value. If a cramp occurs, walking or leg "jiggling" followed by leg elevation may be helpful. Leg stretching, by standing 2 to 3 feet out from a wall, placing hands on the wall, then climbing hands up the wall, keeping the heels on the floor,[16] and use of a warm tub bath may be prophylactic. Judicious use of brandy is a time-honored remedy.

Restless Leg Syndrome

Painless, spontaneous, continuous leg movements are often of psychogenic origin,[18] but may also accompany organic disease states. If accompanied by expressions of exquisite pain, they may be of hysterical origin. The use of low-dose tricyclic antidepressant medication and leg stretching exercises have been helpful.[17] Stretching exercises for the posterior leg muscles should be performed before retiring. (See Fig. 9–10, p. 201.)

Night Starts

Although not limited to the leg, sudden jerking contractures of the limbs that occur shortly after falling asleep are common. They awaken the patient, and the severity of the jerky movements is frightening. Upon falling back to sleep, they seldom recur. No definite cause is known. The condition is self-limited, and treatment is reassurance of the benign temporary nature of the disturbance.

Anterior leg pain and a sensation of swelling, which is lateral and inferior to the tibial tubercle, can result from a contracted or tight hamstring muscle. In any event, the pain is *not* articular. The anterior leg pain is reproduced during straight-leg-raising examination, as the leg is forced straight upward. Pain is relieved by exercises that stretch the hamstring muscles (Fig. 9–10, p. 201).

Reflex Sympathetic Dystrophy

As described previously in Chapter 2, throbbing, burning, aching pain following trauma suggests this disorder. The lower limb is less commonly involved, but when it occurs, diagnosis may be difficult. The pain quality is suggestive of the diagnosis if throbbing and burning occur. The limb is often discolored with dependent rubor or cyanotic mottling noted about the entire foot and lower foreleg. The skin is cool, and hyperhidrosis may be present. Diffuse swelling throughout the ankle and forefoot is noted. Radiographic evidence of spotty osteoporosis is suggestive but not diagnostic. A regional sympathetic nerve block is therapeutic and diagnostic. If transient but significant benefit is noted, a series of lumbar sympathetic nerve blocks should be tried, and concomitantly, sedatives and exercise to mobilize the limb should be employed. A short course of prednisone, beginning with doses of 20 to 30 mg daily, may be beneficial.

NODULES

Pseudorheumatoid nodules have already been mentioned in the discussion of the upper extremity regions; they also occur in the pretibial region in infants and children. No articular abnormalities are seen, and the nodule is painless. Recently, a "hidden" 19 S IgM rheumatoid factor that is complement-fixing has been detected in the sera of such patients.[19] No treatment is necessary. *Surfer's nodules* also may occur in the pretibial foreleg region. They result from activities in which the foreleg and the hyperextended ankle are brought in contact with a hard surface. Recurrent bumping from a surf board is a known cause. The lesions may resemble rheumatoid nodules. Avoiding surface contact is curative. Similar nodules can occur on children's forefeet if they repeatedly sit on their legs with their feet plantarflexed and in contact with hardwood floors.

REFERENCES

1. Baugher WH, Balady GJ, Warren RF, Marshall JL: Injuries of the musculoskeletal system in runners. Contemp Orthop *1*:46–54, 1979.
2. Slocum DB: The shin splint syndrome. Am J Surg *114*:875–881, 1967.
3. Garfin S, Murbarak SJ, Owen CA: Exertional anterolateral-compartment syndrome. J Bone Joint Surg *59A*:404–405, 1977.
4. Matsen FA: Compartmental syndromes. N Engl J Med *300*:1210–1211, 1979.
5. Mubarak SJ, Hargens AR, Owen CA, et al: The wick catheter technique for measurement of intramuscular pressure. J Bone Joint Surg *58*:1016–1019, 1976.
6. Mubarak, SJ, Owen CA: Double-incision fasciotomy of the leg for decompression in compartment syndromes. J Bone Joint Surg *59*:184–187, 1977.
7. Matsen FA: Compartmental syndromes. Hosp Pract *15*:113–117, 1980.
8. Turek SL: Orthopaedics; Principles and Their Application. 3rd Ed. Philadelphia, JB Lippincott, 1977.

9. Norfray JF, Schlachter L, Kernahan WT, et al: Early confirmation of stress fractures in joggers. JAMA *243*:1647–1649, 1980.

9a. Brady DM: Running injuries. Clin Symp 32 *4*:2–36, 1980.

10. Pinals RS: Traumatic arthritis and allied conditions. *In* Arthritis and Allied Conditions. 9th Ed. Edited by DJ McCarty. Philadelphia, Lea & Febiger, 1979.

11. Peterson HA: Leg aches. Pediatr Clin North Am *24*:731–736, 1977.

12. Naish JM, Apley J: "Growing pains": A clinical study of non-arthritic limb pains in children. Arch Dis Child *26*:134–140, 1951.

13. Bates T, Grunwaldt E: Myofascial pain in childhood. J Pediatr *53*:198–209, 1958.

14. Caghan SB, McGrath MM, Morrow MG, Pittman LD: When adolescents complain of pain. Nurse Pract *3*:19–22, 1978.

15. Ayres S, Mihan R: Nocturnal leg cramps (systremma). South Med J *67*:1308–1312, 1974.

16. Daniell HW: Simple cure for nocturnal leg cramps. N Engl J Med *301*:216, 1979.

17. Lee HB: Cramp in the elderly. Br Med J *2*:1259, 1976.

18. Smythe HA: Nonarticular rheumatism and psychogenic musculoskeletal syndromes. *In* Arthritis and Allied Conditions. 9th Ed. Edited by DJ McCarty. Philadelphia, Lea & Febiger, 1979.

19. Moore TL, Dorner RW, Zuckner J: Complement-fixing hidden rheumatoid factor in children with benign rheumatoid nodules. Arthritis Rheum *21*:930–934, 1978.

Chapter *11*

THE ANKLE AND FOOT

From the Madison Avenue slogan "clothes make the man," one should conclude "shoes make the foot." However, although improper shoes may produce a multitude of forefoot and toe problems, they should not be incriminated in all painful soft tissue disorders of the foot. Improper shoes can cause or exacerbate hallux valgus, hammertoes, hard corns, and plantar keratoses. Proper shoes should provide comfort (proper fit) for the weightbearing foot, room for the toes to fully extend, and lack of crowding of the foot.[1] "First and foremost one should remember that the shoe should protect the foot, not disturb it."[2]

Every physician is familiar with problems created by the narrow-toed, high-heeled contemporary female dress shoe. In the last 20 years, greater strides have been made by shoe manufacturers to provide reasonable covering for the foot: a cushion or crepe sole for walking on concrete floors, a toe box with adequate space, and lacing or straps that hold the foot in the shoe.[3] The "earth shoe" relieves metatarsal weightbearing and returns the weightbearing line of vertical force to the more normal position just anterior to the ankle joint (Fig. 11–1). This has been reported to be helpful for a number of painful disturbances of the *forefoot*.[3] Adapting shoes to the patient can be a valuable contribution to the comprehensive treatment of rheumatic diseases of the foot.[4] Because weight should be borne evenly between the heel and the toe and more toward the first metatarsal, shoes may require modification to correct minor structural disorders that change this weightbearing distribution.[5] Some basic features of "specialized" shoes include a heavier rib steel shank that provides rigidity to the forefoot, a long counter to within ⅝ inch of the first metatarsophalangeal joint for support of the longitudinal arch, and a Thomas heel that projects forward on the medial side. These features maintain the arch and prevent the heel from turning out (valgus heel).[6]

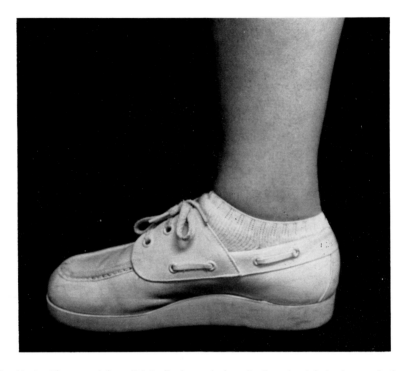

Fig. 11–1. The neutral shoe: Originally the earth shoe distributed weight back upon the heel. Modification of the principle resulted in the neutral shoe, which shifts weight off the metatarsophalangeal joint region toward the ankle. A slightly rounded sole may also act as a rocker bar. The neutral shoe may be helpful for patients with metatarsalgia or rheumatoid arthritis of the forefoot.

A combination last represents a shoe three widths smaller in the heel than in the forefoot area.[6] Shoe modifications, including extra depth to provide insoles or inlays, are discussed throughout this chapter.

The diagnosis of most foot and ankle disorders is aided by the fact that the bones are palpable, the soft tissues can be tested for their supporting functions, and vascular changes are readily apparent.[7] The foot consists of 28 bones and 57 articulations that provide the ability to walk on any surface, to run, or to jump. The intrinsic muscles of the foot provide all the means necessary for grasping. The articulating bones and joints provide the longitudinal arch.[8]

The Examination. Foot complaints must be assessed in a logical sequence in order to determine local versus systemic causes, or traumatic, genetic, or acquired disturbances. The quality of pain should help distinguish neuropathic types of discomfort (burning, tingling) from the more common deep-aching symptoms of tissue strain or injury. When symptoms are intermittent rather than persistent, further inquiry should include the type of flooring in the home or job, any recent change in occupation that might require prolonged standing, or whether recent recovery from a protracted illness has occurred. New activities such as jogging, racquetball, or other impact foot activities should be discussed.

Inspection of the foot while the patient is seated includes noting skin color, hair distribution on the foot and foreleg, presence of a normal arch, forefoot width, and the presence of calluses and other dermatologic features. Next, with the patient standing, the physician looks for spinal curvatures, pelvic tilt, femoral or tibial torsion, patellae rotating away from the midline, and the direction of the weightbearing foot. The flatfoot is accompanied by pronation, a tilting outward of the foot, and valgus deviation of the heel. This can be seen best by inspecting the foot from behind the standing patient. From the frontal view, a line carried from the midpoint of the patella down the anterior spine of the lower tibia should project forward through the web between the second and third toes.

While the patient is standing, the physician should look for toe deformities, particularly hallux valgus, metatarsus primus varus of the

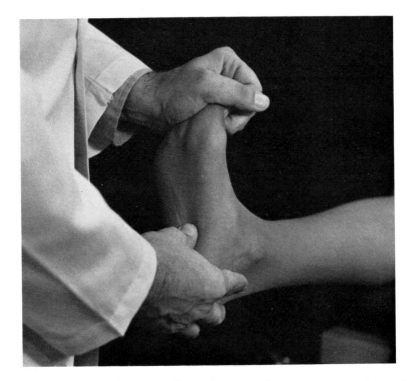

Fig. 11–2. Examination of the plantar fascia: The toes are drawn into extension, thus tensing the bands of the plantar fascia. Palpation reveals points of induration and tenderness. The two feet should be compared.

first toe (the first metatarsus is shortened and deviated to the midline, and the toe is rotated slightly medially as noted by the slant of the toe nail), and for evidence of toe crowding. With the patient lying supine the examiner should next determine the rigidity or softness of the plantar fascia. This is performed by grasping the toes and dorsiflexing them with one hand while palpating the plantar aspect of the foot, particularly the bands comprising the plantar fascia. Only by examining many normal feet can the physician become familiar with the pathologic tightly bound plantar fascia (Fig. 11–2). The assessment of the circulation and neurologic status of the foot should complete the examination.

SOFT TISSUE INJURY OF THE ANKLE

Sprains

The most common problems of the soft tissue-supporting structures of the ankle joint are sprains. The ligamentous structures of the medial side of the ankle are less commonly injured than those of the lateral side. Sprains may be subclassified into 3 types: type 1 is a mild stretching of the ligament with the fibers still intact; type 2 is a more severe injury with partial disruption of the fibers of the ligaments; and type 3 is a complete disruption of the ligament. The more severe sprains should be referred to an orthopedic surgeon.

The lateral-collateral ligaments, composed of the anterior talofibular ligament, the posterior talofibular ligament, and the calcaneofibular ligament are most commonly involved in ankle sprains.[9] Usually the patient notes pain associated with an inverted ankle, and has a sensation of "giving way" of the ankle. Pain is increased upon forced-ankle inversion. The examiner can palpate for tenderness and often determines which portion of the ligament is involved. The medial collateral ligament (the deltoid ligament) can also suffer sprain; gentle eversion accentuates this pain. Swelling, local tenderness, and ecchymosis may occur and weightbearing becomes painful.

Management of type 1 sprain includes immediate application of cold with compression, elevation, and rest for the first 24 to 48 hours. In most cases, radiographic examination to exclude body injury should be carried out. Special radiographic procedures including arthrography and stress roentgenographs may be needed to define the extent of injury.[10] In mild injury when the edema subsides, adhesive strapping or elastic support should be accomplished and continued until symptoms subside. A corticosteroid-anesthetic mixture may be injected into the region of the injury if symptoms persist.[9,11] *Chronic instability of the ankle joint* often results from the additive damage of multiple "turned ankles;" therefore, proper care of the acute injury is essential.[9,11]

Athletic injuries to the ankle may appear to be trivial, but are important in the context of the athlete's future endeavors.[12] Prevention of further injury includes ankle strapping to limit inversion or eversion, use of elastic ankle supports, and shoes with rigid-toe boxes and firm soles. Following recovery from injury, the athlete should progress from walking to jogging, and then to running in figure eights, with gradually tighter circles in order to test the stability of the ankle before competitive activity is resumed. The patient should be referred to physicians who are expert in this area if the injured joint has not improved within 2 to 3 weeks,[12] or if there is any question about the degree of sprain.

Tendinitis

Inflammation of a tendon sheath about the ankle may result from repetitive activity or unaccustomed extraordinary work.[12,13] Other causes include improper footwear resulting in injury, particularly to the extensor hallucis longus or to the Achilles tendon. The shoe vamp may impinge upon the tendons of the dorsum of the ankle and forefoot, and local heat, redness, and tenderness may occur. Severe or repeated traumatic tenosynovitis may result in scarification and require surgical excision of the tendon sheath.

A chronic nonspecific tendinitis may affect several tendons at the ankle, similar to that seen in DeQuervain's tenosynovitis at the wrist.[9,11,14] Tenosynovitis involving the tibialis anterior, tibialis posterior, extensor digitorum longus, or peroneal tendons at the ankle may occur where the tendons become angulated at the ankle; friction can then cause inflammation of the tendon sheath. A bulbous swelling that occurs distally to areas of constriction is helpful in demonstrating points of constriction.[14] Histologic examination of the tendon sheath demonstrates nonspecific inflammation. Occasionally rheumatoid arthritis, and rarely oxalosis, xanthoma, or giant cell tumors are found.[9,15] Tuberculosis is uncommon in this region.[14] Radiographic abnormalities are usually absent, although new bone formation over the posterior aspect of the medial malleolus has rarely been described.[16] Treatment of tendinitis includes partial immobilization of the ankle with bandaging or an elastic ankle support, and physical therapy to maintain range of motion. Sometimes complete immobilization in a cast is helpful. Tendon sheath injection with a corticosteroid-anesthetic mixture may be tried. Excision of the tendon sheath for diagnosis and treatment is rarely necessary.

Tendon Dislocation

The peroneal tendon is the most commonly dislocated leg tendon. It may become taut and dislocate, and the patient may experience an audible painless snapping sensation in this tendon. Such dislocation occurs in older children, and because walking is not affected, may go unrecognized.[11] The dislocated tendon may be seen lying over the lateral malleolus.[9,11] The patient notes the leg or ankle giving way if the peroneus longus muscle goes into spasm with abduction and plantarflexion of the foot.[17] Occasionally the dislocation may result from trauma; more often it results from a congenital shallowness of the tendon groove located on the posterior surface of the lateral malleolus.[9,11] Usually spontaneous reduction occurs; if not, active reduction may be required. After reducing the dislocation, treatment includes immobilization with a cast for 5 to 8 weeks, which usually results in permanent benefit. Occasionally, surgical intervention to reconstruct the sheath or to deepen the groove is necessary.[11,17]

Disorders of the Achilles Tendon Region

A tight Achilles tendon may result from disuse, from complex factors associated with growth, or more often as a problem occurring in women who wear high-heeled shoes. The patient presents with pain over the heel;[11] dorsiflexion of the ankle increases the pain and tenderness. Gentle progressive heel cord stretching exercise is helpful. This exercise is performed by having the patient stand 3 to 4 feet out from a wall with arms extended toward the wall. The heels are kept firmly planted on the ground and the feet are internally rotated 15 to 30 degrees. The patient then "walks" her hands up the wall until a stretching sensation is felt in the region of the heel; this position is maintained for 1 to 2 minutes. These exercises should be performed

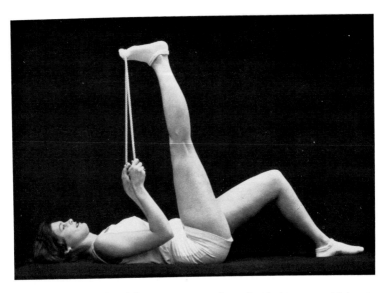

Fig. 11–3. Stretching and mobilizing exercise performed with this non-weightbearing technique is helpful for myofascial disturbances of the lower extremity and foot.

with 10 to 15 repetitions twice daily.[1] The tendon and calf muscles may also be stretched by grasping the forefoot with a loop of rope 3 or 4 feet in length, and then pulling the entire leg straight into the air maintaining the ankle in 90 degrees dorsiflexion. This position can be maintained for 1 minute morning and evening (Fig. 11–3).

Bursitis may involve bursae that lie superficial and deep to the tendon near its insertion onto the calcaneus. Neither deep bursa nor the tendon sheath should be injected because of the possibility of tendon rupture as a result of steroid-induced atrophy. Oral nonsteroidal anti-inflammatory agents are helpful.

Rupture of the Achilles Tendon. Rupture may occur after abrupt calf-muscle contraction. Usually the patient is a male over 30 years of age who sporadically engages in sports. The patient may note an audible snap, followed by pain in the calf as if struck with a baseball. The patient may then be unable to stand up on his toes. The Thompson test may be performed for further evidence of rupture of the Achilles tendon. The patient kneels on a chair with the feet hanging over the edge; when the examiner squeezes the calf muscle on the normal side, the foot responds with plantar flexion. When performing this examination on the suspected side, there is no foot response. Orthopedic consultation for immobilization or surgical repair is necessary.[2]

Adhesive Capsulitis of the Ankle

An adhesive capsulitis may follow an interarticular fracture or other severe injury. Persistent pain and limitation of motion develop. Arthrography is a useful diagnostic test. During arthrography a decreased capacity of the joint is evident. Instillation of a corticosteroid into the ankle and aggressive physical therapy may restore ankle motion.[18]

HEEL PAIN

The following conditions cause heel disturbance or pain: pump bumps, tendinitis, periostitis of the calcaneus, piezogenic papules, apophysitis, retrocalcaneal bursitis, neoplasms, calcaneal spurs, and plantar fasciitis.[9,11,19–22] Referred pain to the heel may result from disease of the subtalar joint or from sciatic nerve impingement.

"Pump bumps" are visible, firm, nodular lesions at the lower end of the tendo Achillis. They are commonly associated with wearing high-heeled pumps or loafers.[9] The bump may be an exostosis of the superior tuberosity of the calcaneus,[2] or may appear as a hatchet-shaped calcaneus with a prominent posterosuperior margin.[21] They often are bilateral and asymptomatic.[2] Occasionally an overlying bursa becomes inflamed.[2] Symptomatic pump bumps are often the result of wearing closely contoured heel counters.[21] The pump bump may also be associated with an adventitial bursitis located at the posterior surface of the calcaneus lateral or medial to the Achilles tendon. Ill-fitting shoes may cause another adventitial bursitis, "last bursitis" located lateral to the heel.[23]

Rheumatoid nodules in this region can be distinguished from pump bumps: the former occur 1 or 2 in. *above* the point of attachment of the tendon to the calcaneus. Conversely, pump bumps are lower down at the superior border of the calcaneus. Treatment includes use of sandals or laced shoes, protective padding, a heel lift, and rarely a corticosteroid injection into the adventitial superficial bursa.[2,9] Conservative therapy is helpful; if not, resection of the posterior prominence of the calcaneus may be necessary.[21] (Table 11–1, p. 233.)

Pain accompanied by exquisite tenderness at the posterior point of the heel may also result from a *bursitis* secondary to calcific tendinitis.[22] Treatment with systemic nonsteroidal anti-inflammatory agents is helpful.

Tenosynovitis or bursitis near the heel are usually acute self-limited disorders. However, if chronic and accompanied by the wearing of boots, the condition is known as "Winter's heel" or "Hagland's disease."[11] Heel pads or molded heel cups are helpful.

Calcaneal periostitis may result from trauma, Reiter's disease, ankylosing spondylitis, psoriatic arthritis, or rheumatoid arthritis.[22] The resulting painful heel may have to be raised 1 to 2 cm with a heel lift for relief.[11] *Calcaneal spurs* develop on the plantar tuberosity, and extend across the entire width of the calcaneum. The apex is imbedded in the plantar fascia. Pain occurs if the apex is angled downward by depression of the long arch.

In the past, an acutely painful heel spur was thought to be a manifestation of gonorrhea. More recent studies have demonstrated the cause to be due to other diseases, such as ankylosing spondylitis, Reiter's syndrome, or rheumatoid arthritis. Heel spurs are more often asymptomatic or innocent bystanders that rarely cause pain themselves. When symptomatic, another mechanical etiology is usually responsible. Plantar fasciitis is a likely cause of heel pain with or without spur formation. Use of shoes with crepe soles, cut-out heels, heel inversion, or arch supports that reduce the forces acting upon the plantar aponeurosis are helpful. A local corticosteroid injection into the point of maximum tenderness is usually helpful.[24]

Herniations of fat that occur as painful papules at the medial inferior border of the heel *(piezogenic papules)* may be noted only upon weightbearing, and are an uncommon cause of painful heels. Weight reduction, use of felt padding, and crepe-soled shoes may provide relief.[20] We have noted these in asymptomatic patients.

In children, heel pain may result from an *apophysitis*, which often follows a change of shoe or increased sports activity. Tenderness at the posterior aspect of the heel and radiographic features of a fluffy, motheaten, flattened, and fragmented apophysis are seen. Treatment includes using a sponge-heel elevation, elastic strapping, avoiding vigorous running, and if necessary, injecting a local corticosteroid.[19]

"Black heel" is a black or bluish-black plaque that usually develops on the heel of the foot. The lesion is oval or circular and may develop on the posterior or posterolateral plantar surfaces of one or both heels. It results from a shearing force during sports that causes intracutaneous bleeding. The lesion is painless, most common in adolescents or young adults, and requires no treatment.[25]

A bursitis at the insertion of the tendo Achillis may also occur in athletes, and requires a change in the heel counter of the athlete's shoe.[9] When an Achilles tendinitis coexists, the heel should be elevated ¼ to ½ inch with heel padding.[1]

PLANTAR FASCIITIS

Plantar fasciitis is one of the most common causes of foot pain.[26] Heel spurs often coexist and may represent a secondary response to an inflammatory reaction. The deep plantar fascia (plantar aponeurosis) is a thick, pearly white tissue with longitudinal fibers intimately attached to the skin. The central portion is thickest and attaches to the medial process of the tuberosity of the calcaneus; distally it divides into five slips, one for each toe.[14] Symptoms include pain in the plantar region of the foot, made worse when initiating walking. A hallmark for diagnosis is local tenderness. Point tenderness along the longitudinal bands of the plantar fascia is best determined by bimanual examination. The examiner dorsiflexes the patient's toes with one hand, pulling the plantar fascia taut. The examiner, with an index finger, palpates along the plantar fascia from the heel to the forefoot (Fig. 11–2). Points of discrete tenderness can be elicited, and may be marked for possible later local corticosteroid injection. The patient should be examined for inflammatory arthritis, the hypermobility syndrome, or pes planus with valgus heel deformity.

Etiology. Strain of the plantar fascia often follows jumping, prolonged standing, or occurs in association with obesity and flatfeet;[9,24] a relation to heel spurs has been noted by most clinicians.[27] In one sizable study of plantar fasciitis,[24] rheumatoid arthritis, gout, and ankylosing spondylitis were diagnosed at the time of the initial examination in 10% of the patients. Subsequently, another 5% developed rheumatoid arthritis or gout. Thus, systemic rheumatic diseases occurred in 15% of the patients. Plantar fasciitis in association with obesity and pes planus was more common. Over half the patients had plantar spurs, but the presence or absence of plantar spurs had no relationship to the outcome. Heel spurs probably are just a further development associated with plantar fasciitis.[27] Plantar fascia pain may also result from use of fluoride for treatment of osteoporosis.[28]

Laboratory and Roentgenographic Examination. Unless systemic disease is also present, tests for inflammation are normal. Radiographic examination will delineate pressure spurs that are usually unrelated to symptoms or outcome. Tumors, fractures, periostitis, and the fluffy-bone change characteristic of Reiter's syndrome and other spondyloarthropathies, Lofgren's syndrome, and sarcoidosis are to be considered in differential diagnosis, and are further reasons for obtaining roentgenographs.

Management. Treatment of obesity, flatfeet, and systemic inflammation is undertaken when the respective conditions are present. Arch-supporting shoes, particularly with a long counter, or shoes with inserted foam-rubber raised arches and rubber or tub heels, rigid shanks, and crepe soles are helpful. Initially the patient may not tolerate wearing the arch-supporting shoes all day. The patient can carry along an older pair of shoes when leaving the house, and after several hours may switch from the new shoes to the old ones. Within a short time the patient can usually tolerate the arch-supporting shoes and is grateful for the benefit received. Points of tenderness along the plantar fascia may be injected with a corticosteroid-anesthetic mixture. A No. 23 or 25 needle inserted ¼- to ½-inch deep into the plantar fascia for deposition of the steroid is utilized (Fig. 11–4).

Outcome and Additional Suggestions. If patients adhere to the program by wearing proper shoes for correction of associated structural foot disorders, benefit often occurs after several weeks in the majority of patients. Wearing slippers or going barefoot may result in recurrence. Patients who work or reside in buildings with concrete floors should use crepe-soled shoes. Rigid inserts are of little value,[1] but heel cups may be helpful. Leather or rubber longitudinal arches may be added in ³/₁₆- to ¼-inch thicknesses. On occasion, patients respond to oral nonsteroidal anti-inflammatory agents. Local strapping of the plantar arch and midfoot may also be helpful.[1] A soft, moldable flexible insert that can be shaped to the foot while it is held in position of correction may be helpful, if structural deformities are also present.[1] In our experience, surgical intervention is rarely needed. Furey reported that only 2% of patients with plantar fasciitis required a Steindler stripping procedure (stripping of the plantar fascia).[24]

MIDFOOT AND METATARSAL PAIN

Following an inversion injury, a *ligamentous sprain* of the calcaneocuboid joint often occurs. Pain, swelling, and tenderness over the lateral border of the foot are noted. For treatment, the midfoot should be taped or wrapped with an elastic bandage or gelocast; following 24 to 48 hours of rest, recovery is the rule.

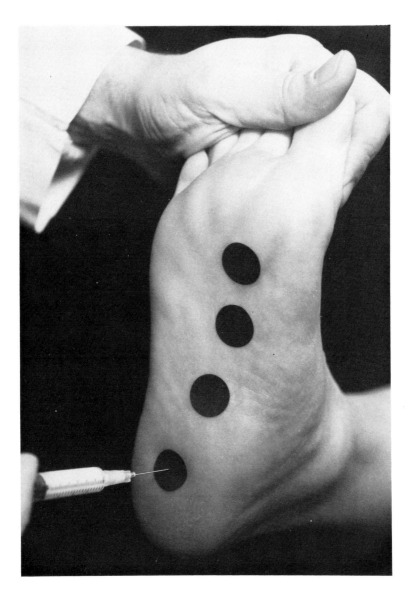

Fig. 11–4. Injection technique for the painful heel and plantar fasciitis. Using a 1-in. No. 23 or No. 25 needle, aliquots of a corticosteroid-local anesthetic mixture are introduced into the painful tissue. Alternatively these sites are approached from a lateral direction.

Tendinitis of the superficial extensor tendons of the foot commonly results from tight lacing, or from ridges on the tongue of the shoe. Frequently, point tenderness and pain follow the use of a new pair of work shoes; swelling is uncommon. To relieve the pressure, a lipstick mark is applied to the point of maximum tenderness, the shoe is replaced and laced; after removing the shoe, the lipstick mark will appear on the undersurface of the tongue of the shoe. A strip of adhesive-backed foam rubber ⅜- to ½-inches wide should be positioned on the undersurface of the tongue at each side of the lipstick mark, thus providing a gap over the point of tenderness. Use of elastic shoe laces may also be helpful.

A painful hard *spur* or *fibroma* on the dorsal aspect of the first tarsometatarsal joint in adults or children may result from tightfitting shoes.[9] Occasionally children suffer a painful disturbance beneath the first metatarsophalangeal joint. In the past this entity was thought to be due to sesamoiditis, but probably represents a *bursitis* associated with physical trauma.[7]

Metatarsalgia

Although Morton's neuroma is a common cause for forefoot pain, many other conditions occur in this region and must be distinguished. The disorders described here are *not* acute in onset, and although they may suggest mild gouty symptoms, they are not as abruptly painful as acute gout.

Disturbances of the metatarsal region may result from congenital structural abnormalities of the foot, weakness of intrinsic foot muscles, arthritis, or trauma.[2,11,14] Upon weightbearing the "metatarsal arch" normally flattens and is therefore not a functioning arch.[2,11] The metatarsal arch created by the transverse metatarsal ligament and the abductor hallucis longus is further supported during push-off by the intrinsic toe flexors, which help to elevate the three central metatarsals.[14]

If a deformity of the first metatarsal is present, the axis of weightbearing may shift to the second metatarsal, with resultant strain upon the normal function of the metatarsal ligaments and musculature.[14] The most common of these deformities is probably metatarsus primus varus, in which the great toe is rotated on its longitudinal axis so that the toenail points medially. Metatarsal pain in the plantar region of the first metatarsal joint may result from a hallux valgus deformity, hallux rigidus (degenerative joint disease), or arthritis of a sesamoid articulation.[29] The second metatarsal bone is tightly fixed between the three cuneiforms and is therefore relatively immobile. The region under the second metatarsal head is easily aggravated by wearing high-heeled shoes, by weakness of the intrinsic foot muscles, or by contracture of the flexor tendons.[30] Congenital ligamentous laxity, particularly if associated with obesity, also may result in metatarsalgia during prolonged standing, and may result in a splay foot[11] with the development of plantar calluses under the second metatarsal head.[14]

A properly fitted shoe with a broad toe box, a metatarsal pad, or a metatarsal bar placed behind the metatarsal heads is helpful.[26] Calluses can be softened with 20% salicylic acid and collodion;[14] the application is removed after 2 or 3 days with warm soaking. Toe flexion exercises, such as crinkling newspaper with the toes, or curling the toes downward while standing on the edge of a phone book should be prescribed. Weight reduction is essential in obese patients. The use of an anterior heel, "earth shoe," running shoe, soft insoles such as Spenco, Plastizote,[3] or comma-shaped inserts[2] are additional methods for relieving weightbearing from the metatarsal region. (See Table 11–1.)

Metatarsal bars may be straight or curved along the inferior surface. The short rocker bar, the most commonly prescribed type, ¼-inch thick, is placed externally behind the metatarsal heads[31] (Fig. 11–5).

Metatarsal bar   Thomas heel

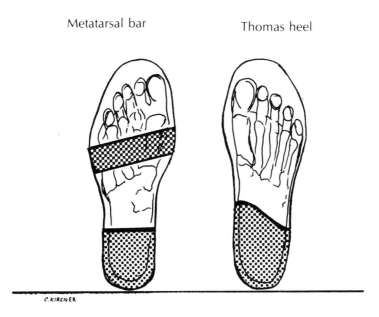

C. KIRCNER

Fig. 11–5. *Left,* An external metatarsal bar distributes weight posterior to the metatarsal region. When standing, the patient should be certain the bar has been placed behind the metatarsophalangeal joints, or the bar should be removed and reattached in the proper location. The bar should be placed on both shoes to allow normal balance. *Right,* The Thomas heel provides support for patients with symptomatic pes planus, valgus heel deformity, or plantar fascia strain.

The metatarsal bar may have a forward curve if the patient has this configuration of the metatarsal heads. A "horseshoe" bar may be used if there is a painful plantar callus. If the metatarsal bar is malpositioned it may aggravate pain and require revision.[1] When positioned properly, symptoms are usually promptly improved.

Plastizote insoles are self-molding but may require an extra-depth shoe with an enlarged toe box[1] (Fig. 11–6). The simple metatarsal foam rubber pad, approximately $3/16$-inch thick, is widely available. The patient can mark the painful area of the foot with lipstick, stand in the shoe, and then place the pad just behind the lipstick mark. Occasionally the pad requires a concave forward edge to accommodate a particularly painful metatarsophalangeal joint. Obviously, the shoe must hold the foot securely and prevent forward slipping. This requires a strap or lacing. The sole should be firm but not rigid, and crepe soles are helpful.[3]

Metatarsalgia of traumatic origin may result from prolonged walking or jumping that results in a sprain of the intermetatarsal ligaments. Dancers may suffer a stress fracture of a sesamoid.[32] Swelling may or may not be present. An intermetatarsal bursitis from tight narrow shoes may also occur.[11,14,33] Sprain of the first metatarsophalangeal joint can incapacitate an athlete; tenderness in the great toe region is aggravated by running when compared to walking; roentgenograms are normal.[9] The adolescent, when engaged in sports, may suffer a stress fracture at the base of the fifth metatarsal, presenting with a painful prominence on the lateral side of the foot.[34] Treatment of the

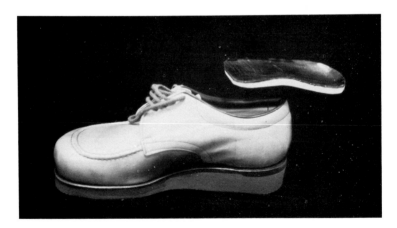

Fig. 11–6. The extra-depth shoe: Often prescribed with the additional feature of the enlarged toe box, this shoe is helpful for patients with metatarsal and metatarsophalangeal joint difficulties, hammertoe, rheumatoid or other inflammatory arthritides with forefoot deformity. If required, the molded soft plastic insert may be provided additionally. Occupational therapists, orthopedists, or podiatrists are skilled in making the mold.

stress fracture includes relief from weightbearing, and if symptoms persist a cast may be necessary.[34]

Fatigue (March) Fracture

A nondisplaced fracture that occurs just proximal to the metatarsal head is often a fatigue fracture. Although frequently seen in military personnel, particularly in new recruits after their first long march, this condition is also seen frequently in women after prolonged shopping, in joggers, in other overuse syndromes, and in persons with a short first metatarsal.[14,32,34,35] The second or third metatarsal shaft is most commonly fractured. These stress fractures rarely occur before age 12.[34] The patient notes tenderness and diffuse forefoot pain accompanied by swelling on the dorsal surface of the metatarsal region. Slight erythema may be present. The onset is subacute and never reaches the intensity of gout. Radiographic evidence of a fracture may be present only after several weeks (Fig. 11–7). A bone callus appears by 3 to 4 weeks and confirms the diagnosis.[36] A molded arch support, snug elastoplast wrapping, or support with a simple external short metatarsal rocker bar provides good results. Sometimes a walking cast is necessary.

Running Injuries

Long-distance runners may have complaints that result from the accumulated impact loading of long-distance running.[37–39] Often these problems relate to biomechanical overuse in patients with

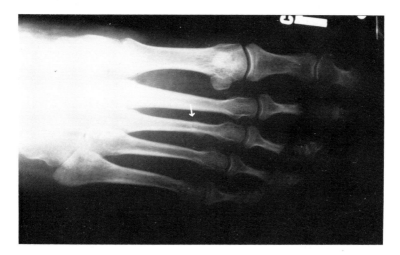

Fig. 11–7. Fatigue (march) fracture: Pain and swelling in the mid-metatarsal region on the dorsal aspect of the foot in a middle-aged patient is suggestive of a fatigue fracture. Roentgenographic examination 2 weeks following the pain should be scrutinized carefully for evidence of fracture and callus (see arrow).

minor structural disorders. Malalignments with mechanical disadvantages, muscle contractures, and use of untrained muscles may lead to biomechanical failure.[38] Physical examination of the runner should include examination of the alignment of the entire lower extremities. The physician should note limb length, range of movement, configuration of the weightbearing foot and heel, and forefoot alignment. The vertical axis of the heel should be parallel to the longitudinal axis of the distal tibia when viewed posteriorly. The plane of the metatarsal head should be perpendicular to the heel.[37]

In a study of 180 injured runners, 232 abnormal structural conditions were noted on careful examination.[37] Of these injuries, 60% were the result of training errors, and of these, 29% were due to the accumulation of excessive mileage not tolerated by the subtle anatomic deformities found in these individuals. Shin splints and knee problems such as chondromalacia patellae and iliotibial tract tendinitis were also common (see Chapts. 9 and 10). Treating running injuries of the foot includes decreasing the runner's mileage, avoiding hard-surface running, changing the runner's stride, stretching the hamstring and calf muscles, and using shoes with waffle soles or orthotics when indicated, with alteration of the heel counter.[37,39]

FLEXIBLE FLATFEET

There are nearly as many terms for flatfeet as there are orthopedists writing about flatfeet. The flexible type is the most common and important type.[5,11,14] Blacks and American Indians normally have flatfeet yet they are not necessarily a precursor of painful feet.[12] Asymptomatic persons with flatfeet should be left alone. Flatfeet, however, do require more intrinsic foot muscle contraction with each step of walking;[40] nevertheless, the degree of flatness or pronation bears no correlation to future foot pain.[2] The flexible flatfoot, by definition, appears normal before it strikes the ground and bears weight; the arch flattens upon weightbearing. Symptoms, when present, include excessive muscular fatigue and aching, and intolerance to prolonged walking or standing. In some patients walking improves symptoms.[11] Symptoms often develop following a change in work habits that require prolonged standing. In addition, symptoms may follow other foot injuries that result in an abnormal gait. In some individuals, symptoms result from prolonged illness with resultant muscular atrophy.[12]

Physical examination reveals loss of the longitudinal arch upon weightbearing, increased prominence of the navicular bone and the head of the talus, or an exostosis on the medial aspect of the foot.[2] The calcaneus is everted (valgus position) as shown in Figure 11-8. The anterior and posterior tibial tendons and plantar muscles become stretched, and the tendo Achillis may become shortened.[14] The

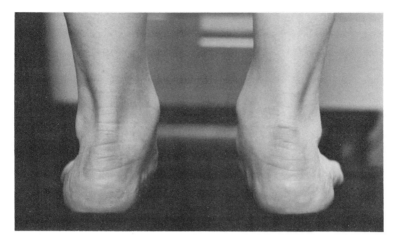

Fig. 11–8. Pes planus (flatfeet) with eversion of the heels is best viewed posteriorly. Examination for pes planus should be part of the examination of any patient with a rheumatologic complaint of the lower extremity.

forefoot swings outward and the foot becomes rotated externally in relation to the leg. Occasionally, edema of the dorsum of the foot and tenderness over the medial aspect of the foot occur.[14]

The determination that the foot (subtalar joint) can be inverted is essential, in order to demonstrate the presence of a flexible rather than a rigid flatfoot.[2] Tenderness may also be noted over the navicular bone, the inferior calcaneonavicular ligament, or the sole of the foot.[11] While walking, the flatfooted patient raises the heel and toe together rather than using a heel-to-toe gait and demonstrates a splay foot with the toes turned outward. This results from an attempt to prevent strain on the tarsal or metatarsal ligaments.[11] The patient's gait has no "spring" to it. The shoe wears down more on the medial side of the sole than on the lateral sides. A corn on the fifth toe is further evidence of altered weightbearing. If the flatfoot is not evident from the frontal view, then it should become evident from a posterior view.

Etiology. The infant is born flatfooted and acquires an arch after a year or so of ambulation. The symptomatic flexible flatfoot may result from general hypermobility and a failure of postural muscle function to maintain the arch.[11] In any event, it is probably not a result of improper footwear. Of patients with flatfeet, 70% have an inherited predisposition to flatfeet.[11]

Laboratory and Radiographic Examination. Flatfeet may be a late manifestation of any inflammatory rheumatic disease, and other features of that disease should be manifest at the time of examination. When confronted with a *rigid* flatfoot, special roentgenographic techniques are required to demonstrate bony bridging due to inflammatory or congenital defects of the tarsal region.

Differential Diagnosis. The rigid flatfoot also results from congenital or acquired infection, or from inflammatory or traumatic disturbances of the tarsal region.[14] Painful reflex spasm of the peroneal muscle[14] can result from a rigid flatfoot.[40]

Management. The most important rule in this chapter is not to treat asymptomatic flatfeet with a rigid arch support. Basic to the treatment of the symptomatic flatfoot is to move the center of gravity of the foot more to the outside of the foot and to remove points of pressure that are causing symptoms.[11] This can be accomplished by the use of a firm heel counter and a tight well-fitted instep with a low heel.[14] The physician may recommend a Thomas heel and a gradual shoe correction, and should not hastily order an expensive plastic rigid molded insert.[1] The Thomas heel for the symptomatic flatfoot should provide a varus tilt to the heel in order to put the ankle in a more vertical alignment. The Thomas heel can extend to the mid-part of the navicular so that it intersects the longitudinal axis of the fibula.[1] The shank of the shoe should remain flexible unless an appliance is being added to the shoe, or if a hallux rigidus coexists. Most patients require only a firm long-countered oxford shoe, and only a few require an insert. The examiner must determine whether the foot can be inverted, and if so an arch support can be tried. Such a support should not be rigid and should seldom exceed ⅛ of an inch rise in the longitudinal arch.[2] Felt-type padding is not a permanent insert as it packs down. However, it is inexpensive and can be used to determine whether an insert will provide relief. If so, a permanent type should be prescribed for relief of pressure.[1] Only after failure of proper shoes without inserts, followed by a trial of flexible leather inserts, should moldable soft plastic inserts be considered. More often the latter inserts are used to treat structural foot disorders, such as forefoot or hindfoot varus, or valgus deformities. In general, the molded insert is not necessary in patients suffering from flexible flatfeet.

Recognition of aggravating symptomatic factors such as work on concrete floors, prolonged standing, obesity, or coexisting plantar fasciitis is essential for effective management. Grasping exercises for intrinsic foot muscles and mobilizing exercises that plantarflex the foot and invert the ankle are helpful. Crinkling newspaper with the feet on the floor, and ankle rotation performed with the foot constantly cupped, first clockwise, then counterclockwise, may help maintain mobility in the involved soft tissues (Fig. 11–9).

Outcome and Additional Suggestions. In our experience, patients with flexible flatfeet have self-limited episodes of pain brought about by prolonged weightbearing in improper shoes, excessive weight gain, carrying heavy objects, or moving to a home or job with a

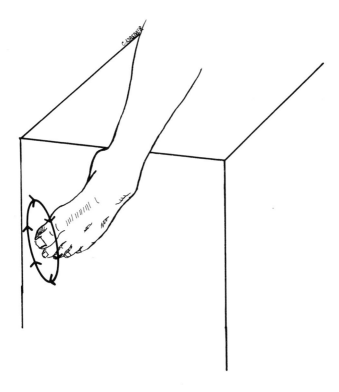

Fig. 11–9. Mobilizing exercise for the foot and ankle: While the toes are kept in downward flexion, the ankle is drawn to 90 degrees, and then a circular motion of the entire foot and ankle in one direction and then another is accomplished.

concrete floor. Often such episodes of pain are due to plantar fasciitis rather than flatfeet per se. Patients with chronic foot pain must be examined for systemic disorders mentioned in association with plantar fasciitis. If symptoms have persisted despite conscientious use of proper foot gear, and no other underlying cause has been found, the clinician should carefully reexamine the entire lower extremity and lumbar spine for evidence of other disorders, such as peripheral neuropathy, gout, or lumbar disc disease.

TOE DISORDERS

The term "bunion" refers to soft tissue swelling over the first metatarsophalangeal joint. It is often mistakenly used to describe all disorders that enlarge the first metatarsophalangeal joint.[12] Several of the more common disorders of this joint region as well as disorders affecting the other toes are discussed.

Hallux Valgus Deformity

The patient with this common foot deformity presents with medial deviation of the head of the first metatarsal and lateral deviation of the great toe, often accompanied by a painful soft adventitial bursa. Because of this disorder, the second toe is forced dorsally and may develop into a hammertoe.[14] Displacement of a sesamoid bone is often associated with this deformity. The condition occurs more commonly in cultures where shoes are worn and in females. Generally the large toe is rotated so that the nail faces medially. The bursa overlying the medial bony prominence may become secondarily infected or acutely inflamed from the pressure of ill-fitting shoes.[2,9,14] The patient often sees the physician not because of pain, but rather because of the inability to wear "dress shoes."

Hallux Rigidus

Progressive loss of motion of the great toe joint is associated with arthritis of the first metatarsophalangeal joint. This condition may follow hallux valgus deformity[14] or trauma, or may be associated with pes planus, the pronated foot, or metatarsus varus primus deformity.[41] Hallux rigidus is usually more disabling than hallux valgus deformity.[29]

Treatment of hallux valgus without rigidus includes the use of shoes with an enlarged toe portion, the use of a felt ring, or the use of a plastic cap.[14] Occasionally we have had a shoemaker remove the dorsal portion of the shoe and replace it with a wide roomy vinyl covering. Additional measures include pads of felt or rubber behind the first metatarsophalangeal joint, or arch supports with lateral and medial flanges to fit over medial and lateral bunions.[2] High-heeled or soft flexible shoes are not well-tolerated. Surgical intervention should be performed only for symptoms and not for cosmetic reasons.[14] Bunion surgery is 85% effective, yet 12,000 unsatisfactory operations are estimated to occur each year.[2] Use of joint replacement is still in the experimental stage.

If the bursa over a hallux valgus deformity is swollen and tender, measures to keep the shoe covering from rubbing against it are imperative. In summer months the use of an open sandal may be helpful. When a shoe must be worn, the vamp should be cut with a linear slit through the lining just above the sole and over the bunion.[42] We have found it advantageous for patients to cut a wide half-circle throughout the medial portion of an old laced shoe. This allows support for the hind foot, provides a rigid sole for the forefoot, and reduces friction across the medial surface of the first metatarsophalangeal joint.

In addition to the measures previously mentioned, treatment of hallux rigidus requires the use of a thick and rigid shoe sole.[11,12] The clinician may also try a long rocker bar to add rigidity to the sole.[31] On occasion, a local corticosteroid-anesthetic injection into the region of a dorsal exostosis at the first metatarsal joint line is helpful.[2,12] Stretching the toe downward for a moment or so, morning and evening, has also been helpful.[2] Joint fusion, debridement arthroplasty, or other surgical procedures may be necessary.[11]

Hammertoe Deformity

This disorder is usually acquired as a result of pressure from hallux valgus,[14] from tight shoes,[1,14] or it may be congenital in origin. It is usually a bilateral deformity with the second toe nearly always involved. The toe is flexed at the proximal interphalangeal (PIP) joint and the tip of the toe points downward.[14] Thus the middle and distal phalanges of the second toe are flexed on the proximal phalanges.[1] A painful bursa and callus often form over the dorsal aspect of the flexed proximal interphalangeal joint. The toe tip becomes broadened and thick.[14] In children with congenital hammertoe, treatment is best handled with adhesive strapping and use of shoes with an adequate depth of toe box.[14] An "X" incision in the shoe vamp over the pressure

Table 11–1.   Common Shoe Modifications[43,44]

Problem Area	Possible Shoe Modification
Great Toe	Broad toe box, shoe cut-out around bunion, vinyl patch to enlarge toe box, thicker or more rigid sole, broad external rocker bar, felt ring, and plastic cap.
Other Toes	"X" incision above toe, wider shoe size, metartarsal pads, and extra-depth shoes.
Metatarsal Area	Pads, excavation of innersole beneath lesion, "closed cell" foam pad (Spenco), molded flexible insert with "open cell" foam (Plastizote), short external metatarsal bar (1 inch wide), longer external rocker bar, vinyl covering to widen toe box, and anterior placed heel.
Plantar region of midfoot, flexible flatfoot, plantar fasciitis	Long-counter shoe, Thomas heel, scaphoid pad, flexible arch support, cutout under heel spur, scaphoid pad, 3/16-inch foam medial arch insert, and wedging of the medial sole.
Dorsal Midfoot	Strips of foam rubber cemented to inner tongue to lift tongue off of lesion, and elastic shoe laces.
Heel	Heel lift, heel pad, cutout heel pad, excavation of innersole beneath heel spur or lesion, plastic heel cup, and "V" incision into rim of counter.

point is helpful.[42] When keratoses are also present, surgical correction is often necessary.[12]

None of these toe disorders result in soft tissue swelling of the toe. When swelling occurs, sepsis (felon or whitlow), systemic rheumatic disease (e.g., rheumatoid arthritis, psoriatic arthritis), and other disease entities (e.g., gout, tumors) are considerations.

Table 11–1 provides possible shoe modifications for various foot problems. Combinations of these modifications may be indicated depending upon careful assessment of the individual problem.

Information for moldable plastics or extra depth shoes may be obtained from the following sources:

AliMed, 138 Prince St., Boston, Mass. 02113; P.W. Minor & Son Inc., Batavia, New York 14020; and Alden Shoe Company, Taunton St., Middleborough, Mass. 02346.

ENTRAPMENT NEUROPATHIES

With the increased use of high boots with high heels and with the popularity of activities such as jogging, entrapment neuropathies of the foot and ankle are being seen more often. When the patient complains of burning paresthesia day and night, this disorder should be suspected. However, that history is often not volunteered and must be sought. Any nocturnal foot symptoms and foot pain that radiates out to the toes should suggest an entrapment neuropathy.

The Tarsal Tunnel Syndrome

This syndrome refers to an entrapment neuropathy of the posterior tibial nerve as it passes through the tunnel beneath the flexor retinaculum on the medial side of the ankle.[26,45,46] Beneath this retinaculum (or lancinate ligament)[47,48] lies a tunnel containing the tendons of the flexor digitorum longus and flexor hallucis longus, the vascular bundle, the posterior tibial nerve, and the medial and lateral plantar nerves[14] (Fig. 11–10). Most commonly the patient presents with aching, burning, numbness, and tingling involving the plantar surface of the foot, the distal foot, the toes, and occasionally the heel. The pain may also radiate up to the calf or higher.[14,49] The discomfort is often nocturnal, and may be worse after standing; the discomfort sometimes leads to removal of the shoe even while driving. Physical examination seldom reveals swelling or atrophy. Sensory nerve loss is variable and often is not found.[14] The Tinel test, in which the nerve is tapped with the finger or reflex hammer, is often positive at the flexor retinaculum located posterior and inferior to the medial malleolus. To be complete, tapping must be performed over the entire course of the posterior tibial nerve or one of its branches.[50] Occasionally, firm-rolling pressure across the nerve may be required to reproduce the symptoms. A tourniquet applied just above the ankle may reproduce

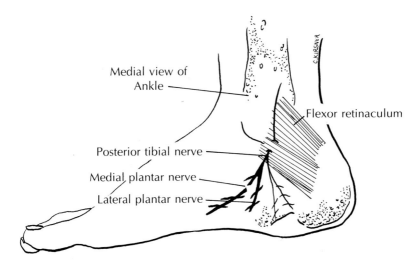

Fig. 11-10. Tarsal tunnel: Posterior tibial nerve is often trapped beneath the flexor retinaculum on the medial side of the ankle. Entrapment may also include the two branches, the medial and lateral plantar nerves.

these symptoms by creating venous engorgement of the tarsal tunnel.[14]

Most often the tarsal tunnel syndrome results from a compression neuropathy in which the tarsal tunnel has been compromised by a tenosynovitis of one or more of the tendons passing through the region. This may result from injury, from rheumatoid arthritis, or from other sources of inflammation[14] or tumors.[51] Perhaps the most common cause for a tarsal tunnel syndrome is a fracture or dislocation involving the talus, calcaneus, or medial malleolus.[47,48] Previous involvement of a *carpal* tunnel has been described in patients who later develop a *tarsal* tunnel syndrome.[1,52] Most often the tarsal tunnel syndrome occurs in the absence of inflammatory rheumatic disease, but if other features are suggestive, the erythrocyte sedimentation rate and tests for rheumatic disease, including rheumatoid factor and antinuclear factor should be performed. Diabetic neuropathy may cause similar symptoms unrelated to tarsal tunnel involvement.

Diagnosis of tarsal tunnel syndrome may be confirmed by electrodiagnostic tests. Tibial nerve conduction velocity normally is 49.9 ± 5.1 msec, and latency from the malleolus to the abductor hallucis normally is 4.4 ± 0.9 msec . Prolonged latency in excess of 6.1 msec for the medial plantar nerve and 6.7 msec for the lateral plantar nerve is indicative of disease;[14,48,53,54] however, normal values do not exclude the syndrome. Perhaps the best diagnostic test is response to a local

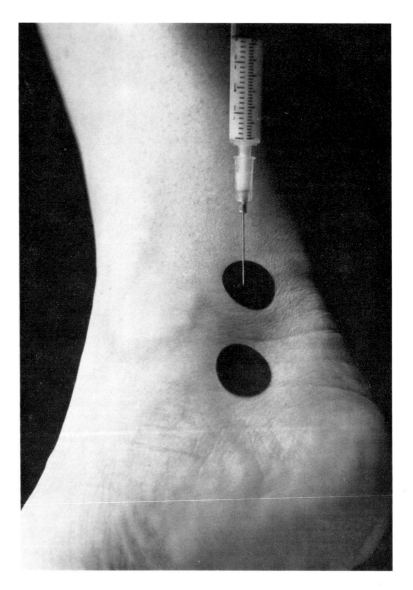

Fig. 11–11. Sites for injection of the tarsal tunnel or posterior tibialis tendinitis on the medial aspect of the ankle. A 1-in. No. 23 needle should be used, and the medication instilled in a fan-like manner.

corticosteroid-anesthetic injection into the region of the tarsal tunnel, with relief confirming the presence of the syndrome.

In most cases a local corticosteroid-anesthetic mixture injected once or twice into the region inferior and posterior to the medial malleolus and injected in a fan-like manner provides relief (Fig. 11–11). Others report only a 30% response and recommend decompression surgery.[14,49,50] It may be that surgical intervention is most often required when the tarsal tunnel syndrome follows fracture or dislocation. If symptoms persist, local or systemic underlying disorders causing a tarsal tunnel or similar symptomatic syndromes must be considered. These include vascular disease with venous stasis, diabetes mellitus with neuropathy, rheumatoid arthritis, myxedema, pregnancy, and amyloidosis.[53]

Compression Neuropathy of the Common Peroneal Nerve

Footdrop (inability to dorsiflex the foot) often results from peroneal nerve compression due to crossing the leg, hanging the leg over a constricting rigid object, or from direct trauma. A tight boot or cast may also result in sensory or motor peroneal nerve loss, and a partial or complete footdrop. A footdrop brace with a spring action that returns the foot to a 90-degree angle may be required for many months following injury.[46,47]

Plantar Nerve Entrapment

Forced overpronation or pressure associated with a hallux rigidus, tenosynovitis, or venous engorgement of the posterior tibial veins may compress the plantar nerve on the medial aspect of the foot below the calcaneonavicular ligament.[46] The patient may present with a painful heel as well as numbness or tingling across the sole of the foot. A local corticosteroid injection at the site of compression and correction of abnormal foot mechanics with a medial shoe wedge, a scaphoid pad, or molded soft flexible inserts should provide relief.[47]

Interdigital Plantar Neuroma (Morton's Neuroma)

Entrapment neuropathy with or without an associated plantar neuroma often develops between the third and fourth toes on the plantar surface. This involves the anastomoses of the medial and lateral plantar nerves. Pain radiates forward from the metatarsal heads to the third and fourth toes. Similar involvement of other interdigital plantar nerves may occur. This entity, commonly called Morton's neuroma, has neuropathic features of hyperesthesia of the toes, numbness and tingling, and aching and burning in the distal forefoot. It is aggravated by walking on hard surfaces and wearing tight or high-heeled shoes.[14,46,47,50]

Physical examination reveals tenderness in the plantar aspect of the distal foot over the third and fourth metatarsals; compressing the forefoot reproduces the symptoms. The tenderness is occasionally aggravated by direct pressure to the plantar aspect of the third and fourth metatarsophalangeal joints. There should be a concomitant sensation of burning distally. Possible causes include excessive mobility of the fourth metatarsal,[50] nerve impingement between flattened metatarsal heads,[46,47] or compression of the nerve as it is angulated over the transverse tarsal ligament.[14,46,47,55] Chronic compression leads to neuroma formation.

Conservative treatment requires increased plantar flexion at the metatarsal heads obtained by use of a metatarsal support, metatarsal bar, or a comma-shaped metatarsal shoe insert.[47] Although symptoms are unilateral in 85% of cases, external appliances should be placed on both shoes so that the patient walks evenly.[1] A broad-toed shoe that allows spreading of the metatarsal heads is helpful. A local corticosteroid injection into the site of compression may be beneficial. Surgical removal of the neuroma *and nerve* may be required in patients who are resistant to nonoperative therapy.[14,47]

Joplin's Neuroma

Perineural fibrosis of the plantar proper digital nerve may follow a bunionectomy or trauma to the first metatarsophalangeal joint.[2] This results in pain and paresthesia at the plantar aspect of the first metatarsophalangeal joint of the great toe. A Tinel test may be positive beneath the first metatarsophalangeal joint. Relief occurs with foot rest or removal of the shoe. Surgical excision of the nerve may be necessary.

NIGHT CRAMPS

Benign nocturnal cramps in the legs and feet may be a distressing complaint (for detailed explanation see Chapt. 10). Acute symptoms may be prevented by prophylactic use of quinine, or at times, diphenhydramine (Benadryl). A warm bath or foot soaks at bedtime may be helpful. Structural disorders of the feet should be sought and treated appropriately in an effort to prevent recurrences.

REFERENCES

1. Mann RA: Conservative treatment and office procedures. *In* DuVries' Surgery of the Foot. 4th Ed. Edited by RA Mann. St. Louis, CV Mosby, 1978.
2. Giannestras NJ: Foot Disorders; Medical and Surgical Management, 2nd Ed. Philadelphia, Lea & Febiger, 1973.
3. Miller WE: Nonoperative approach to foot problems. Orthop Rev 7:19–21, 1978.
4. Dagnall JC, Calabro JJ: Chiropody (podiatry) and arthritis. Bull Rheum Dis 23:692–695, 1972.

5. Jahss MH: The abnormal plantigrade foot. Orthop Rev 8:31–34, 1978.
6. Cracchiolo A: The use of shoes to treat foot disorders. Orthop Rev 8:73–83, 1979.
7. Raymakers R: The painful foot. Practitioner 215:61–68, 1975.
8. Mayer PJ: Pes cavus: A diagnostic and therapeutic challenge. Orthop Rev 7:105–116, 1978.
9. Glick JM: Traumatic injuries to the soft tissues of the foot and ankle. In DuVries' Surgery of the Foot. 4th Ed. Edited by RA Mann. St. Louis, CV Mosby, 1978.
10. Harrington KD: Degenerative arthritis of the ankle secondary to long-standing lateral ligament instability. J Bone Joint Surg 61:354–361, 1979.
11. Duthie RB, Ferguson AB: Mercer's Orthopedic Surgery, 7th Ed. Baltimore, Williams & Wilkins, 1973.
12. Mann RA, DuVries HL: Acquired nontraumatic deformities of the foot. In DuVries' Surgery of the Foot, 4th Ed. Edited by RA Mann. St. Louis, CV Mosby, 1978.
13. Lipscomb PR: Nonsuppurative tenosynovitis and paratendinitis. Am Acad Orthop Surg Instructional Course Lectures, Vol 7. Ann Arbor, 1950.
14. Turek, SL: Orthopaedics; Principles and Their Application. 3rd Ed. Philadelphia, JB Lippincott, 1977.
15. Johnston JO: Affections of the foot. In DuVries' Surgery of the Foot, 4th Ed. Edited by RA Mann. St. Louis, CV Mosby, 1978.
16. Norris SH, Mankin HJ: Chronic tenosynovitis of the posterior tibial tendon with new bone formation. J Bone Joint Surg 60:523–526, 1978.
17. Inman VT, Mann RA: Major surgical procedures for disorders of the ankle, tarsus, and midtarsus. In DuVries' Surgery of the Foot, 4th Ed. Edited by RA Mann. St. Louis, CV Mosby, 1978.
18. Goldman AB, Katz MC, Freiberger RH: Posttraumatic adhesive capsulitis of the ankle: arthrographic diagnosis. Am J Roentgenol 127:585–588, 1976.
19. Sorrells RB: Heel pain. J Arkansas Med Soc 74:494–497, 1978.
20. Shelley WB, Rawnsley HM: Painful feet due to herniation of fat. JAMA 205:308–309, 1968.
21. Dickinson PH, Coutts MB, Woodward EP, Handler D: Tendo achillis bursitis. J Bone Joint Surg 48:77–81, 1966.
22. Gerster JC, Saudan Y, Fallet GH: Talalgia; a review of 30 severe cases. J Rheumatol 5:210–216, 1978.
23. Layfer LF: "Last" bursitis—a cause of ankle pain. Arthritis Rheum 23:261, 1980.
24. Furey JG: Plantar fasciitis; the painful heel syndrome. J Bone Joint Surg 57:672–673, 1975.
25. Siebert JS, Mann RA: Dermatology and disorders of the toenails. In DuVries' Surgery of the Foot, 4th Ed. Edited by RA Mann. St. Louis, CV Mosby, 1978.
26. Moskowitz RW: Clinical Rheumatology. Philadelphia, Lea & Febiger, 1975.
27. Campbell JW, Inman VT: Treatment of plantar fasciitis and calcaneal spurs with the UC-BL shoe insert. Clin Orthop 103:57–62, 1974.
28. Riggs BL, Hodgson SF, Hoffman DL, et al: Treatment of primary osteoporosis with fluoride and calcium. JAMA 243:446–449, 1980.
29. Baxter DE, Mann RA: Bones of the foot and their afflictions. In DuVries' Surgery of the Foot, 4th Ed. Edited by RA Mann. St. Louis, CV Mosby, 1978.
30. Inmann VT, Mann RA: Principles of examination of the foot and ankle. In DuVries' Surgery of the Foot, 4th Ed. Edited by RA Mann. St. Louis, CV Mosby, 1978.
31. Milgram JE, Jacobson MA: Footgear; therapeutic modifications of sole and heel. Orthop Rev 7:57–62, 1978.
32. Epps CH: Fractures of the forepart and midpart of the adolescent foot. Orthop Rev 7:63–69, 1978.
33. Bossley CJ, Cairney PC: The intermetatarsophalangeal bursa—its significance in Morton's metatarsalgia. J Bone Joint Surg 62:184–187, 1980.
34. Gross RH: Foot pain in children. Pediatr Clin North Am 24:813–823, 1977.
35. Chapman MW: Fractures and fracture-dislocations of the ankle and foot. In DuVries' Surgery of the Foot, 4th Ed. Edited by RA Mann. St. Louis, CV Mosby, 1978.
36. Garcia A, Parkes JC: Fractures of the foot. In Foot Disorders: Medical and Surgical Management, 2nd Ed. Edited by NJ Giannestras. Philadelphia, Lea & Febiger, 1973.

37. James SJ, Bates BT, Osternig LR: Injuries to runners. Am J Sports Med 6:40–50, 1978.
38. Baugher WH, Balady GJ, Warren RF, Marshall JL: Injuries of the musculoskeletal system in runners. Contemp Orthop 1:46–54, 1979.
39. Brady DM: Running injuries. Clinical Symposium (CIBA) 32(No. 4)2–36, 1980.
40. Mann RA: Biomechanics of the foot and ankle. Orthop Rev 7:43–48, 1978.
41. Giannestras NJ: Principles of bunion surgery. Orthop Rev 7:83–86, 1978.
42. Jacobson MA: Simple footgear corrections useful in office emergencies. Orthop Rev 8:63–68, 1979.
43. Shields MN, RPT: Disorders of the foot. Postgraduate Clinical Seminar, 44th Annual Meeting, Am Rheum Assoc, Atlanta, May 28, 1980.
44. Goodwin C, OTC: Personal communication.
45. Keck C: The tarsal tunnel syndrome. J Bone Joint Surg 44:180–182, 1962.
46. Kopell HP, Thompson WAL: Peripheral Entrapment Neuropathies. Huntington NY, RE Krieger, 1976.
47. Curtiss PH: Neurologic diseases of the foot. In Foot Disorders; Medical and Surgical Management, 2nd Ed. Edited by NJ Giannestras. Philadelphia, Lea & Febiger, 1973.
48. Goodgold J, Kopell HP, Spielholz NI: The tarsal-tunnel syndrome. N Engl J Med 273:742–745, 1965.
49. Wilemon WK: Tarsal tunnel syndrome. Orthop Rev 8:111–118, 1979.
50. Mann RA: Diseases of the nerves of the foot. In DuVries' Surgery of the Foot, 4th Ed. Edited by RA Mann. St. Louis, CV Mosby, 1978.
51. Janecki CJ, Dovberg JL: Tarsal-tunnel syndrome caused by neurilemoma of the medial plantar nerve. J Bone Joint Surg 59:127–128, 1977.
52. McGill DA: Tarsal tunnel syndrome. Proc R Soc Med 57:23–24, 1964.
53. Gretter TE, Wilde AH: Pathogenesis, diagnosis, and treatment of the tarsal-tunnel syndrome. Cleve Clin Q 37:23–29, 1970.
54. Fu R, DeLisa JA, Kraft GH: Motor nerve latencies through the tarsal tunnel in normal adult subjects. Arch Phys Med Rehabil 61:243–248, 1980.
55. Lassmann G, Lassmann H, Stockinger L: Morton's metatarsalgia. Virchows Arch [Pathol Anat] 370:307–321, 1976.

Chapter *12*

FIBROSITIS SYNDROME

The fibrositis syndrome is the epitome of the soft tissue rheumatic pain disorders. The term "fibrositis syndrome" refers to a disorder with variable features that includes wide-spread aching and stiffness accompanied by localized sites of deep myofascial tenderness, sleep disturbance, a characteristic personality, and chronicity.[1] "Fibrositis" should not be used merely to describe widespread soft tissue pain symptoms.[3] Essential to the diagnosis are the localized firm tender trigger points first described over a century ago.[2] The syndrome often begins in mid-life, although persons of any age may become symptomatic. Fibrositis may follow a precipitating life stress, such as an automobile accident.

The myofascial origin of these pain symptoms was popularized by Travell and co-workers,[4] who advocated procaine injections into the localized deep tender places, later termed "trigger zones"[5] or "trigger points." The procaine provided relief whereas similar injections into more distant areas were not beneficial. Trigger points have been the subject of extensive investigation since that time and were extensively reviewed by Simons.[2,6]

The term "fibrositis," introduced by Gowers in 1904,[7] was applied to regional painful conditions thought to arise at the points of fascial and tendinous attachment. The tissues were thought to have suffered irritation and inflammation, perhaps from overstretching. Gowers used the term "inflammation" in a broad sense (see Chapt. 13). He applied "fibrositis" as a descriptive term that included "traumatic fibrositis" or "cervical fibrositis." At first the term was used to imply any pain of muscle origin and was to some extent used interchangeably with fasciitis, myofibrositis, myofasciitis, muscular rheumatism, and muscular strain.[8]

Presently, the term fibrositis syndrome is reserved for a specific soft tissue pain syndrome with the following characteristics:

Aching, Stiffness, and Paresthesia. Soft tissue aching is widespread in broad regions of the cervical and lumbar spinal segments. The symptoms are aggravated by fatigue, tension, excessive work activity, immobilization, and chilling.[1] Heat, massage, programmed activity, and vacations are helpful in symptom relief. Although these symptoms may vary from day to day, they are nevertheless always present, and these patients rarely have "normal" days. Trunk pain usually is bilateral and symmetric, although use may cause one side to be more tender than the other. Leg cramps are frequent. Stiffness occurs more diffusely than in specific joint areas. (This differs from the pattern of morning stiffness in rheumatoid arthritis in which stiffness is maximally localized to joints.) Neck pain and stiffness, and muscle contraction headache often occur in the early morning hours. Paresthesia of the lower extremities occurs commonly after prolonged sitting, or after performing any prolonged activity. Paresthesia and the *sensation* of swelling of the hands and arms are common. Rings feel tight in the morning. *Visible swelling does not occur*, at least to the physician observer.

Trigger Points. Essential to the diagnosis of fibrositis are the presence of trigger points, usually three or more.[1,3,6,9,10] Similar *but painless* areas of firmness have been noted in normal persons,[11,12] but the key finding is *pain reproduction* after trigger-point palpation. Upon rolling the trigger point, the muscle[10] or the patient may jump.[13] The "jump sign" reaction is considered by some to be essential to recognizing a true trigger point.[14] The muscle containing the trigger point often contracts violently when injected.

Trigger points are reproducible areas of induration that occur in precise locations. Common sites for trigger points are deep cervical points near the transverse processes of cervical vertebrae 4, 5, 6; within the muscle belly of the right and left trapezius muscles; at the second costochondral junction of either side, approximately 1 cm lateral to the junction or on the superior surface of the rib; at the origin of the supraspinatus muscle near the medial border of the scapula of either side; within the muscle belly of the rhomboids, levator scapulae, or infraspinatus muscles of the scapulae; 1 to 2 cm distal to the lateral epicondyle of the elbow in the extensor communis tendons; the upper lateral quadrant of the buttocks in the gluteal fascia; the lumbar interspinous ligaments to either side of lumbar vertebrae 4, 5, S1; the medial fat pad proximal to the joint line overlying the collateral ligament of the knee; and bony points, particularly the tip of the acromion or at the greater trochanter[3] (Figs. 12–1, 12–2).

Sleep Disturbance. If the patient does not volunteer that she suffers sleep disturbance, the patient's spouse often volunteers that the patient "moves all over the bed all night long." The patient may

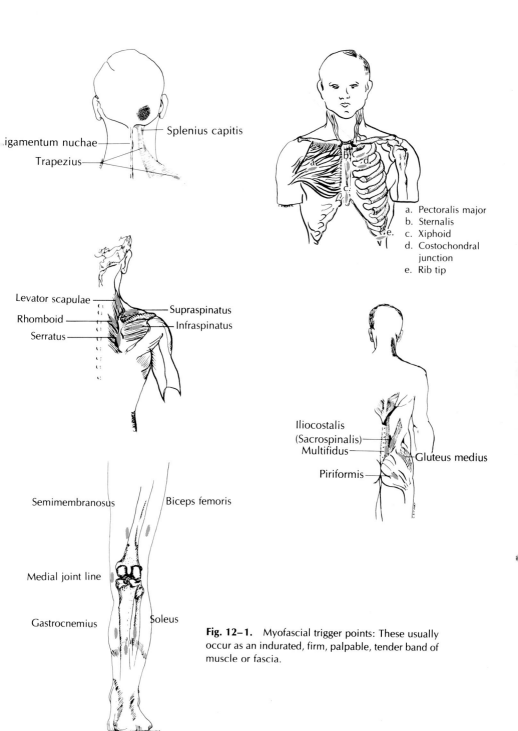

Splenius capitis

Ligamentum nuchae

Trapezius

a. Pectoralis major
b. Sternalis
c. Xiphoid
d. Costochondral
   junction
e. Rib tip

Levator scapulae

Rhomboid

Serratus

Supraspinatus

Infraspinatus

Iliocostalis
(Sacrospinalis)

Multifidus

Gluteus medius

Piriformis

Semimembranosus

Biceps femoris

Medial joint line

Gastrocnemius

Soleus

Fig. 12–1. Myofascial trigger points: These usually occur as an indurated, firm, palpable, tender band of muscle or fascia.

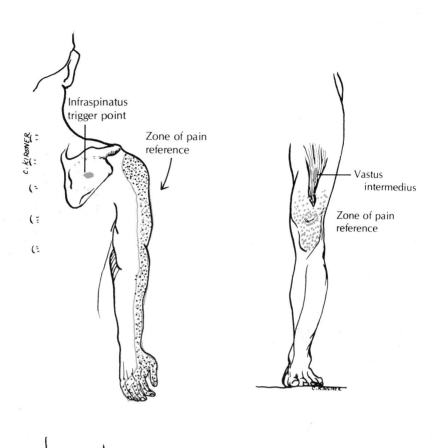

Infraspinatus trigger point

Zone of pain reference

Vastus intermedius

Zone of pain reference

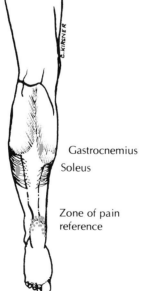

Gastrocnemius

Soleus

Zone of pain reference

Fig. 12–2. Zones of reference: Upon palpating the trigger point, pain is produced at some distant point. This zone of reference is quite characteristic for each trigger point.

fall asleep promptly but then awakens frequently throughout the night. Characteristically, the patient feels more tired in the morning than when she went to bed. Sleep is not restful. Moldofsky noted that non-rapid eye movement (non-REM) sleep was disturbed and contaminated by alpha rhythms in patients with the fibrositis syndrome.[15] Furthermore, by depriving volunteers of non-REM sleep, the characteristic trigger points were produced.[15,16] Patients with fibrositis do not enter deep sleep (stage 4 sleep); they often feel that if they could keep moving and not stop, they would be better off. However, fatigue develops quickly.

Perfectionistic Personality. The patients tend to be compulsive at work, at home, at hobbies, or at social activities. They live with rigid time deadlines. When presented with an appointment, they are characteristically conscientiously prompt. They dislike tranquilizers and are sparse users of drugs or alcohol.[1] Features of compulsive grooming may be evident including precise hair arrangement, plucked eyebrows, and fastidious nail care. They are rarely obese. They tend to be of above-average intelligence. Living the compulsive life often leads to depression, particularly at midlife. Migraine headaches are often noted in the patients' family or in the patients themselves.

Normal Laboratory Tests. Studies that are characteristically normal include complete blood counts, erythrocyte sedimentation rate, serum proteins, muscle enzyme studies, and antinuclear and rheumatoid factor determinations.[1] Laboratory abnormalities are inconsistent with a diagnosis of primary fibrositis.

When making a diagnosis of fibrositis, the physician should consider all of the five features outlined. Additional features that may occur include autonomic dysfunction with dermographism,[14] cutis anserina ("goose skin"—contraction of the arrectores pilorum muscles that causes elevation of hair follicles),[8] or cutis marmorata (a transitory purplish mottling of the skin), and excessive sweating.[9] Skinfold tenderness with hyperesthesia over the upper scapular region may be noted. Following testing for skinfold tenderness performed by rolling the patient's skin in a gentle pinching fashion, a marked hyperemia sometimes occurs.[1]

During the physical examination the patient appears unhappy, but is generally not overtly depressed and usually is forthright without much grossly evident neurotic behavior. Joint examination reveals normal range of active and passive motion. However, general musculoskeletal discomfort is evident. Grip testing is approached hesitantly and is carried out slowly, but usually the patient demonstrates full or low normal levels of strength.[1]

The five criteria previously defined serve to distinguish fibrositis from pain that is a malingering pretense or that is neurotically symbolic.[1] The fibrositis syndrome can be added upon other systemic disease; the compounded symptoms then may lead to more complex, inappropriate, and at times, hazardous medical or surgical treatment than the primary systemic disease would have required. If fibrositis is identified as a concomitant problem, therapy should be directed toward both disorders.[1] For example, the addition of features of the fibrositis syndrome to patients suffering from rheumatoid arthritis or systemic lupus erythematosus often results in treatment with drugs far stronger than signs of inflammation would warrant. Following treatment of the fibrositis syndrome, the anti-inflammatory drugs or corticosteroids can be significantly reduced or even eliminated.

Etiology. Fibrositis syndrome may be the result of an interaction of local factors, reflex phenomena associated with chronic pain of deep origin, disturbed sleep, or factors involved in the "gate theory" of pain persistence.[1]

Local lesions have been suspected, but are found inconsistently. In these patients, the episacroiliac lipoma (described in Chapt. 7) is not likely responsible for the widespread pain in the lumbar region.[1] Histopathologic changes described in uncontrolled studies of trigger points include a metachromatic substance in interfibrillar spaces,[17] masses of mucoid amorphous substances between muscle fascicles, platelet clots or clusters, and mast cells discharging granules into intercellular spaces.[18] In one report,[19] the lactic dehydrogenase isoenzymes, LD 3-5 fractions were found to be increased in tissue and blood.[19]

Reflex phenomena as contributing factors in pathogenesis have been the subject of much speculation since Travell's mapping of the trigger point locations. She suggested a reflex pain cycle,[9] further elaborated as a pain-spasm-pain cycle by Bonica.[8] A concept of a circular physiologic mechanism in which emotional stress enhances muscle spasm with local vasoconstriction and with further induced muscle spasm has been the subject of intense speculation.[20] Following "misuse injury,"[21] a trigger point becomes established. Electromyographic findings of bursts of motor-unit action potentials support a reflex nature of such trigger points.[22,23] The persistence of pain and reflex muscle spasm are associated with inhibition of voluntary movement, increased blood flow, and cutaneous or deep hyperalgesia. These changes may be found in sites far removed from the area of deep pain.[1]

In a controlled study utilizing a standardized task, patients suffering from chronic muscle tension produced 50% more electrical activity in performing the task than did normal controls. The patients' estimations of the degree of muscle tension were lower than measured. This misperception of muscle tension may require a reeducation program.[24]

The persistence of the reflex phenomenon thought to be involved in the trigger point pathogenesis may involve features of the gate theory of pain discussed in Chapter 13. Myofascial trigger points are thought to correlate with acupuncture points.[25] Enkephalins, endorphins, and related neurochemicals may relate to these phenomena.[1]

The sleep disturbance seen in patients with the fibrositis syndrome may not simply be the result of pain. Rather, Moldofsky has provided evidence that deprivation of stage 4 non-REM sleep may induce lesions comparable to trigger points.[3,15,16] These investigations suggest that an endogenous arousal system is activated by stressful life situations. In turn, this disturbed sleep, pain, and fatigue become locked into a self-perpetuating cycle.[3,13]

Although osteoarthritis is found in many patients with the fibrositis syndrome,[14] symptoms do not appear to correlate with degenerative changes of the spinal apophyseal joints, or disc degeneration.[26,27] Although most persons over the age of 40 will have developed osteoarthritis, these radiographic features should be interpreted with caution. This caveat has been discussed in previous chapters.

Laboratory and Radiographic Examination. As mentioned earlier, a requirement for the diagnosis of primary fibrositis is the finding of normal laboratory tests. In addition to the erythrocyte sedimentation rate, complete blood count, urinalysis, and muscle enzymes, we commonly utilize a chemical battery or profile that includes tests of thyroid function. Metabolic disorders such as hypo- or hypercalcemia, diabetes mellitus, thyroid dysfunction, and hyperlipidemias are ruled out at small cost. Dysproteinemia and hematologic malignancies can similarly be excluded. Radiographic examination of patients with fibrositis sometimes reveals calcification of the lower costal cartilages; the association to fibrositis is unclear.[28] Straightening of the cervical spine may also be noted.

Differential Diagnosis. The fibrositis syndrome is not synonymous with psychogenic rheumatism. It differs significantly from the latter by the presence, the location, and the constancy of trigger points. The fibrositic patient often relates symptoms to changes in her *external* environment including weather, heat, cold, humidity, rest, or exercise. These external factors influence the patient's symptoms for better or for worse. Conversely, the patient with psychogenic rheumatism is at the mercy of changes in her *internal* environment; symptoms vary with mood, psyche, pleasure, excitement, mental distraction, worry, or fatigue. A problem exists when a patient with the fibrositis syndrome also has a marked neurosis. The patient with psychogenic rheumatism frequently exhibits the "touch me not" reaction when a physical examination is performed.[29] Such patients react excessively to the examiner's touch anywhere on the body.

Secondary fibrositis has been described in association with metabolic, hematologic, neuropathic, and occult or overt malignant disorders.[14] Occult early connective tissue disease must also be excluded.[11] One of the common causes for secondary fibrositis is a hypothyroid myopathy (Hoffman's syndrome).[21] These patients have painful muscle spasm and the characteristic slow relaxation phase of myxedema reflexes in addition to features of fibrositis; myoedema presumably underlies these features. Occasionally the use of laxatives may result in a similar constellation of findings, as they may induce hypokalemia and give rise to a state of muscle irritability.[30]

Five other conditions that can be confused with the fibrositis syndrome deserve more detailed consideration and are described here.

Polymyalgia Rheumatica. This syndrome occurs in older persons, is characterized by pain and stiffness in the neck, shoulder, and pelvic girdle, and is accompanied by a rapid erythrocyte sedimentation rate.[31] Temporal arteritis must be excluded. The older age and the abnormal tests of inflammation distinguish polymyalgia or temporal arteritis from the fibrositis syndrome.

Rheumatoid Arthritis. Symptoms of fatigue, myalgia, and malaise may develop before the onset of joint symptoms in patients with rheumatoid arthritis[32] or other connective tissue diseases.[14] The test for rheumatoid factor may be positive despite the absence of evident articular inflammation. Careful inquiry for morning stiffness in true joint locations, particularly in the fingers and toes, careful palpation of digits for joint synovitis, and examination for finger flexor tendinitis should be carried out. Although response to aspirin therapy is nonspecific, patients with fibrositis secondary to rheumatoid arthritis generally show a better response than do patients with primary fibrositis.

The Hypermobility Syndrome. Hypermobility has been found in approximately 7% of school children[33] and 4% of adults;[34] such hypermobile individuals occasionally develop a generalized pain state. This may begin upon resuming increased physical activity after a period of illness or sedentary activity. These patients require more muscle tone to maintain joint function than do others. Most patients with the hypermobility syndrome have true joint pain,[34] and this may help to distinguish the hypermobility syndrome from the fibrositis syndrome (see Chapt. 5).

Idiopathic Edema. These patients often present with morning stiffness and swelling of the hands, and with aching, warmth, and purplish discoloration of the legs after they have been dependent for some time. They suffer periodic extreme fatigue. Nocturia, awakening with puffy eyes and face, marked fluctuation in body weight, and lower extremity edema that develops toward evening should suggest idiopathic edema. Although these patients have general tenderness they do not have true trigger points. They may have subtle nonpitting edema. Treatment with salt restriction, diuretics, and in the occasional patient, use of dextroamphetamine is beneficial and assists in distinguishing idiopathic edema from the fibrositis syndrome.[35]

Dyskinetic Phase of Parkinsonism. Stiffness associated with this condition may be confused with fibrositis, particularly if Parkinsonism develops in the fourth or fifth decade of life.[36] Other evidences of Parkinsonism, such as tremor at rest, cog-wheel movements, absence of associated arm movement, nocturnal drooling of saliva, or a positive blink test in which the patient blinks synchronously with tapping over the bridge of the nose should be sought.

Management. Identification of trigger points that reproduce the patient's pain is a great moral victory for the patient. Family members, tired of hearing the patient complain without seeing evidence of disease, have usually inferred a psychogenic pain state. The clinician may now direct the patient away from a purely psychologic cause for the symptomatology.[1]

The patient comes to the physician feeling threatened by her illness. Treatment should begin with reassurance, explanation, and relief from mechanical stress to the neck and low-back areas.[1] Initial therapy should include proper sleep position with support under the arch of the neck, use of a firm mattress, and development of strong abdominal muscles to provide back support.

Pain relief enables the patient to enter a general mobilization-exercise program. Identifying trigger points and injecting them with a corticosteroid-anesthetic mixture is helpful and can often be advised on the first visit.[10,14] Narcotics do not play a role in the treatment of the fibrositis syndrome, and indeed they don't work. Drugs that are useful include meprobamate, carisoprodol, and diazepam to depress the brainstem activating systems and provide a sedative effect. Furthermore, they may act centrally as skeletal muscle relaxants.[37] Nocturnal sedation with amitriptyline, 25 to 100 mg at bedtime, is helpful for sleep disturbance.[1]

Attitudinal changes should be approached with the patient. The clinician should urge the patient to recognize perfectionistic features and impatience with activities of daily living, since these patients tend to complete a task no matter what the physical cost. These patients should be taught to pace physical activity, housekeeping, or hobbies. They should pursue a physical fitness activity such as swimming, roller skating, tennis, and racquetball depending on overall assessment. These activities tend to involve considerable muscular stretching as well as toning up. Tension should be dealt with by rest, programmed exercise, and emotional escape. Biofeedback relaxation and learning to appreciate tension perception are often helpful.[24]

Physical therapy with mobilizing exercises should be part of the regimen of every patient with the fibrositis syndrome. Patients often find a hot bath or ice pack rewarding. A vapocoolant spray has been helpful for thoracic trigger points.[10] Such measures should be utilized immediately before performing a stretching-mobilizing exercise program. Additional exercises for posture correction, and exercises to correct any functional deficit should be individually tailored to the patient's needs.[13] We recommend that a 10- to 15-minute exercise regimen be performed in the morning before dressing and be repeated in the evening following undressing.[1,38] If the fibrositis syndrome overlies another associated disease, the fibrositis must be managed concomitantly with the basic disease.[14]

Outcome and Additional Suggestions. The patient should know at the onset that a multidisciplinary approach as outlined will take several months before significant benefit is realized. Loss of all symptoms is unusual,[1] and the longer the patient has suffered before entering treatment, the less favorable the outcome.[14] It is wise for the clinician to inform the patient that during the first month the pain may actually seem worse. This can result from vigorous stretching, or simply from changing the patient's routine.

If the exercises are done with a gradual prolonged initiation of the stretching portion of each exercise, less irritation will occur. On occasion amitriptyline may result in a stimulating rather than a sedative effect and patients should be warned that if this occurs, amitriptyline should be discontinued and another tricyclic tried (see Chapt. 13).

Interruption of employment can be a disaster. The patient should be kept both psychologically and physically active, keeping in mind the value of a job as a positive distraction. If fired or forced to resign because of failure to perform as a result of pain and exhaustion, these patients seldom return to full productive capacity.[1] After an interval of 4 to 6 weeks, night pain or persistent regional pain reproduced by trigger-point palpation may indicate the need for another corticosteroid trigger-point injection. Some clinicians prefer multiple repeated injections with only a local anesthetic. No controlled observations are available comparing the results of a corticosteroid-anesthetic injection to results obtained when a local anesthetic is used alone. A total maximum of 40 mg of methylprednisolone or equivalent can be administered into multiple sites at any one time. The steroid may be suspended in 1 to 10 ml of a local anesthetic, depending on the amount of corticosteroid used.

The expertise of the Bureau of Vocational Rehabilitation may be utilized for the purpose of evaluating the effect of chronic pain on the job performance and the psychosocial makeup of the patient. We have had good results when the patient is brought in contact with a knowledgeable vocational counselor. Work should not require prolonged sitting or standing. Rather, these patients should be provided jobs that require variation in body positions. They seem to function better as secretaries, store managers, hostesses, or teachers, and less well as bookkeepers, accountants, and physicians!

In our experience many of these patients do obtain gratifying relief of symptoms. We have followed hundreds of these patients for many years; we remain amazed at their diligence in performing the exercise program twice daily, and often they no longer require drug therapy. A subgroup requires amitriptyline during stressful situations. Total cures are rare. This is in sharp contradistinction to the results of rheumatoid arthritis and other connective tissue disease in which a significant minority have remissions.[1] The young woman who develops the fibrositis syndrome shortly after the establishment of a family has a less satisfactory outlook for remission than a similar patient with lupus or rheumatoid arthritis.[1] Current research into endorphins, antipain regions in the central nervous system, and gate controls may lead to more satisfactory solutions.

REFERENCES

1. Smythe HA: Nonarticular rheumatism and psychogenic musculoskeletal syndromes. *In* Arthritis and Allied Conditions. 9th Ed. Edited by DJ McCarty. Philadelphia, Lea & Febiger, 1979.
2. Simons DG: Muscle pain syndromes—Part II. Am J Phys Med 55:15–41, 1976.
3. Smythe HA, Moldofsky H: Two contributions to understanding of the "fibrositis" syndrome. Bull Rheum Dis 28:928–931, 1977.
4. Travell J, Rinzler S, Herman M: Pain and disability of the shoulder and arm. JAMA 120:417–422, 1942.
5. Edeiken J, Wolferth CC: Persistent pain in the shoulder region following myocardial infarction. Am J Med Sci 191:201–210, 1936.
6. Simons DG: Muscle pain syndromes—Part I. Am J Phys Med 54:289–311, 1975.
7. Gowers WR: Lumbago: Its lessons and analogues. Br Med J 1:117–121, 1904.
8. Bonica JJ: Management of myofascial pain syndromes in general practice. JAMA 164:732–738, 1957.
9. Travell J, Rinzler SH: The myofascial genesis of pain. Postgrad Med 11:425–434, 1952.
10. Travell J: Myofascial trigger points: clinical view. *In* Advances in Pain Research and Therapy, Vol. I. Edited by JJ Bonica, D Albe-Fessard. New York, Raven Press, 1976.
11. Slocum CH: Fibrositis. Clinics 2:169–178, 1943.
12. Copeman WSC: Aetiology of the fibrositic nodule: a clinical contribution. Br Med J 2:263–264, 1943.
13. Smythe HA: 'Fibrositis' as a disorder of pain modulation. Clin Rheum Dis 5:823–832, 1979.
14. Kraft GH, Johnson EW, LaBan MM: The fibrositis syndrome. Arch Phys Med Rehabil 49:155–162, 1968.
15. Moldofsky H, Scarisbrick P, England R, Smythe H: Musculoskeletal symptoms and non-REM sleep disturbance in patients with "fibrositis syndrome" and healthy subjects. Psychosom Med 37:341–351, 1975.
16. Moldofsky H, Scarisbrick P: Induction of neurasthenic musculoskeletal pain syndrome by selective sleep stage deprivation. Psychosom Med 38:35–44, 1976.
17. Brendstrup P, Jespersen K, Asboe-Hansen G: Morphological and chemical connective tissue changes in fibrositic muscles. Ann Rheum Dis 16:438–440, 1957.
18. Awad EA: Interstitial myofibrositis: hypothesis of the mechanism. Arch Phys Med Rehabil 54:449–453, 1973.

19. Ibrahim GA, Awad EA, Kottke FJ: Interstitial myofibrositis: serum and muscle enzymes and lactate dehydrogenase isoenzymes. Arch Phys Med Rehabil 55:23–28, 1974.
20. Bonica JJ: Neurophysiologic and pathologic aspects of acute and chronic pain. Arch Surg *112*:750–761, 1977.
21. Fowler WM, Taylor RG: Differential diagnosis of muscle diseases. *In* Musculoskeletal Disorders. Edited by RD D'Ambrosia. Philadelphia, JB Lippincott, 1977.
22. Simons DG: Electrogenic nature of palpable bands and "jump sign" associated with myofascial trigger points. *In* Advances in Pain Research and Therapy, Vol I. Edited by JJ Bonica, D Albe-Fessard. New York, Raven Press, 1976.
23. Cobb CR, deVries HA, Urban RT, et al: Electrical activity in muscle pain. Am J Phys Med *54*:80–87, 1975.
24. Fowler RS, Kraft GH: Tension perception in patients having pain associated with chronic muscle tension. Arch Phys Med Rehabil 55:28–30, 1974.
25. Melzack R, Stillwell DM, Fox EJ: Trigger points and acupuncture points for pain: correlations and implications. Pain 3:3–23, 1977.
26. Lawrence JS, Bremner JM, Bier F: Osteoarthrosis: prevalence in the population and relationship between symptoms and x-ray changes. Ann Rheum Dis 25:1–24, 1966.
27. Lawrence JS: Disc degeneration: its frequency and relationship to symptoms. Ann Rheum Dis 28:121–138, 1969.
28. Lovshin L: Personal communication.
29. Hench PS, Boland EW: The management of chronic arthritis and other rheumatic diseases among soldiers of the United States army. Ann Rheum Dis 5:106–114, 1946.
30. Kahn MF: Joint pain complaints linked to three commonly used medications. Orthop Rev 4:73, 1975.
31. Healey LA: Polymyalgia rheumatica. *In* Arthritis and Allied Conditions. 9th Ed. Edited by DJ McCarty. Philadelphia, Lea & Febiger, 1979.
32. Williams RC: Clinical picture of rheumatoid arthritis. *In* Arthritis and Allied Conditions. 9th Ed. Edited by DJ McCarty. Philadelphia, Lea & Febiger, 1979.
33. Carter C, Wilkinson J: Persistent joint laxity and congenital dislocation of the hip. J Bone Joint Surg *46*:40–45, 1964.
34. Kirk JA, Ansell BM, Bywaters EGL: The hypermobility syndrome; musculoskeletal complaints associated with generalized joint hypermobility. Ann Rheum Dis 26:419–425, 1967.
35. Pinals RS, Dalakos TG, Streeten DH: Idiopathic edema as a cause of nonarticular rheumatism. Arthritis Rheum *22*:396–399, 1979.
36. St John Dixon A: Soft tissue rheumatism: concept and classification. Clin Rheum Dis 5:739–742, 1979.
37. Domino EF: Centrally acting skeletal-muscle relaxants. Arch Phys Med Rehabil 55:369–373, 1974.
38. Lewit K: The needle effect in the relief of myofascial pain. Pain 6:83–90, 1979.

Chapter *13*

CHRONIC PERSISTENT PAIN

Pain is a suffering of the body and mind[1] that can only be known to an individual in his consciousness.[2] Like hunger, pain is an awareness-of-a-need state. It is a drain upon the physical, the emotional, and the economic resources of the patient.[3]

When a person is injured, pain is not always perceived.[4] Consider a football player whose rib is fractured during a tackle; during subsequent active play, the football player may feel no pain. The pain is experienced after play when his attention returns to himself. Thus, pain perception and pain thresholds appear alterable.[5] The phenomena of persistent pain in phantom limbs, or magnification of pain by emotion have stimulated researchers to look beyond a simple conduction system within the central nervous system. Experiments to quantify pain thresholds are actively being pursued.[6-8] Anti-pain impulses from the brain areas that descend to the spinal cord have recently been discovered. These and other factors that influence pain are described in this chapter.

MYOFASCIAL PAIN

Myofascial "trigger points" have been the subject of considerable investigation. These trigger points, located in muscle and fascia,[9] correlate with many acupuncture points.[10] Painful hard places in muscles of patients with rheumatism have been noted for nearly two centuries. In 1904, Gowers,[11] in a thoughtful discussion of lumbago, stated that myalgia, like neuralgia, occurred as a spontaneous, painful condition. He coined the term "fibrositis" for a generalized myofascial pain state associated with the characteristic trigger points. This term was chosen because Gowers broadened the concept of inflammation to include conditions that predispose to induration *or* suppuration.

Gowers presented supporting evidence for his concept of inflammation based on the indurated nature of the trigger point, the sensitivity of muscles to cold, the patient's awareness of morning stiffness, and the histologic feature of increased vascularity. He recognized that there was no hyperplasia or suppuration.

Although the initial trigger point may be of traumatic origin, the persisting discomfort of myofascial pain syndromes is thought to arise from a pain-cycle mechanism. Reflex spasm in response to pain contributes to a barrage of sympathetic impulses. These result in vasospasm and augmented firing of small sensory nerve fibers.[11] The emotional stress of persistent pain can further result in muscle spasm. This pain-spasm-pain cycle[12] has been extensively studied. Electromyographic studies of trigger points suggest continuous firing or bursts of motor-unit action potentials and muscle contraction.[13,14] Recent electrophysiologic research in myofascial pain supports the pain-spasm-pain cycle as originally proposed.[14] For those interested in further detail relative to trigger-point mechanisms, an extensive review of the subject is recommended.[15,16]

GATE CONTROL THEORY UPDATED

Melzack and Wall in 1965 suggested that *modulation* of nerve synapses within the dorsal horn of the spinal cord occurs with a feedback control system from other parts of the nervous system. They suggested that each synapse or "gate" may be closed or open to the pain impulses. Thus pain perception is subdued or enhanced by "gates" all along the nerve pathway.[17]

Nerve impulses produced by noxious injury excite "central transmission cells," which receive both excitatory and inhibitory messages from other parts of the nervous system. Descending anti-pain impulses come from the brainstem and higher centers, such as the analgesic center in the mesencephalon.[5,8,18-23] The analgesic center and its descending anti-pain controls to the spinal cord "gates" are stimulated by non-noxious impulses such as a gentle breeze, love stroking, soft speech, or other soothing sensations. Pain perception results from an interplay of all these influences and is perceived only if the "gates" allow the message to reach the brain.[24] The gate theory has provoked much criticism, debate, and research in the past decade.[25] The criticism was that the system was too simple. Mechanical, thermal, and other sensory systems were probably also involved.

The search for neurotransmitter substances involved in anti-pain transmission led researchers to the discovery of *endogenous* morphine-like peptides, the enkephalins and the endorphins,[26-28] which arise within the central nervous system.[29-32] The morphine-like action of these substances is blocked or suppressed by morphine antagonists (e.g., naloxone).[22] Endorphins provide not only a naturally-occurring analgesia but are also involved in regulation of mood and affect. Thus the perception of pain and its modification by emotion have been related to a complex and fascinating neurochemistry.[33]

Pain is associated with abnormal firing patterns or after-discharges both in spinal cord cells and in cells of the brainstem reticular formation. Transmitter cells then set up a "pattern-generating mechanism" *for continued bursts of firing*[8] or reverberating circuits in the internuncial pool.[34] These cells and synapses can be modulated by changes in emotion and behavior (e.g., "rest can relieve pain"). Furthermore, emotional factors may provoke liberation of substances that enhance sympathetic nervous system reflexes.[3] Pain can be modulated further by brainstem inhibitory anti-pain areas. Imbalance in the feedback regulation of the central nervous system results in changes in the sensitivity of pain receptors.

Pain occurs when the number of nerve impulses per unit of time carried from peripheral nerves to the brain areas exceeds a critical level, or when there is a *decreased* input of anti-pain impulses from the analgesic centers located in the mesencephalon. The mesencephalon requires *stimulation* by non-noxious stimuli in order to respond with analgesia.

Because of the intimate relation of stress to illness and the suggestion that stress is linked to ACTH, corticosteroids, enkephalins, and endorphins, we may someday recognize associations of a patient's basic temperament to a specific disease.[32] Quantitative and qualitative determinations of these anti-pain substances perhaps may lead to a better understanding of the relation of tension and anxiety to stress reactions.

PSYCHOLOGIC FACTORS IN CHRONIC PAIN

Pain may cause temporary changes in personality.[35] Psychologic evaluation of persons who suffer from chronic pain reveals several common deviations including neuroticism and depression. These personality patterns do not, however, relate to future disability or disease outcome.[36-39] In fact, these deviations tend to normalize following relief of the pain.[35] Anxiety, hostility, denial, fear, guilt, hysteria, and depression are associated with changes in pain perception.[40]

In one study, six different personality patterns were defined, yet none of these related to chronicity or to "illness behavior patterns."[38] In another study, examining patients who were undergoing surgery for treatment of painful disorders, affirmative answers to two questions were useful as predictors of a poor outcome: (1) "Has your appetite decreased recently?", and (2) "Has your sexual interest lessened?"[41] In other reports of patients treated nonsurgically, certain other characteristic features were also found that were predictive of an unsuccessful outcome. These included guilt, particularly if related to a supernatural reason given for the illness; projection of guilt onto others, particularly the therapist;[42,43] and pretreatment medication dependency, accident proneness, and expressed dissatisfaction with previous therapy.[44] During care in a comprehensive pain center, these patients opposed psychologic approaches, used circumscribed delusions, and resisted many attempts at treatment. The pain center utilized formal and informal psychologic approaches in an effort to alleviate a "negative—resigned" attitude in such patients.[42]

Pain of purely psychologic origin is rare. Such pain includes hysteria, phobic pain (pain that prevents the hand from doing harm), assertive pain (e.g., a compulsive rebel who uses pain to assert control over others),[40] or delusional pain (a psychosis with a well circumscribed delusional system and with pain as the central complaint).[45]

ANTI-PAIN MODALITIES

It has been stated that if *acute* painful disorders were managed more astutely, there would be less *chronic* pain.[46] Pain centers must often deal with the results of less than adequate prior management in these patients. An institution or pain center that provides only one modality of care for these patients is doomed to failure; this inadequate care may likely exhaust the patient's emotional and financial resources.

Oral Drug Therapy

We have emphasized throughout this book that oral medication often plays a minor role in the management of many musculoskeletal soft tissue pain syndromes. When inappropriately used, drug dependence may be as great a problem as the underlying pain disorder. In addition to analgesics and nonsteroidal anti-inflammatory agents, we generally use two additional classes of oral medication. First are the skeletal muscle relaxants such as meprobamate, carisoprodol, and diazepam. These agents are thought to depress the brainstem activating system, to provide a sedative effect, and to have central-acting skeletal muscle relaxant properties.[47] Often they are used only when initiating an exercise program.

The second class of drugs, the tricyclic anti-depressants such as amitriptyline, imipramine, desipramine, doxepin, and protriptyline are beneficial for selective patients, particularly those with chronic pain or the fibrositis syndrome. These agents may provide increased relief from pain and reduced need for analgesics.[48-50] It is difficult to separate the pain-sparing effects from the anti-depression effect.[51] The tricyclic drugs are generally well tolerated. However, drug interactions have been reported. These include an increased anti-depressant effect with thyroxin, decreased anti-depressant effect as well as marked sedation with alcohol, additive anti-cholinergic effect with anti-Parkinsonism drugs, increased anti-coagulant effect with dicumarol, increased hypotensive effect with guanethidine, and decreased anti-depressant effect with propranolol or methyldopa.[52] Contraindications include glaucoma, urinary retention, and previous hypersensitivity to the drug. They should not be given concomitantly with a monoamine oxidase inhibitor. Central nervous system stimulation with nervousness, insomnia, and heart palpitations occur but are infrequent. Appetite stimulation is a definite problem. These drugs are generally given in small doses before retiring. The initial starting dose should be low, followed by gradual increases until restful sleep is noted. The dose may then be reduced to the lowest effective maintenance dosage; every-other-day dosage may maintain the beneficial effect.

Transcutaneous Electrical Nerve Stimulators (TENS)

Patients with persistent soft tissue rheumatic pain and spasm may respond to transcutaneous nerve stimulation; however, many investigators remain skeptical. One author states that use of percutaneous currents has been resurrected by the desire for alternatives to traditional physical therapy and to provide a market for the electronics industry.[53] Another author states that transcutaneous stimulation is a safe placebo.[54] If so, it is expensive. Yet transcutaneous nerve stimulation, if successful, does allow the patient to participate in treatment (Fig. 13–1). Instructions regarding the proper variation of the electric current and frequencies, and the regions of application such as to painful areas, dermatomes, or distal sites must be provided.[53,55]

Studies have attempted to quantify the role of TENS units in pain therapy. Although they do suggest that use of a TENS unit modifies pain, well demonstrated placebo effects complicate interpretation of the data. Studies are further complicated by the large number and types of TENS units available and the types of pain problems being evaluated.[55–61] Whether the effect is real or placebo, TENS use may at times be beneficial in the treatment of persistent soft tissue rheumatic pain if the patient supplements this modality with a total therapeutic program. Placebo response may represent a specific therapeutic modality in that stimulation of endogenous endorphins results.[62,63]

Implantable (dorsal spinal column) stimulators have been the subject of interest, debate, concern, and guarded enthusiasm and should be considered only in very select patients.[56,64]

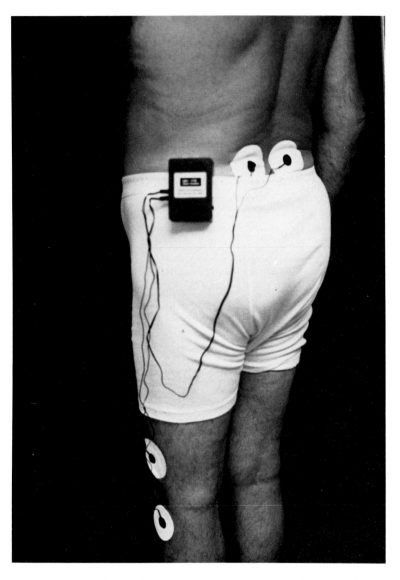

Fig. 13–1. One of several types of transcutaneous electric nerve stimulators with electrodes in place for sciatica.

Acupuncture

Acupuncture and electro-acupuncture received initial enthusiasm in the lay press a few years ago. As previously noted, acupuncture sites often overlap myofascial trigger points. Some 365 acupuncture points have been reported.[65] Pain thresholds may be raised by acupuncture.[5] In some studies, short-term pain relief was associated with acupuncture treatment; similar relief occurred in patients treated with placebo acupuncture.[65-67] The initial enthusiasm for acupuncture in myofascial and soft tissue pain syndromes has waned.

Biofeedback Training

The application of biofeedback training to relieve muscle tension has been the subject of considerable interest over the last two decades.[53,68] A visual feedback method to facilitate muscle relaxation was first reported a decade ago.[69] Biofeedback training is essentially a reinforcement of muscle reeducation. It attempts to modify autonomic functions, pain, and motor disturbances by acquired volitional control.[53] The technique employs sequential voluntary muscle contraction and relaxation. Electromyography (EMG) provides audible or visible feedback to the patient.[70] Biofeedback training is generally used only as an adjunct to another treatment in order to enhance that therapy.[71] A controlled study of EMG monitored biofeedback for relaxation training recognized that the taking of frequent rest breaks by the anxiety-tension-prone individual may be of equal importance to that of the biofeedback training.[72] Biofeedback training for reinforcement of muscle reeducation is also helpful in cases of hysterical paralysis, in modifying autonomic nervous system function and pain, and in developing control of motor disturbances.[53] Using biofeedback training for raising skin temperature in patients with Raynaud's phenomenon has been noted (see Chapt. 5).

Another simple relaxation technique uses a meditation procedure that can be practiced independent of a therapist.[73] The patient is taught how to relax body segments by deep concentration. This technique facilitates rehabilitation, particularly in patients with features of hopelessness and depression.

Transcutaneous nerve stimulators, acupuncture, biofeedback training, and psychotropic drugs are still undergoing clinical evaluation and are to be considered only as adjuncts to a comprehensive treatment plan.[74]

DMSO

Dimethyl sulfoxide (DMSO) provides local analgesia when used by topical application.[75] A garlic odor imparted to the user's breath has limited the ability to test this agent in double-blind controlled trials.

Although ocular toxicity in animals led to removal of the agent from the market, DMSO may soon be released as a controlled drug, to be dispensed only by prescription. Skin sensitivity and irritation may result from its use. At present, use of this product remains investigational.

Further Measures

The decade following the publication of the "gate control" theory has been fruitful. The therapeutic measures described in preceding chapters will help the vast majority of patients. For the present, the physician can often *prevent* a chronic pain state by following the six points of management presented in the Introduction. When pain has become chronic (defined as longer than 6 months in duration),[40] the clinician should seek factors that compensate the patient for having pain. Occasionally a state of conflict and anxiety may produce a self-destructive injury-producing act ("the accident process").[76] Such patients may respond best to a group psychotherapy program including role changes in home and work, acquiring new social or personal skills, and other measures to improve the patient's "self image."[77] Biofeedback relaxation or transcutaneous nerve stimulation may improve pain:antipain imbalance. Such measures can succeed only if the physician and patient cooperate in a comprehensive therapeutic endeavor.

Chronic pain may require efforts to correct abnormal learned behavior. Operant conditioning, or behavior modification, as recommended by Fordyce[78] has been helpful in reducing the patient's awareness of pain and in allowing the patient to return to a more natural social existence. Operant conditioning refers to the recognition and removal of anything that enforces or encourages pain. Provision of rewards for proper attitude and behavior may prod a poorly motivated patient.[79]

Most patients with chronic pain can achieve relief and become effective members of their community and family. To achieve this, the patient, clinician, therapist, vocational counselor, insurance personnel, and other "third-party" persons must work together by communicating, trying, and trusting one another.

REFERENCES

1. Webster: The New American Webster Handy College Dictionary. New York, New American Library, Inc., 1972.
2. Merskey H: Psychiatric aspects of the control of pain. *In* Advances in Pain Research and Therapy, Vol I. Edited by JJ Bonica, D Albe-Fessard. New York, Raven Press, 1976.
3. Bonica JJ: Neurophysiologic and pathologic aspects of acute and chronic pain. Arch Surg 112:750–761, 1977.
4. Wall PD: On the relation of injury to pain: The John J Bonica lecture. Pain 6:253–264, 1979.

5. Mayer DJ, Price DD: Central nervous system mechanisms of analgesia. Pain 2:379–404, 1976.
6. Lynn B, Perl ER: A comparison of four tests for assessing the pain sensitivity of different subjects and test areas. Pain 3:353–365, 1977.
7. Sternbach RA: Evaluation of pain relief. Surg Neurol 4:199–201, 1975.
8. Melzack R, Loeser JD: Phantom body pain in paraplegics: Evidence for a central "pattern generating mechanism" for pain. Pain 4:195–210, 1978.
9. Travell J: Myofascial trigger points: clinical view. *In* Advances in Pain Research and Therapy, Vol. I. Edited by JJ Bonica, D Albe-Fessard. New York, Raven Press, 1976.
10. Melzack R, Stillwell DM, Fox EJ: Trigger points and acupuncture points for pain: Correlations and implications. Pain 3:3–23, 1977.
11. Gowers WR: Lumbago: Its lessons and analogues. Br Med J 1:117–121, 1904.
12. Travell J, Rinzler S, Herman M: Pain and disability of the shoulder and arm. JAMA 120:417–422, 1942.
13. Cobb CR, deVries HA, Urban RT, et al: Electrical activity in muscle pain. Am J Phys Med 54:80–87, 1975.
14. Simons DG: Electrogenic nature of palpable bands and "jump sign" associated with myofascial trigger points. *In* Advances in Pain Research and Therapy, Vol. I. Edited by JJ Bonica, D Albe-Fessard. New York, Raven Press, 1976.
15. Simons DG: Muscle pain syndromes—Part 1. Am J Phys Med 54:289–311, 1975.
16. Simons DG: Muscle pain syndromes—Part 2. Am J Phys Med 55:15–42, 1976.
17. Melzack R, Wall PD: Pain mechanisms: A new theory. Science 150:971–979, 1965.
18. Reynolds DV: Surgery in the rat during electrical analgesia induced by focal brain stimulation. Science 164:444–445, 1969.
19. Dennis SG, Melzack R: Pain-signalling systems in the dorsal and ventral spinal cord. Pain 4:97–132, 1977.
20. Bloom F, Segal D, Ling N, Guillemin R: Endorphins: Profound behavioral effects in rats suggest new etiological factors in mental illness. Science 194:630, 1976.
21. Liebeskind JC: Pain modulation by central nervous system stimulation. *In* Advances in Pain Research and Therapy, Vol. I. Edited by JJ Bonica, D Albe-Fessard. New York, Raven Press, 1976.
22. Adams JE: Naloxone reversal of analgesia produced by brain stimulation in the human. Pain 2:161–166, 1976.
23. Procacci P: A survey of modern concept of pain. *In* Handbook of Clinical Neurology, Vol. 1. Edited by PJ Vinken, GW Bruyn. Amsterdam, North-Holland, 1969.
24. Wall PD: Modulation of pain by nonpainful events. *In* Advances in Pain Research and Therapy, Vol. I. Edited by JJ Bonica, D Albe-Fessard. New York, Raven Press, 1976.
25. Nathan PW: The gate-control theory of pain. Brain 99:123–158, 1976.
26. Pert CB, Pasternak G, Snyder SH: Opiate agonists and antagonists discriminated by receptor binding in brain. Science 182:1359–1361, 1973.
27. Simon EJ, Hiller JM, Edelman I: Stereo-specific binding of the potent narcotic analgesic (^{3}H) etorphine to rat-brain homogenate. Proc Natl Acad Sci USA 70:1947–1949, 1973.
28. Terenius L: Characteristics of the receptor for narcotic analgesics and a synaptic plasma membrane fraction from rat brain. Acta Pharmacol Toxicol 33:377–384, 1973.
29. Guillemin R: Beta-lipotropin and endorphins: Implications of current knowledge. Hosp Pract 13:53–60, 1978.
30. Guillemin R: Endorphins, brain peptides that act like opiates. N Engl J Med 296:226–228, 1977.
31. Basbaum AI, Fields HL: Endogenous pain control mechanisms: Review and hypothesis. Ann Neurol 4:451–462, 1978.
32. Rosch PJ: Stress and illness. JAMA 242:427–428, 1979.
33. Bunney WE, Pert CB, Klee W, et al: Basic and clinical studies of endorphins. Ann Intern Med 91:239–250, 1979.
34. Luce JM, Thompson TL, Getto CJ, Byyny RL: New concepts of chronic pain and their implications. Hosp Pract 14:113–123, 1979.

35. Bond MR: Pain and personality in cancer patients. *In* Advances in Pain Research and Therapy, Vol. I. Edited by JJ Bonica, D Albe-Fessard. New York, Raven Press, 1976.
36. Crown S: Psychological aspects of low back pain. Rheumatol Rehabil *17*:114–122, 1978.
37. Waring EM, Weisz GM, Bailey SI: Predictive factors in the treatment of low back pain by surgical intervention. *In* Advances in Pain Research and Therapy, Vol. I. Edited by JJ Bonica, DG Albe-Fessard. New York, Raven Press, 1976.
38. Pilowsky I, Spence ND: Is illness behavior related to chronicity in patients with intractable pain? Pain 2:167–173, 1976.
39. Pheasant HC: The problem back. Curr Pract Orthop Surg 7:89–115, 1977.
40. Millman BS: Managing intractable pain: Resources and recourses. Drug Ther 8:65–80, 1978.
41. Forrest AJ, Wolkind SN: Masked depression in men with low back pain. Rheumatol Rehabil *13*:148–153, 1974.
42. Khatami M, Rush AJ: A pilot study of the treatment of outpatients with chronic pain: symptom control, stimulus control and social system intervention. Pain 5:163–172, 1978.
43. Diamond MD, Weiss AJ, Grynbaum B: The unmotivated patient. Arch Phys Med Rehabil *49*:281–284, 1968.
44. Swanson DW, Swenson WM, Maruta T, Floreen AC: The dissatisfied patient with chronic pain. Pain *4*:367–378, 1978.
45. Swanson DW, Swenson WM, Maruta T, McPhee MC: Program for managing chronic pain. Mayo Clin Proc *51*:401–408, 1976.
46. Cailliet R: Chronic pain: is it necessary? Arch Phys Med Rehabil 60:4–7, 1979.
47. Domino EF: Centrally acting skeletal-muscle relaxants. Arch Phys Med Rehabil 55:369–373, 1974.
48. Halpern LM: Analgesic drugs in the management of pain. Arch Surg *112*:861–869, 1977.
49. Duthie AM: The use of phenothiazines and tricyclic antidepressants in the treatment of intractable pain. S Afr Med J *51*:246–247, 1977.
50. Beaumont G: The use of psychotropic drugs in other painful conditions. J Int Med Res *4*:56–57, 1976.
51. Ward NG, Bloom VL, Friedel RO: The effectiveness of tricyclic antidepressants in the treatment of coexisting pain and depression. Pain 7:331–341, 1979.
52. Rosenbaum AH, Maruta T, Richelson E: Drugs that alter mood; tricyclic agents and monoamine oxidase inhibitors. Mayo Clin Proc *54*:335–344, 1979.
53. Rusk HA: Rehabilitation Medicine, 4th Ed. St. Louis, CV Mosby, 1977.
54. Swezey RL: Rehabilitation aspects in arthritis. *In* Arthritis and Allied Conditions, 9th Ed. Edited by DJ McCarty. Philadelphia, Lea & Febiger, 1979.
55. McKelvy PL: Clinical report on the use of specific TENS units. Phys Therapy 58:1474–1477, 1978.
56. Eriksson MBE, Sjolund BH, Nielzen S: Long term results of peripheral conditioning stimulation as an analgesic measure in chronic pain. Pain 6:335–347, 1979.
57. Thorsteinsson G, Stonnington HH, Stillwell GK, Elveback LR: The placebo effect of transcutaneous electrical stimulation. Pain 5:31–41, 1978.
58. Sternbach RA, Ignelzi RJ, Deems LM, Timmermans G: Transcutaneous electrical analgesia: a follow-up analysis. Pain 2:35–41, 1976.
59. Timmermans G, Sternbach RA: Human chronic pain and personality: A canonical correlation analysis. *In* Advances in Pain Research and Therapy, Vol. I. Edited by JJ Bonica, D Albe-Fessard. New York, Raven Press, 1976.
60. Schuster GD, Infante MC: The efficacy of TENS; noninvasive postoperative analgesia. Orthop Rev 8:143–149, 1979.
61. Serrato JC: Pain control by transcutaneous nerve stimulation. South Med J 72:67–71, 1979.
62. Levine JD, Gordon NC, Fields HL: The mechanism of placebo analgesia. Lancet 2:654–657, 1978.
63. Benson H, Epstein MD: The placebo effect: A neglected asset in the care of patients. JAMA 232:1225–1227, 1975.

64. Long DM: Electrical stimulation for the control of pain. Arch Surg *112*:884–888, 1977.
65. Murphy TM, Bonica JJ: Acupuncture analgesia and anesthesia. Arch Surg *112*:896–902, 1977.
66. Kepes ER, Chen M, Schapira M: A critical evaluation of acupuncture in the treatment of chronic pain. *In* Advances in Pain Research and Therapy, Vol. I. Edited by JJ Bonica, D Albe-Fessard. New York, Raven Press, 1976.
67. Waylonis GW: Long-term follow-up on patients with fibrositis treated with acupuncture. Ohio State Med J *73*:299–302, 1977.
68. Peck CL, Kraft GH: Electromyographic biofeedback for pain related to muscle tension. Arch Surg *112*:889–895, 1977.
69. Jacobs A, Felton GS: Visual feedback of myoelectric output to facilitate muscle relaxation in normal persons and patients with neck injuries. Arch Phys Med Rehabil *50*:34–39, 1969.
70. Kottke FJ: Therapeutic exercise. *In* Handbook of Physical Medicine and Rehabilitation, 2nd Ed. Edited by FH Krusen. Philadelphia, WB Saunders, 1971.
71. Shapiro D, Schwartz GE: Biofeedback and visceral learning: clinical applications. Semin Psychol *4*:171–183, 1972.
72. DeVries HA, Burke RK, Hopper RT, Sloan JH: Efficacy of EMG biofeedback in relaxation training. Am J Phys Med *56*:75–81, 1977.
73. Grzesiak RC: Relaxation techniques in treatment of chronic pain. Arch Phys Med Rehabil *58*:270–272, 1977.
74. deJong RH: Central pain mechanisms. JAMA *239*:2784, 1978.
75. Penrod DS, Bacharach B, Templeton JY: Dimethyl sulfoxide for incisional pain after thoracotomy. Ann NY Acad Sci *141*:493–495, 1967.
76. Hirschfeld AH, Behan RC: The accident process: etiological considerations of industrial injuries. JAMA *186*:193–199, 1963.
77. Steinhart MJ: Conversion hysteria. Am Fam Pract *21*:125–129, 1980.
78. Fordyce WE: An operant conditioning method for managing chronic pain. Postgrad Med *53*:123–128, 1973.
79. Licht S: History. *In* Therapeutic Exercise. 3rd Ed. Edited by JV Basmajian. Baltimore, Williams & Wilkins, 1978.

Chapter 14

SOFT TISSUE INJECTION

Over two decades of experience in the use of local anesthetics or corticosteroid suspensions for soft tissue injection have established both its safety and its effectiveness in therapy.[1] Although it has been stated by some that no statistically valid data are available to support the use of local injection of corticosteroids in the treatment of musculoskeletal disorders,[2] observations by other clinicians support the safety and prolonged benefit of this therapy.[2-4] Furthermore, in this era of concern for cost containment, soft tissue injection is recognized for its value in reducing the need for more complex prolonged medical measures and for surgical intervention.[5-7] For example, over 70% of patients with stenosing tenosynovitis, "trigger finger," can be successfully treated with this modality without resorting to surgical intervention.[6,7] Hollander reported on the safety of local soft tissue and joint injection therapy in over 100,000 injections in 4000 patients.[3] The incidence of infection was less than 1 per 16,000 injections. Others report 3000 or more injections per year (Mayo Clinic) with no untoward reactions.[2,4] In the past 20 years we too have performed thousands of *soft tissue* injections with few complications.

The technique of soft tissue injection has been presented in each chapter. We recommend combining a corticosteroid with a local anesthetic. Some package inserts accompanying the corticosteroid agents suggest that other agents should not be mixed with them; in our experience no untoward reactions have occurred when local anesthetics are mixed in the same syringe with the corticosteroid suspension. The addition of the local anesthetic has the advantage of providing immediate symptomatic relief and also dilutes the steroid preparation, allowing a more diffuse distribution of the drug with less hazard of local tissue atrophy. The total amount of local anesthetic administered to the patient should be kept to less than 6 to 8 ml if

264

possible. Use of local anesthetics without corticosteroids has been advocated by some; this requires more frequent injections[8,9] and is less often effective in subacute or chronic disorders. Recently introduced longer-acting local anesthetic agents, such as bupivacaine and etidocaine, may prove more effective and improve injection technique.[10]

The addition of a corticosteroid suspension is recommended for the following reasons: (1) benefit is often longer lasting and in most cases one injection suffices, (2) the safety of infrequent injections has been established by time, (3) more frequent injections with a local anesthetic alone increase the risk of inadvertent intravenous instillation of the anesthetic, (4) reactions to local anesthetics are proportional to the number of sites injected as well as the volume and total dosage utilized at any one time, and (5) the addition of the corticosteroid reduces the necessity to locate and inject every trigger point; rather, only the most prominent trigger point need be injected; the less significant lesions usually also improve.

A local anesthetic-corticosteroid injection facilitates an exercise and physical therapy regimen. It is one of the few regional analgesic-anti-inflammatory techniques that is suitable for everyday practice and requires little special training.[1,8] In the treatment of entrapment neuropathies, tendinitis, tenosynovitis, or bursitis, the local anesthetic-corticosteroid injection results in such predictable benefit that diagnosis is assisted by the resulting benefit.

INDICATIONS

Use of soft tissue injection is indicated in traumatic, inflammatory, or degenerative processes of the musculoskeletal system, especially when associated with local tenderness or trigger points;[4,8] to assist in confirming the diagnosis of bursitis, tendinitis, and entrapment neuropathies; and in certain periarticular soft tissue conditions that can lead to limitation of motion. In these situations, injection is helpful in providing a more rapid resumption of active range of motion, thus preventing more serious sequelae.[2]

CONTRAINDICATIONS

Hypersensitivity to any anesthetic preparation is rare but can occur.[11] Dermal allergy is less common with lidocaine and its derivatives.[11] Soft tissue injection is obviously contraindicated in the vicinity of infections. A relative contraindication is an extremely apprehensive or neurotic patient.[8] Injections into tendon areas are contraindicated in anyone who tends to overuse these structures, which may result in tendon rupture.[12]

HAZARDS

A corticosteroid agent for soft tissue injection should be used with some caution in patients who have had previous peptic ulcers or diabetes, or who are using anticoagulants. The diabetic who is taking insulin may be advised to use a sliding scale of increased insulin dosage for 1 or 2 days following the injection based upon the result of fractional urine sugar determinations. Aggravation of the diabetic state is rarely a problem. Application of local compression following soft tissue injection avoids significant hematomas in most patients receiving anticoagulants. An *active* peptic ulcer is a relative contraindication to a local corticosteroid injection. Local injections with corticosteroids should also be used with caution, if at all, in patients with recent thromboembolic disease, pneumonia, or active systemic infection.[8] Introducing infection has become remarkably rare since the introduction of disposable needles and syringes.[3]

The complications of systemic corticosteroids are widely recognized. The interval between injections as recommended in this chapter should prevent systemic complications known to result from prolonged corticosteroid use. Furthermore, the problem of corticosteroid pseudorheumatism will be avoided.[13]

Certain hazards are related to the specific site of injection. A pneumothorax may result when soft tissue injections are made into the chest or trapezius regions.[14] Intravascular injection or hematoma formation is a risk following injection of the popliteal, antecubital, or groin regions. Reflex sympathetic dystrophy and nerve injury with paralysis may follow inadvertent injection of a neurovascular bundle, but are rare complications.

Although tendon rupture following local steroid injection may occur, this complication is infrequent if injections are made around, rather than directly into the tendon, and if overexertion is avoided for a week or longer. Most research supports the finding that harmful effects of corticosteroids on tendons generally result from use of massive corticosteroid doses.[15] Bowstring deformity of a digit following corticosteroid injections for flexor tenosynovitis has been described but is rare.[16] Corticosteroid injections into the region of the Achilles tendon should never be performed, since tendon rupture at this site is a disastrous complication. Patellar tendon rupture following a corticosteroid injection is a distinct hazard in athletes.[17] Experimental studies of corticosteroid injections into rabbit tendons using usual therapeutic doses revealed disorganization of collagen and a 35% loss of tendon strength; this healed within 14 days.[15]

The use of these agents as described here may be associated with specific pharmacologic or hypersensitivity reactions:

Local Anesthetics. (See Table 14–1.) Accidental intravenous introduction of the local anesthetic agent may result in central nervous system or cardiovascular reactions. These effects may depend on the blood levels of the agents, which in turn depend upon the site of the injections, the number of sites injected, and the dose. A linear relationship exists between reactions and the total dose of the local anesthetic.[11]

Central nervous system effects include lightheadedness, dizziness, visual or auditory (tinnitus) complaints, slurred speech, muscle twitching, or muscle tremors, particularly about the face.[11] Cardiovascular effects include prolongation of the conduction time with resultant bradycardia, and stimulation of vascular smooth muscle contractions. Another rare hazard of local anesthetics is anaphylaxis.[11] More severe reactions following intravenous injection include clonic and tonic convulsions, shallow respirations, diminished blood pressure and pulse rate, and finally, cardiorespiratory collapse. These reactions may begin 5 to 15 minutes or even several hours following the injections.[8] Serious hypersensitivity or toxic reactions are more likely

Table 14–1.   Local Anesthetics in Current Use[11]

Anesthetic agents	Concentrations available	Duration of action (Min)
Procaine (Novocaine)	1–2 mg/ml	50
Lidocaine (Xylocaine) (Dilocaine) (L-Caine) (Nervocaine) (Nulicaine) (Ultracaine)	10–15–20 mg/ml	100
Chloroprocaine (Nesacaine)	10–20 mg/ml	60
Mepivacaine (Carbocaine)	10–20 mg/ml	100
Prilocaine (Citanest)	10–20–30 mg/ml	60
Bupivacaine (Marcaine)	2.5–5 mg/ml	175
Etidocaine (Duranest)	2.5–5–10 mg/ml	200

to occur when large amounts of local anesthetic are used alone for soft tissue injection therapy.

The clinician should have an airway, oxygen, intravenous diazepam, short-acting parenteral barbiturates, phenylephrine, epinephrine, and rapid-acting intravenous corticosteroids available for emergency use.[8,11]

More common than the serious reactions described is the more immediate vasovagal reaction seen in patients with vasomotor instability. The vasovagal reaction occurs within seconds following the injection. The patient becomes pale, sweaty, and lightheaded, and may faint. The pulse rate is slow but blood pressure remains normal. A crushable ampule of ammonia is helpful for use in such patients.

Focal muscle injury, which is proportional to the potency and duration of action of the local anesthetic agent, may occur and is usually reversible.[11] Localized nerve damage has not been seen following use of a local anesthetic agent unless the injection is inadvertently made into a nerve.

Corticosteroids. Systemic toxicity from local injections of corticosteroids is infrequent if the interval between subsequent injections is longer than 6 weeks and the number of injections is less than 8 per year.[18] Adrenal suppression may occur but is usually transient.[19] Local complications include infections, which will be rare if the clinician uses disposable equipment and careful aseptic technique.[18] Although infection is a rare complication, the patient should report any post-injection development of pain, redness, or swelling.[8] Local cutaneous

Table 14–2.   Corticosteroids in Current Use

Corticosteroids	Concentrations available	Dose range
Prednisolone tebutate (Hydeltra TBA)	20 mg/ml	5–15 mg
Betamethasone acetate and disodium phosphate (Celestone Soluspan)	6 mg/ml	1.5–3 mg
Methylprednisolone acetate (Depomedrol)	20–40–80 mg/ml	10–20 mg
Triamcinolone acetonide or diacetate (Kenalog, Aristocort)	10–25–40 mg/ml	5–15 mg
Triamcinolone hexacetonide (Aristospan)	5–20 mg/ml	5–20 mg
Dexamethasone acetate suspension (Decadron-LA)	8 mg/ml	0.8–3.2 mg

atrophy or depigmentation may occur;[8,20] the atrophy usually resolves but may require weeks or months to regress. A postinjection "flare" or local crystal reaction occurs in 1 to 2% of patients receiving steroid injections, and is ameliorated with ice packs.[21] When triamcinolone preparations are used for injection in women, menstrual irregularity, breast tenderness, and skin flushing can occur.

Corticosteroids used for local injections should be the repository preparations in suspension.[8] We generally use the dose ranges given in Table 14–2 for any given injection site depending on the size of the area and the total number of sites to be injected.[1] Although we prefer to use procaine or lidocaine in a 1% solution and the methylpred-nisolone acetate or triamcinolone acetonide, the preparations, cost, availability, and personal experience will assist each clinician in choosing the most suitable agents. The addition of epinephrine to the local anesthetic is not recommended.

TECHNIQUE

Prior to injection the point of maximum tenderness should be located by palpation. Then the clinician can use the open end of the needle container cover to indent and mark the trigger point location.[22] Strict skin sterilization is essential. If iodine is used, a history of iodine sensitivity should be sought prior to skin preparation. We do not routinely use sterile gloves, although the clinician may feel more comfortable doing so. The use of a sterile finger cot may be helpful. Raising a skin wheal before deep injection is not as essential since the introduction of disposable needles that are sharp and without barbs. A vapocoolant spray such as ethylchloride may provide surface anesthesia if desired.

A No. 20 spinal needle 4 inches long may be necessary for injecting the piriformis muscle, the trochanteric bursa, or the low back region. On the other hand, a No. 25, No. 26, or No. 27 dermal needle ½ inch long is most appropriate for a "trigger finger" tendon injection. Between these extremes is carpal tunnel injection with a No. 22 or No. 23 needle, 1 inch long. In myofascial pain disorders, the needle point may be used as a probe to reproduce the patient's pain.

Although we much prefer use of a corticosteroid-anesthetic mixture, some clinicians may wish to use a local anesthetic agent alone. A total of 1 to 20 ml of a local anesthetic repeated daily or as required for relief has been recommended.[8] Reportedly, 5% of persons are refractory in response to procaine and similar local anesthetic compounds.[8] Use of jet injectors or similar devices has been limited by the necessity for daily care and cleaning of the delivery instrument.[8]

Pitfalls to Injection Therapy. These injections are not solvents for hypertrophic or degenerated tissue.[8] The injection must be part of a comprehensive program for soft tissue rheumatic pain as described throughout each section of this book. Among the pitfalls leading to failure are the following:[8] (1) a wrong diagnosis or incorrect localization of the soft tissue rheumatic pain site, (2) advanced or irreversible changes, (3) uncorrected contributory factors such as poor body mechanics, or systemic factors that are unrecognized or untreated, (4) multiple lesions that are unrecognized, (5) refractoriness to "caine" drugs if used alone, (6) treatment of subjective complaints without findings, and (7) persons who are hypersensitive or who have low pain thresholds.

If infection is suspected, local injection therapy should not be used until infection has been excluded. A previous mild crystal reaction or a vasovagal reaction is not an absolute contraindication to future reinjection.

Frequency of Injections. How often and how many times a soft tissue lesion should be injected requires common sense. Disorders known to be occasionally stubborn in their response, such as a carpal tunnel syndrome or a thickened olecranon bursitis, may best be treated by surgery rather than by many repeated local injections.

Repeated need for injection of the same site should raise the possibility of continued strain or aggravation. Review of work, hobby, sport, or homemaking activity should be undertaken. In general, more than 3 corticosteroid-anesthetic injections over a short period of time into the same site should be avoided.

REFERENCES

1. Moskowitz RW: Clinical Rheumatology. Philadelphia, Lea & Febiger, 1975.
2. Fitzgerald RH: Intrasynovial injection of steroids; uses and abuses. Mayo Clin Proc 51:655–659, 1976.
3. Hollander JL, Jessar RA, Brown EM: Intra-synovial corticosteroid therapy: A decade of use. Bull Rheum Dis 11:239–240, 1961.
4. Finder JG, Post M: Local injection therapy for rheumatic diseases. JAMA 172:2021–2030, 1960.
5. Alexander SJ: Cost containment in carpal tunnel syndrome. Arthritis Rheum 22:1415–1416, 1979.
6. Phalen GS: Soft tissue affections of the hand and wrist. Hosp Med 7:47–59, 1971.
7. Clark DD, Ricker JH, MacCollum MS: The efficacy of local steroid injection in the treatment of stenosing tenovaginitis. Plast Reconstr Surg 51:179–180, 1973.
8. Steinbrocker O, Neustadt DH: Aspiration and Injection Therapy in Musculoskeletal Disorders. New York, Harper and Row, 1972.
9. Swezey RL: Rehabilitation aspects in arthritis. In Arthritis and Allied Conditions. 9th Ed. Edited by DJ McCarty. Philadelphia, Lea & Febiger, 1979.
10. Brown BB: Diagnosis and therapy of common myofascial syndromes. JAMA 239:648, 1978.
11. Covino BG, Vassallo HG: Local Anesthetics: Mechanisms of Action and Clinical Use. New York, Grune and Stratton, 1976.
12. Sweetnam R: Corticosteroid arthropathy and tendon rupture. J Bone Joint Surg 51:397–398, 1969.
13. Rotstein J, Good RA: Steroid pseudorheumatism. Arch Intern Med 99:545–555, 1957.

14. Shafer N: Pneumothorax following "trigger point" injection. JAMA 213:1193, 1970.
15. Kennedy JC, Willis RB: The effects of local steroid injections on tendons: A biomechanical and microscopic correlative study. Am J Sports Med 4:11–21, 1976.
16. Gottlieb NL, Riskin WG: Complications of local corticosteroid injections. JAMA 243:1547–1548, 1980.
17. Ismail AM, Balakrishnan R, Rajakumar MK: Rupture of patellar ligament after steroid infiltration. J Bone Joint Surg 51B:503–505, 1969.
18. Hollander JL: Arthrocentesis and intrasynovial therapy. In Arthritis and Allied Conditions. 9th Ed. Edited by DJ McCarty. Philadelphia, Lea & Febiger, 1979.
19. Reeback JS, Chakraborty J, English J, et al: Plasma steroid levels after intra-articular injection of prednisolone acetate in patients with rheumatoid arthritis. Ann Rheum Dis 39:22–24, 1980.
20. Cassidy JT, Bole GG: Cutaneous atrophy secondary to intra-articular corticosteroid administration. Ann Intern Med 65:1008–1018, 1966.
21. McCarty DJ, Hogan JM: Inflammatory reaction after intrasynovial injection of microcrystalline adrenocorticosteroid esters. Arthritis Rheum 7:359–367, 1964.
22. Finkel RI: Personal communication.

Chapter *15*

THE EXERCISE PLAN

Patients with soft tissue rheumatic pain syndromes often become sedentary as a result of their chronic symptoms. Frequently they have poor muscle tone, or they have used muscles inappropriately. However, myofascial pain can also occur in active people and athletes. The goal of an exercise program is to correct local or general body pathophysiology that has resulted in loss of normal function.[1,2] The specific exercise program must be individualized, based on a prior appropriate evaluation of the musculoskeletal system in each patient.[3]

There is much to learn in the science of conditioning exercise. Whether exercises are performed for correction of a postural disorder or for development of endurance, a fundamental knowledge of the basic aspects of rehabilitation are necessary. For example, stretching exercises cannot be performed effectively without first providing for relaxation of the involved muscles. Sometimes assisted stretching exercise must be augmented by using brief contractions of agonist muscles in order to induce relaxation of antagonists.[2] More simply, we tell patients that they must obtain increased muscle length before they can accomplish muscle strength.

Ligamentous and capsular structures tend to shorten when normal tension or stretching forces are interrupted.[2] The strength and length of flexor muscles should be in balance with opposing extensor muscles. An exercise program must also provide proper posture and proper rest positions in order to prevent muscle fatigue.

Flexibility is the ability to yield to passive stretch and then to relax; flexibility helps to facilitate action with minimal resistance to the tissues. Flexibility in boys increases from ages 6 to 10 and then declines at age 16. In girls flexibility peaks at age 12. In studies of 16-year-old athletes, swimmers and baseball players had greater flexibility, whereas wrestlers were least flexible.[4] After age 25 there is a general and steady loss of flexibility. Stretching exercises designed to produce a greater range of motion have resulted in significant improvement in flexibility; the improvement continues for many weeks after the cessation of exercises. Lack of flexibility may lead to muscle "brittleness" and soft tissue rheumatic complaints.

GOALS OF THERAPEUTIC EXERCISE

The obvious overall goal is to obtain maximum independent function and efficiency within the limits imposed by the musculoskeletal condition.[1] The specific objectives may be listed as follows:[3]

1. Develop a sense of good body alignment.
2. Relax unneeded musculature to permit smooth coordinated efficient motion.
3. Increase muscular strength as needed to attain and maintain good alignment and function.
4. Achieve flexibility within a normal range.
5. Maintain and increase joint range of motion.

EVALUATION FOR AN EXERCISE PLAN

Therapists should determine the potential response capabilities of the patient's musculoskeletal system. This potential is based on an assessment of strength, range of movement, functional ability, and any abnormal skeletal motion.[1] Range of motion determination has already been described. Numerous methods and standards for range of motion determination have been critically analyzed, and the interested reader should refer to the chapter "Clinical Assessment of Joint Motion" by Margaret L. Moore in Basmajian's excellent text, *Therapeutic Exercise.*[5]

THE TYPE OF EXERCISE

Most likely the clinician will refer the patient to a qualified physical therapist. The clinician should provide the therapist with the diagnosis, which body regions are of concern, and what goals the clinician and patient have established. The physical therapist should evaluate the patient and then develop an exercise plan which should be communicated to the clinician. Most of the exercises we are concerned with in soft tissue rheumatic pain conditions involve mobilizing and stretching exercises.

Exercises are categorized as passive, active, active assisted, and resistive. These terms refer to the amount of effort the patient undertakes in performing a therapeutic exercise. If the therapist alone performs a movement of the patient's musculoskeletal system, the activity is "passive." If the patient performs the activity with some help by the therapist, the exercise is "active assisted." If the patient performs without assistance, the exercise is "active." And if the exercise is performed against weight, it is defined as "resistive."[2]

Strengthening as opposed to mobilizing exercise has been the subject of much research in recent years. This modality may be added to the exercise program once the muscles have responded favorably to the mobilizing exercise plan. Strengthening exercises may be categorized as static or isometric, dynamic or isotonic, or isokinetic. These refer to the performance of a resistive exercise without joint motion (static-isometric); exercise with joint motion and against resistance (dynamic or isotonic); or exercise against a machine that provides a defined time and rate of movement of the joint (isokinetic).[6]

Recommendations regarding the pace of exercise vary. In the DeLorme system,[7,8] a gradually increasing amount of resistance is applied to achieve strength; in the modified DeLorme (Oxford) technique,[9] a maximum resistance weight is determined for a given exercise, and then after performing with maximum weight, the load is gradually reduced. The number and duration of repetitions of resistance exercise are further components of the specifically prescribed program. The isokinetic exercise machine is helpful because it provides a quantitative evaluation of the patient's progress.[6]

Throughout this text, certain brief exercises utilizing activities of 5 to 10 seconds' duration with momentary rest between efforts have been described. We wish to stress that muscle training is an extremely complex process; there is no one right way. Different techniques have been effectively utilized to achieve the same goal for a given condition. It is wise to urge the patient to allow the therapist to develop an exercise plan unique for that patient. This can seldom be provided on a single visit. Some clinicians prefer to take the time to teach the patient the exercise program themselves, rather than depend upon a physical therapist. If this is done, we recommend the patient return and demonstrate the exercises after several weeks of unsupervised therapy at home. A planned graduated exercise program must be based on periodic reevaluation.[1]

Therapeutic exercise can be overdone. Pain may result from improper performance, improper diagnosis, or too vigorous a program. We ask the patient to accept discomfort that lasts no longer than 20 minutes following the exercise performance. Others will allow up to 3 hours of discomfort.[1] Short periods of exercise repeated during the day are preferred to a prolonged single daily session.[1] We recommend that the exercise program take no more than 20 to 30 minutes per session. Most of our patients require less than 10 minutes of exercise twice daily. An overly prolonged muscle contraction is self-defeating since ischemia induced by the contraction reduces the muscle's own blood supply.[10] When strength is desired, the exercise should eventually be carried to the point of muscle fatigue.[6] Strengthening exercises are not nearly as painful as are mobilizing exercises of tissues that suffer from adhesions, such as in adhesive capsulitis or frozen shoulder.

ADJUNCTS TO AN EXERCISE PROGRAM

In order to provide increased blood flow, reduce muscle irritability, and raise the pain threshold, either moist heat or ice may be applied before performing the exercise.[2] Diathermy is a rather expensive form of heat. Ultrasound, also a heat modality, may facilitate extensibility of soft tissues.[11] Biofeedback training and transcutaneous nerve stimulation may increase general relaxation before performing an exercise. Probably the most important adjunct to physical therapy is the relationship developed between the therapist and the patient. A therapy program achieves success only after a proper evaluation, the establishment of reasonable goals, individualization of the exercise prescription, proper pacing of the exercise program, and last and most importantly, motivation of the patient to the performance of a diligent exercise plan. If a patient is looking for a "magic bullet," less effective results are to be anticipated. We can help best those patients most willing to help themselves.

REFERENCES

1. Rusk HA: Rehabilitation Medicine. 4th Ed. St Louis, CV Mosby, 1977.
2. Swezey RL: Rehabilitation aspects in arthritis. *In* Arthritis and Allied Conditions. 9th Ed. Edited by DJ McCarty. Philadelphia, Lea & Febiger, 1979.
3. Daniels L, Worthingham C: Therapeutic Exercise for Body Alignment and Function. 2nd Ed. Philadelphia, WB Saunders, 1977.
4. Allman FL: Exercise in sports medicine. *In* Therapeutic Exercise. 3rd Ed. Edited by JV Basmajian. Baltimore, Williams & Wilkins, 1978.
5. Moore ML: Clinical assessment of joint motion. *In* Therapeutic Exercise. 3rd Ed. Edited by JV Basmajian. Baltimore, Williams & Wilkins, 1978.
6. DeLateur BJ: Exercise for strength and endurance. *In* Therapeutic Exercise. 3rd Ed. Edited by JV Basmajian. Baltimore, Williams & Wilkins, 1978.
7. DeLorme TL: Restoration of muscle power by heavy-resistance exercises. J Bone Joint Surg 27:645–667, 1945.
8. DeLorme TL, Watkins AL: Techniques of progressive resistance exercise. Arch Phys Med 29:263–273, 1948.
9. Zinovieff AN: Heavy-resistance exercises; the "Oxford technique." Br J Phys Med 14:129–132, 1951.
10. Liberson WT: Brief isometric exercises. *In* Therapeutic Exercise. 3rd Ed. Edited by JV Basmajian. Baltimore, Williams & Wilkins, 1978.
11. Gersten JW: Effect of ultrasound on tendon extensibility. Am J Phys Med 34:362–369, 1955.

APPENDIX OF
ILLUSTRATIONS

SOFT TISSUE INJECTION

Indications, contraindications, hazards, and general techniques for soft tissue injection are provided in detail in Chapter 14. This component of the Appendix provides a composite review of sites for injection, duplicating figures provided throughout the text in appropriate chapters where details for injection of specific sites are given.

THERAPEUTIC EXERCISES

An overall philosophy of exercise plans, including goals of therapeutic exercise, evaluation for an exercise plan, type of exercise, and adjuncts to an exercise program are provided in Chapter 15. This component of the Appendix provides a composite review of postural, mobilizing, and resistive exercises, the details of which are given in appropriate chapters where these same figures are utilized throughout the book.

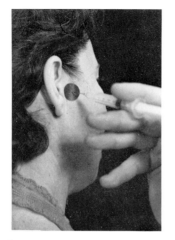

Fig. 1–3   p. 17

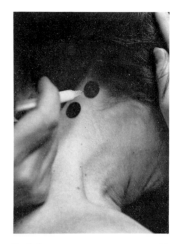

Fig. 1–9   p. 24

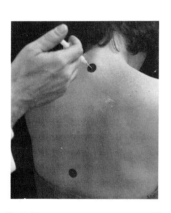

Fig. 1–12   p. 29

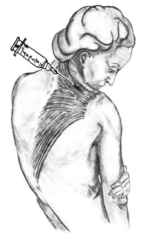

Fig. 1–8   p. 23

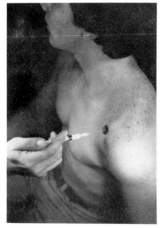

Fig. 3–10   p. 65

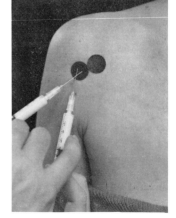

Fig. 3–11   p. 66

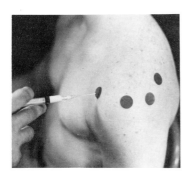

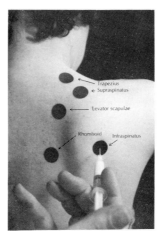

Fig. 3–17   p. 73   Fig. 3–19   p. 77

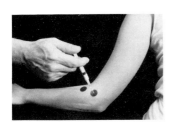

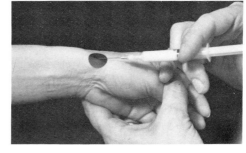

Fig. 4–2   p. 84   Fig. 5–6   p. 101

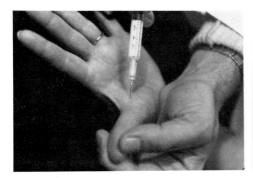

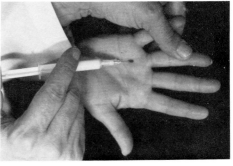

Fig. 5–7   p. 102   Fig. 5–8   p. 102

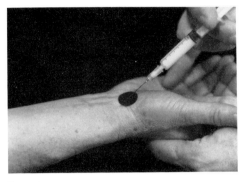

Fig. 5–12   p. 107

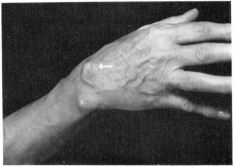

Fig. 5–15   p. 112

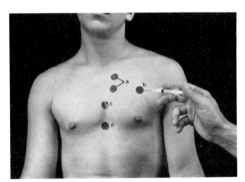

Fig. 6–4   p. 123

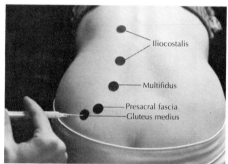

Fig. 7–15   p. 161

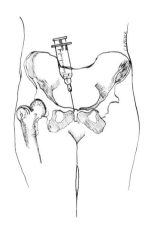

Fig. 7–17   p. 166

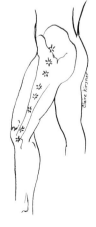

Fig. 8–5   p. 177

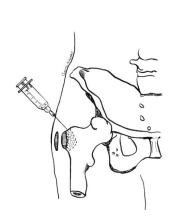

Fig. 8–6   p. 179

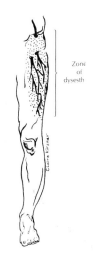

Zone of dysesth

Fig. 8–7   p. 181

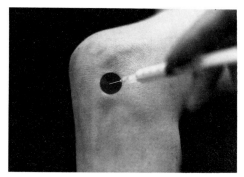

Fig. 9–7   p. 196

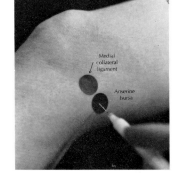

Medial collateral ligament

Anserine bursa

Fig. 9–8   p. 199

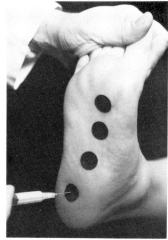

Fig. 11–4   p. 223

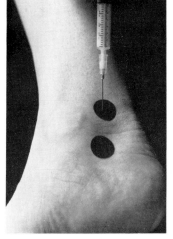

Fig. 11–11   p. 236

THERAPEUTIC EXERCISES
Posture Exercises (A to C)

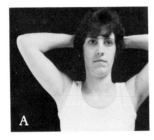

Fig. 1–6   p. 21

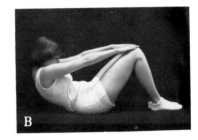

Fig. 7–8   p. 156

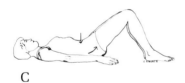

Fig. 7–9   p. 157

Mobilizing Exercises (A to D)

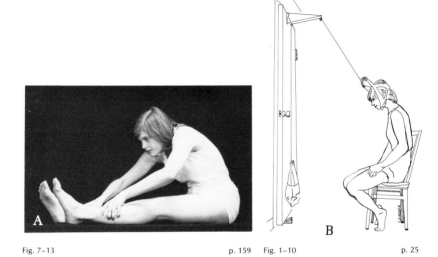

Fig. 7–13   p. 159   Fig. 1–10   p. 25

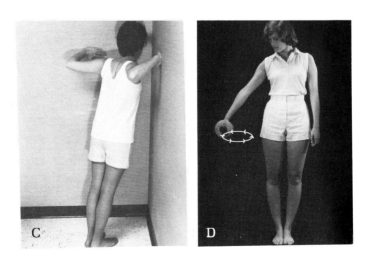

Fig. 6–3   p. 122   Fig. 3–12   p. 67

Mobilizing Exercises (Continued)
(E to H)

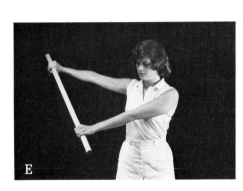

E

Fig. 3–16   p. 72

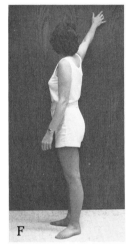

F

Fig. 3–15   p. 71

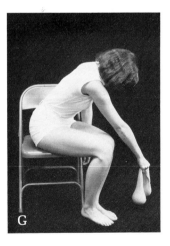

G

Fig. 3–18   p. 75

H

Fig. 4–3   p. 86

Mobilizing Exercises *(Continued)*
(I to L)

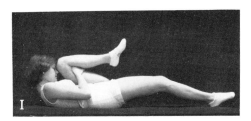

Fig. 7–10   p. 157

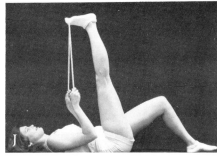

Fig. 7–12   p. 159

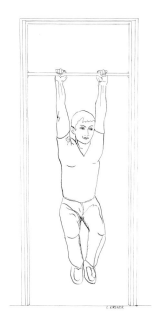

K

Fig. 7–14   p. 160

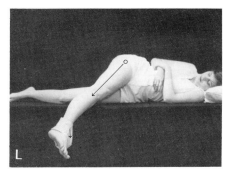

Fig. 8–4   p. 176

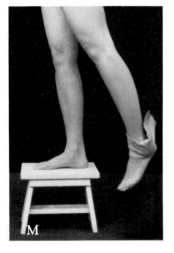

Fig. 8–8   p. 182

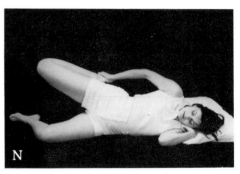

Fig. 8–3   p. 175

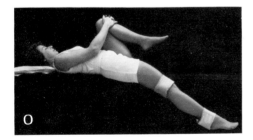

Fig. 9–6   p. 193

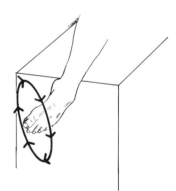

P

Fig. 11–9   p. 231

Resistive Exercises (A to E)

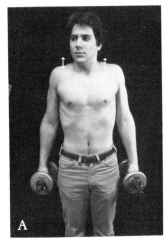 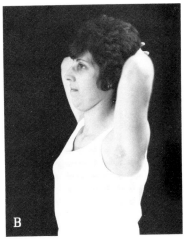

Fig. 2–5   p. 41   Fig. 2–6   p. 42

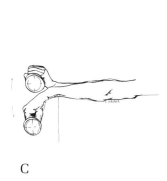 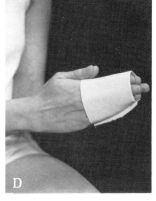

Fig. 4–4   p. 87   Fig. 5–4   p. 99

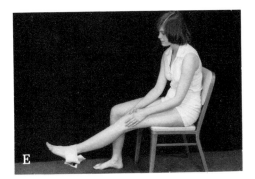

Fig. 9–5   p. 192

INDEX

289